Handbook of
Rodent and Rabbit Medicine

Edited by

KATHY LABER-LAIRD
Charleston, South Carolina, USA

M. MICHAEL SWINDLE
Charleston, South Carolina, USA

PAUL FLECKNELL
Newcastle Upon Tyne, UK

PERGAMON

U.K.   Elsevier Science Ltd, The Boulevard, Langford Lane, Kidlington, Oxford, OX5 1GB, UK

U.S.A.   Elsevier Science Inc., 660 White Plains Road, Tarrytown, New York 10591-5153, U.S.A.

JAPAN   Elsevier Science Japan, Tsunashima Building Annex, 3-20-12 Yushima, Bunkyo-ku, Tokyo 113, Japan

First edition 1996

Library of Congress Cataloging-in-Publication Data

Handbook of rodent and rabbit medicine/edited by Kathy Laber-Laird, M. Michael Swindle, Paul Flecknell. 1st ed.
p. cm — (Pergamon veterinary handbook series)
Includes index.
1. Rodents —Diseases — Handbooks, manuals, etc.
2. Rabbits — Diseases — Handbooks, manuals, etc.
3. Rodents —Handbooks, manuals, etc. 4. Rabbits — Handbooks, manuals etc. I. Laber-Laird, Kathy. II. Swindle, M. Michael. III. Flecknell P. A. IV. Series. SF997.5.R64H36 1995
636'. 932-dc20   94-45569

British Library Cataloguing-in-Publication Data

A catalogue record for this book is available from the British Library

ISBN 0-08-0425054 (Hardcover)
ISBN 0-08-0425046 (Flexicover)

Disclaimer

Whilst every effort is made by the Publishers to see that no inaccurate or misleading data, opinion or statement appear in this book, they wish to make it clear that the data and opinions appearing in the articles herein are the sole responsibility of the contributor concerned. Accordingly, the Publishers and their employees, officers and agents accept no responsibility or liability whatsoever for the consequences of any such inaccurate or misleading data, opinion or statement.

Drug and Dosage Selection: The Authors have made every effort to ensure the accuracy of the information herein, particularly with regard to drug selection and dose. However, appropriate information sources should be consulted, especially for new or unfamiliar drugs or procedures. It is the responsibility of every veterinarian to evaluate the appropriateness of a particular opinion in the context of actual clinical situations, and with due consideration of new developments.

Printed in Great Britain by BPC Wheatons Ltd, Exeter

Contents

List of Contributors

Kenneth R. Boschert, DVM, Diplomate, American College of Laboratory Animal Medicine, Associate Director, Division of Comparative Medicine, Washington University School of Medicine, St. Louis, Missouri, USA.

Laura A. Davis, DVM, Associate Veterinarian, Division of Comparative Medicine, Washington University School of Medicine, St. Louis, Missouri, USA.

Michael T. Fallon, DVM, PhD, Diplomate, American College of Laboratory Animal Medicine, Director, Veterinary Medical Unit, Veteran's Medical Center, Atlanta, Georgia, USA.

Paul Flecknell, MA, VetMB, PhD, DLAS, MRCVS, Director, Comparative Biology Centre, Medical School, Framlington Place, Newcastle Upon Tyne, UK

Charmaine Foltz, DVM, Diplomate, American College of Laboratory Animal Medicine, Clinical Veterinarian, Division of Comparative Medicine, Massachusetts Institute of Technology, Cambridge, Massachusetts, USA.

Michael J. Huerkamp, DVM, Diplomate, American College of Laboratory Animal Medicine, Chief, Laboratory Animal Medicine, Division of Animal Resources, Emory University, Atlanta, Georgia, USA.

Kathy Laber-Laird, DVM, MS, Diplomate, American College of Laboratory Animal Medicine, Assistant Professor, Department of Comparative Medicine, Medical University of South Carolina, Director, Veterinary Medical Unit, Veteran's Medical Center, Charleston, South Carolina, USA.

Marie La Regina, DVM, Diplomate, American College of Laboratory Animal Medicine, Associate Veterinarian, Division of Comparative Medicine, Washington University School of Medicine, St. Louis, Missouri, USA.

Neil S. Lipman, DVM, Diplomate, American College of Laboratory Animal Medicine, Director, Animal Resources, University of Chicago, Chicago, Illinois, USA.

Kathleen A. Murray, DVM, Diplomate, American College of Laboratory Animal Medicine, Associate Director of Professional Services, Charles River Laboratories Inc., Wilmington, Massachusetts, USA.

Susan E. Orosz, DVM, Associate Professor of Avian and Exotic Animal Medicine, College of Veterinary Medicine, University of Tennessee, Knoxville, Tennessee, USA.

Paul M. Shealy, DVM, MS, Diplomate, American College of Veterinary Surgeons, Chairman, Department of Surgery, The Animal Medical Center, New York, New York, USA.

Susan Stein, DVM, MS, Diplomate, American College of Laboratory Animal Medicine, Clinical Veterinarian, University Laboratory Animal Resources, Michigan State University, East Lansing, Michigan, USA.

James G. Strake, DVM, Clinical Veterinarian, Abbott Laboratories, Abbott Park, Illinois, USA.

M. Michael Swindle, DVM, Diplomate, American College of Laboratory Animal Medicine, Professor and Chairman, Department of Comparative Medicine, Professor, Department of Surgery, Medical University of South Carolina, Charleston, South Carolina, USA.

Sally Walshaw, MA, VMD, Associate Professor, University Laboratory Animal Resources, East Lansing, Michigan, USA.

Acknowledgements

We would especially like to thank Kathy Carr for her unconditional support during the entire process of researching, writing, and editing the manuscript. She made it possible for Kathy Laber-Laird to be in two places at once! Thanks also to Debra Allston and Beth Powell for giving up many evenings to work with the formatting nightmare of multiple-author chapters. The major contribution from Paul Flecknell was aided by internet and electronic mail, which greatly speeded transatlantic communications. Gratitude to the Swindle family members Paula, Katelyn and Ashley. Finally, thanks to Diane, Earl, Scott and Hank for being wonderful cheerleaders.

Preface

The biology, behaviour, disease and treatment of rodents and rabbits are subjects that are not traditionally emphasized in veterinary schools. Historically, these animals were not viewed as pets or significant contributors to the human food chain. However, with the continued population growth resulting in an increase in the number of people living in smaller spaces, these animals are now increasingly being kept as pets. Private practitioners need a working knowledge of these species and their diseases.

Most of the knowledge gathered about these species has been from veterinarians who have specialised and worked with these species in a biomedical research environment. In this setting, emphasis is placed on herd health and diagnosis of subclinical diseases that can significantly interfere with research results. Placing these animals in a 'pet' environment can alter the incidence and presentation of certain diseases, especially those affected by husbandry. Therefore, having a thorough understanding of the animal's environment, be it in a laboratory or a home, is critical when attempting to diagnose the diseases that afflict these species.

This book attempts to provide the basic information necessary for veterinarians, practicing in either a research setting or private practice to diagnose and treat the symptomatic diseases more commonly seen in these animals. To do that effectively, the reader also needs to have an understanding about the animals' unique biology, behaviour and husbandry requirements. For quick reference, tables that summarise the diseases are included for each species as well as tables covering treatment, anaesthetic, and analgesic drug dosages. Separate chapters cover the topics of surgery and anaesthesia/analgesia.

On a final note, it is especially important to remember that for these species, good husbandry is the best form of preventive medicine and preventive medicine is more effective in keeping rabbits and rodents alive than attempting to treat them once they've become ill.

1

Rats and Mice

MICHAEL T. FALLON

Introduction

Mice and rats make good pets for children and adults alike. They are entertaining to watch, fairly easy and inexpensive to maintain, take up little space and are very docile when familiar with human contact. Mice tend to be more active than rats, but rats tend to exhibit more individual personality. Both species demonstrate amusing and endearing social behaviour when in stable groups and enjoy being transported around on human shoulders. They may urinate initially when handled (their normal alarm reflex), but this behaviour usually stops as they grow more accustomed to human handling.

Although there is evidence that mice were used in Chinese religious rituals 3000 years ago, it was not until the 17th century that mice were used experimentally in Europe. At that time mice were used by William Harvey in reproductive and blood circulation studies, by Joseph Priestley in studies leading to the discovery of oxygen and by Antoine Lavoisier in respiratory physiology studies. Over the next few hundred years there was a proliferation of breeding mice by scientists throughout Europe and Asia, resulting in a profusion of varieties (Foster *et al.*, 1981).

Although obscure, the origins of the laboratory rat, *Rattus norvegicus,* appear to be in Asia. The opportunities to share human grain and habitat allowed rapid expansion into continental Europe by the 1700s, England by about 1730 and America by about 1775. The term 'Norway' rat has little known significance beyond reflecting the species name. One account attributes domestication to the Western European sport of 'rat baiting' in the early to mid 19th century.

This involved gambling on how fast trained terriers could kill trapped rats in a pit. Finally stopped by decree, unusual albino mutants saved by breeders apparently ended up as pets or show animals, thus providing the potential source of albino rats used in European research laboratories in the mid to late 19th century. American laboratories began to use albino rats from stock which was probably provided by a visiting German scientist (Adolf Meyer) in the 1890s, but the exact origins of the albino rats used in America today are unclear (Baker *et al.*, 1979).

In the modern research facility, rodent medicine usually resembles large animal herd medicine rather than companion animal medicine, in the sense that the major emphasis is on prevention, rather than examination and diagnosis of unique diseases of individual animals. Because of the absolute need for healthy, disease-free animals that allow proper reproducibility and interpretation of biomedical experiments and the relatively low cost of most mouse or rat strains, humane sacrifice instead of treatment is often the appropriate course of action. However, when presented with a pet mouse or rat, the situation is very different. The most likely diagnosis and reasonable treatment, if any, should be offered.

The goals of this chapter are to present general information on the biology, behaviour, husbandry, housing and nutrition of rats and mice and to provide a concise discussion of the clinical signs, diagnosis, treatment and control of the more common diseases. Zoonotic agents will also be covered, even though most are expected to have a very low prevalence in laboratory or pet mice and rats.

Unique Biology

The mouse (*Mus musculus*) and rat (*Rattus norvegicus*) species are rodents in the order Rodentia, family Muridae. They are grouped with hamsters and gerbils (family Cricetidae) in the suborder Myomorpha. The lifespan of a mouse is about 1.5–2.5 years, and for a rat 2.5–3.5 years (at least one rat has lived to an age of 4 years 8 months (Baker *et al.*, 1979)). The dentition for both consists of 16 teeth, an incisor and 3 molars per quadrant, with a prominent space (the diastema) separating the incisors from the molars. The incisors grow continuously throughout life, are self-sharpening and wear down by mastication. Like most rodents, mice and rats have two pairs of opposing incisors, (the presence of a third pair of incisors in the maxilla of rabbits, the peg teeth, was one of the criteria used to move them out of Rodentia into their own order, Lagomorpha). The teeth normally have a yellowish colour.

Sexing of young animals can be performed by contrasting the shorter anus-to-vulva distance in females with the longer anus-to-penis distance in the male. The inguinal canals remain open, allowing the testes to be retracted out of the scrotum throughout life. Males have an os penis and preputial glands that occasionally become abscessed or neoplastic. Older male rats often have brownish sebaceous particles at the base of the hairs over the dorsum which can appear on first impression to be mites. The amount of coat affected and particle density are enhanced by testosterone and inhibited by oestrogen. Male mice and rats have highly developed paired accessory sex glands, including preputial glands near the penis, seminal vesicles, coagulating glands (or anterior prostate), dorsal, lateral and ventral prostates, and ampullary glands (or the glands of the ductus deferens) in the area of the bladder and the bulbourethral glands (also called Cowper's glands), which are found adjacent to the urethra as it exits the pelvic area. Females have paired clitoral glands near the vulva which are considered to be homologues of the male preputial glands. Tails are very long in relation to body size (slightly more so in females), very

sensitive to pain and act as a balancing aid (as well as a thermoregulatory organ, see below).

A histopathologist can identify the sex of a mouse by looking at the glomeruli in the renal cortex. The parietal layer of Bowman's capsule is cuboidal in the female and columnar in the male. Also, in male mice, a zone in the adrenal gland called the 'X' zone (located between the cortex and medulla) degenerates during puberty whereas female mice usually retain it (Foster and Small, 1983).

As is typical of rodents, mice and rats do not have sweat glands and do not pant. Mice salivate a little in response to high temperatures, but rats do not. These adaptations preserve body water. Unlike most animals, high ambient temperatures actually inhibit water consumption. In response to high ambient temperature they seek cool shelter and in the wild, burrow. In general they cannot regulate body temperature as well as most other mammals and do not tolerate heat (they begin to die at an environmental temperature of about 37°C). The tail and ears are important for heat dispersion (Baker *et al.*, 1979; Foster and Small, 1983).

Female mice and rats usually have 5 and 6 pairs of teats, respectively. The mammary tissue has an extensive distribution that includes areas as far dorsal as the shoulder blades along the length of the trunk. This distribution should be kept in mind because mammary tumours are relatively common in both mice and rats.

The average gestation period is 19–21 days for mice and 21–23 days for rats. Both species exhibit a postpartum fertile oestrus within 24 h of parturition. Hence, the tremendous reproductive potential of rodents; females may give birth to a second litter even before the first litter is completely weaned. Pups do not acquire thermoregulatory capabilities until the end of the first week (they are kept warm by each other in the nest and by their mother). They are weaned at 3–4 weeks, but will begin nibbling on solid food by the third week if it is accessible. Litter size varies tremendously depending on genetic background, but litters of more than 10 are not uncommon. Unlike hamsters, male mice and rats are larger than females. Female mice and rats experience a continuous 4–5 day oestrus cycle until pregnant. To prevent unwanted litters, pups should be separated by sex before they reach puberty at about 6–9 weeks.

Harderian glands, present behind the eyes, produce secretions containing porphyrin, a reddish fluorescent pigment. In rats, Harderian hypersecretion during stress can result in a blackish staining of the periocular and perinasal fur. The secretion will turn a reddish colour if cleaned with a moist gauze pad. This is a clear indication of stress, but should not be confused with blood.

Rat bone ossification is not complete until after the first year of life which is later, in relation to puberty, than most mammalian species. This should be taken into consideration when interpreting radiographs.

Like most rodents, mice and rats cannot vomit. Rats do not have a gall bladder. The stomach of both species is divided by a limiting ridge into a non-glandular proximal forestomach and a distal glandular body. The well developed caecum in the left lower abdominal quadrant should be avoided when intraperitoneal (IP) injections are given.

The senses of smell, hearing and touch are well developed in mice and rats whereas visual acuity is generally marginal. True albinos (white fur, pinkish to reddish tint in eyes) have very poor eyesight due to degenerative retinas and rely instead on their acute sense of smell and facial vibrissae to navigate their surroundings.

Figures 1.6–1.9 contain expanded selected normal values.

Behaviour

Both mice and rats are very inquisitive, social animals. Although they quickly adapt to feeding and husbandry routines, novel situations always interest them. They indicate curiosity by moving toward the novel stimulus. Both species will rear up or climb up to the cage lid and push their noses as high as possible, trying to sample the air at the top of the cage. All rodents are naturally tidy, spending hours each day grooming themselves and their cagemates. Although a specific area for defaecation and urination is not always clearly established in the cage, the communal sleeping areas that form at the periphery of the cage are rarely soiled. Both species practice coprophagy, which can be quite surprising to observers unfamiliar with this practice. The faeces may be eaten even as they come out of the anus (a typical practice for rabbits).

When faced with a human hand both species give behavioural clues as to how the interaction is likely to proceed. Rats that rear up, carefully follow the course of the hand, press their ears against their heads and position a forepaw to fend off the handler are likely to put up a struggle and bite. Likewise, mice that face the hand and rear up are also more likely to try to bite.

Although both mice and rats are basically nocturnal, mice usually display more daylight activity than rats, exhibiting cycles of activity and rest throughout the day and night. Both rodents tend to sleep for 5–10 min, wake up, adjust posture and drift back to sleep again (White, 1994). When in groups both rodents sleep in communal piles, with individuals gradually exchanging positions over time. Both mice and rats enjoy clean bedding, often playing in it with great enthusiasm.

Mouse and rat littermates raised together from birth usually coexist peacefully. However, the females and especially the males of some laboratory strains of mice (e.g. C57BL/6, BALB/c) are notorious for their tendency to fight. Sometimes the only solution is to place one mouse per cage. Whenever a group of mice or rats is assembled, or when new animals are added to a stable group, the group should be observed carefully to prevent injury from fights (fighting animals must be separated). Mice usually inflict bite wounds from behind on the tail or over the rump area. In cages where a dominant male or female is continually biting the other mice, outright deaths may occur in some cases. But more likely, lower ranking mice will lose weight because the continual attacks make feeding difficult. In contrast, rats usually face each other when settling disputes and the bite wounds tend to be around the head and shoulders. Fights between rats are rare. Fighting between males of both species is more likely when the males have been used as breeders and postparturient dams housed communally may also fight on occasion (White, 1994). Because of their relatively even temperament, DBA mice and Fisher (F344) rats can be recommended as good choices of laboratory strains for pets.

Pet mice and rats are not equipped behaviourally to survive in the wild. As with any pet, clients should be encouraged to find homes for unwanted mice or rats.

Reproduction

Sexual Development and Mating

Female mice and rats usually reach puberty at 6–8 weeks of age, although some strains (e.g. C57BL/6 mice) can reach puberty at about 5 weeks of age. Within a given strain, males tend to reach puberty a week or two later than females. The vagina opens a few days before the first oestrus occurs. Mature females are poly-oestrous and usually exhibit a 4–5 day oestrous cycle. When female mice are isolated in groups from male mice, their cycle tends to lengthen to 5–6 days. The light cycle can have marked effects on the oestrous cycle of mice and rats. For instance, the timing of luteinising hormone release prior to ovulation is strongly influenced by the diurnal cycle (Foster and Small, 1983). In general, a 12 h light/12 h darkness schedule is recommended (Baker *et al.*, 1979; Foster and Small, 1983).

The oestrous cycle of mice and rats is commonly divided into pro-oestrus, oestrus, met-oestrus and dioestrus phases. If necessary, vaginal smears can be evaluated to determine the oestrous phase. One way to obtain a vaginal smear is to put a drop of sterile saline into the vagina with an eyedropper (tip should be smooth), then aspirate the fluid back out. The fluid can be transferred to a slide, stained with dilute (0.1%) methylene blue to make the nuclei easier to visualise, then covered with a cover slip (Rugh, 1990). Alternatively, a small metal spatula with rounded edges dipped in saline can be

used to scoop moist scrapings gently onto a slide for staining (Waynforth and Flecknell, 1992). The oestrous cycles for both the mouse and rat are similar and can therefore be described together.

During pro-oestrus, the reproductive tract is rapidly enlarging and the vaginal smear shows leucocytes and nucleated epithelial cells in approximately equal numbers, with a few cornified cells. The vulva becomes swollen and congested during oestrus and the female is sexually receptive to the male. In a vaginal smear, clearly defined epithelial cells (with or without nuclei) are replaced by cornified cells and nuclei become rare. If a fertile mating does not occur, metoestrus follows. In the vaginal smear, cornified cells appear with leucocytes. Finally, dioestrus occurs in which leucocytes and epithelial cells dominate the smear (Baker *et al.*, 1979; Fox *et al.*, 1984; Rugh, 1990).

For timed breedings, the female is commonly placed in the male's cage, then removed the next morning. Fights are extremely rare. Female mice and rats will copulate only during oestrus. Acting on olfactory and other cues such as lordosis, the male will inspect the female genitalia, then make multiple mountings and intromissions over a period of 5–20 min (males of the C57BL/6 strain may copulate so frequently when multiple females in oestrus are present that trauma to the penis can result). In both mice and rats, a gelatinous copulatory plug produced by the male accessory sex glands can often be seen in the vagina after mating, or occasionally underneath in the bedding (Fox *et al.*, 1984). When lodged in the vagina, the plug prevents leakage of semen from the vagina.

Pheromones appear to play a role in reproduction in both mice and rats. Exposure to sexually mature male and female mice or their urine can cause an acceleration and delay, respectively, in the onset of female puberty in mice and the presence of mature males can delay puberty in male mice. Grouping small numbers of mature female mice in the absence of a male can cause pseudopregnancy (the Lee–Boot effect) (Foster *et al.*, 1983) or, in larger groups, anoestrus. But when the group is exposed to a male or his urine, the female mice will exit from pseudopregnancy and synchronously go into oestrus about 3 days later (the Whitten effect) (Baker *et al.*, 1979; Foster *et al.*, 1983; Fox *et al.*, 1984). This effect can be used to advantage if multiple litters of the same age are desired. The implantation of embryos in a recently mated mouse can be halted when she is exposed to a strange male mouse or his urine, resulting in a premature return to oestrus (the Bruce effect) (Foster *et al.*, 1983).

In rats, there is evidence that pheromones play a role in reproductive physiology, but less work on this has been performed. Oestrus suppression in grouped female rats and oestrus synchronisation in the presence of a male or his excreta have been described (the Whitten effect), but the effect is not as pronounced as that seen in mice (Fox *et al.*, 1984).

Breeding Systems

Two major systems are used to breed mice and rats. In the monogamous system, one male and one female are placed together in a cage. The litters are born and weaned in the same cage in the presence of the male. Because the male can breed with the female during the postpartum oestrus, this breeding system produces the most pups in the shortest period of time. It also allows accurate record keeping of male and female reproductive performance as well the age of pups, but requires one male for each female.

In the polygamous mating system, one male and 2–5 female mice (up to 8 or 9 female rats) are placed in a large cage. If accurate records of reproductive performance must be maintained or the age of the pups must be known, the females are removed from the communal cage when pregnant and placed in a smaller cage to give birth and wean the pups. Because the male is not present during the postpartum oestrus, not as many pups will be obtained per time period. In the 'harem' polygamous system, the females are left in the cage to give birth, so the postpartum oestrus is productive and more pups are produced. However, it is difficult to keep track of the age of the pups in the multiple litters and

it is more difficult to monitor individual reproductive performance (Foster *et al.*, 1983; Fox *et al.*, 1984).

Gestation and Birth

Parturition occurs most commonly between midnight and 4 a.m. A vaginal discharge may be present a few hours before parturition and the mother signals the onset of birth with pronounced stretching movements. The pups are normally born within 1 or 2 h and any pups born dead are usually eaten by the mother. The first litter is usually the smallest and the fourth or fifth the largest. Litter size begins to drop off slowly after 6–7 months of age and breeding usually stops somewhere around 1–1.5 years of age in females (later in males). Parturition can be delayed if the mother is lactating (Fox *et al.*, 1984).

Mouse and rat mothers make a small depression in the bedding for the pups, often in a cage corner. The blind pups find the teats by pheromone clues secreted by the ventral skin and receive maternal antibodies in milk until they are weaned at about 3 weeks. When large litters are involved, the mother may actually rest completely off the bedding on top of the pups while nursing. Soft nesting materials will be used to hide the pups, if made available. It is best not to disturb the pups for at least 2 weeks, but if it is necessary to disturb them, it must be ensured that the pups are not touched with bare human skin. In a research setting, latex-gloved hands can be moistened with urine in the cage bedding before the pups are handled to reduce the likelihood of cannibalism by the mother. Alternatively, the pups can be scooped up with a layer of bedding beneath them if they must be transferred to a new cage. Pets used to the smell of humans are less likely to cannibalise their young if handled. If the nest is disturbed and the pups are scattered in the cage, the mother will carefully retrieve each pup back to the nest in her mouth. Mothers with litters require additional floor space.

Pups are born hairless with closed eyes and ears. The ears open within 4 days, the incisors erupt in the second week and eyes open by the end of the second week. By 7–10 days of age the pups are fully haired.

Husbandry

Housing

Although pet rodent cages can be constructed from materials readily available from hardware stores, the best results are usually obtained by purchasing any of a variety of commercial rodent cages. The lid or door should be tight-fitting to prevent escape. The cage design should allow good ventilation and no surfaces accessible to the animals should harbour sharp edges that could produce injury. Although fish aquaria are often used as examples of caging in popular guides, they are difficult to clean and the high solid sides limit ventilation. Ideally, the cage should be constructed of non-porous lightweight material such as plastic or metal that can easily be cleaned. Rodents gnaw on any and all surfaces so cage surfaces should not be coated with any sealers or paint that would be toxic if ingested. The *Guide for Care and Use of Laboratory Animals* (USDHHS, 1985) recommends at least 97 cm^2 (15 in^2) of space for each mouse over 25 g and 453 cm^2 (70 in^2) for each rat over 500 g. Mouse cages should be at least 13 cm (5 in) high and rat cages should be 18 cm (7 in) high.

When housed in contact with bedding at the bottom of the cage, a semi-absorbent material such as wood chips or sawdust should be used that prevents urine contact with skin; very absorbent materials like newspaper allow too much moisture to remain in contact with the animal. Corn cob bedding must be checked carefully to make sure it is not mouldy and potentially adulterated with mycotoxins. Cedar, pine and other aromatic wood chips are often used at home to mask odours, but such bedding is inadvisable in a research setting because the aromatic hydrocarbons cause physiological changes such as the induction of liver microsomal enzymes. The bedding level should not be so high as to come into contact with the water bottle sipper tube (clogging or flooding can result).

As discussed previously, mice and rats are very social animals and will usually be physically and psychologically healthier when kept in groups. A sensible recommendation for clients is to house two or three females together in a large cage. Females are smaller, produce less urine (and secondary microbial ammonia) and tend to be more gentle. By grouping them, they are socially enriched and their charming interactive grooming and play behaviour comes out.

Both rats and mice enjoy using soft bedding material, such as wood shavings, for nesting. They also delight in playing with empty toilet paper or paper towel rolls or other small enclosures that allow them some opportunity to hide. Indeed, studies show that rats prefer to sleep and rest under a shelter (White, 1994), so a small cardboard box with one or two open ends or the end of a waxpaper milk carton might be provided. Some animals enjoy an exercise wheel, more commonly provided for hamsters. Perishable items like cardboard tubes should be replaced periodically as they become wet or soiled and permanent items such as exercise wheels should be cleaned in hot soapy water every second week. Soaps, detergents and disinfectants should always be thoroughly rinsed from any surface in contact with the animals.

The importance of maintaining adequate sanitation should be strongly emphasised to the client. For instance, high ammonia levels dramatically predispose rodents to severe respiratory disease caused by mycoplasms (National Research Council, 1991). Foot and tail sores, ventral dermatitis, stress and overall poor health can result when cages are not cleaned on a regular basis. Foot lesions are particularly common when wire-bottomed cages are used without good sanitation practices. Many recommendations in the *Guide for Care and Use of Laboratory Animals* formulated for research settings are useful for home settings. Bedding should be changed as often as needed to keep animals dry and clean, usually one to three times a week. Shoe box-type cages (in which the animal lives directly on the bedding) should be cleaned in hot, soapy water at least once a week. Cages with wire mesh bottoms should be similarly cleaned at least every second week, as should all cage surfaces.

Particular attention should be paid to maintaining clean sipper tubes and water bottles, which should be cleaned at least every other week. Mice are particularly fond of pushing bedding into the sipper tube, which causes rapid fouling of the water and potentially lethal dehydration due to sipper tube clogs. It is a good idea to ask the client to bring the pet in its cage so that the general sanitation of the cage can be assessed and the sipper tube can be checked. Open watering bowls are not appropriate for mice or rats and sipper tubes should be metal, not plastic or glass. During transportation, the water bottle can be removed from the cage to prevent it from spilling into the cage and soaking the bedding as it is jarred.

The ammonia that characterises cages in need of a bedding change is produced by the action of microbial urease on urea in the urine. Some vendors offer antibiotic-impregnated non-contact bedding materials that reduce ammonia production by reducing microbial numbers.

Rats and mice tolerate cool temperatures much better than heat (see Unique Biology above). A relative humidity of 40–70% and an ambient temperature range of 18–26°C (65–79°F) are suggested, but at least 50% humidity and a temperature between 18 and 22°C (65–72°F) will be closer to optimal.

Nutrition

The nutritional requirements of the omnivorous mouse and rat are well known and with the availability of well balanced commercial pelleted diets, nutritional problems should be rare. A diet with at least 20% protein is generally recommended, although less is probably necessary for non-breeding animals (Baker *et al.*, 1979; Foster *et al.*, 1982). Food should be stored in a cool, dry place and should not be used past the expiration date if available. Mice and rats effectively store fat-soluble vitamins, synthesise vitamin C and, through the practice of coprophagy, efficiently recover many B vitamins. Small treats of well washed raw fruits, vegetables, grains and

nuts can be a good source of environmental and nutritional enrichment, but pets fed primarily on table scraps are likely to develop any number of nutritional diseases. Chocolate or sugar treats should be used very sparingly because they promote obesity, poor health and reduced lifespan. To prevent dietary problems, clients should be encouraged to rely primarily on commercial chow, with periodic treats for variety. Mouldy chow should never be used because of the lowered nutritional value and the potential for mycotoxicosis. *Ad libitum* feeding is recommended, but dietary restriction is an option for obese animals. Mice will consume about 15 g of balanced chow and drink about 15 ml of water per 100 g body weight. Rats will consume about 5 g of balanced chow and drink about 10 ml of water per 100 g body weight (Harkness and Wagner, 1989). Hard food satisfies the need of rodents to gnaw and helps to keep incisors properly trimmed.

Although mice and rats are primarily nocturnal animals and will consume most of their food at night, they will eat periodically around the clock. The forepaws of both species are used to grab large chunks of chow, which are chipped to a smaller size by the incisors in preparation for grinding by the molars.

Handling, Injection, Specimen Collection

Handling

Remember that rodents have an acute sense of smell and any carnivore scents on your clothing or skin may upset them and make handling difficult. Pet mice and rats used to handling can be manipulated easily without protective gloves. Mice can be removed from the cage in cupped hands for examination. Rats can be removed for examination by grasping the body gently over the shoulders and lifting. To avoid struggles, immediately place the rat on your arm or on a solid surface. Many pet rat owners will appreciate it if you can carefully trim the toenails with a small human-style fingernail clipper. The nails are very sharp and can cause irritating scratches during forays on human skin (nail trimming is also recommended therapeutically to prevent skin damage from scratches while pruritic mite infections are treated). Although not painful, rats do not usually like to have their paws (particularly the front ones) manipulated and hence patience is required. To minimise the chance of damaging the quick, compress the paw gently between your thumb and forefinger to spread the digits out and extend the nails before trimming.

Although time pressures frequently make this difficult, the animal husbandry staff in a large colony setting can tame both rats and mice effectively by picking them up as described above during bedding changes. The rodents quickly become accustomed to being handled, which benefits both the animal (less stress) and the eventual human handler.

Personnel exposed to large numbers of mice and rats in a research or breeding setting should consider the use of disposable examination gloves and a surgical mask when routinely handling the animals. These precautions are recommended to limit aerosol and contact exposure to potent rodent urine and dander (particulate skin and coat) allergens. Allergies to rodents are a serious occupational hazard for personnel who must handle or care for rodents. Because allergies can become more serious over time with repeated exposure, respirators instead of surgical-type masks should be considered for allergic individuals who will be exposed.

Even the friendliest rodent is likely to bite if subjected to painful procedures. In these situations, mice handled without a protective glove can at most deliver a modest bite that infrequently penetrates the skin. In contrast, rats can deliver a severe bite and require more careful consideration. In a practice situation, remember that the client may be upset at the sight of a large handling glove being used on their relatively small pet, so it may be wise to ask the client to leave if such handling is necessary. Although many experienced rodent handlers feel comfortable handling untamed rats without a protective glove, this is inadvisable for most people when potentially painful manipulations are

planned. A leather or less-bulky chain-mesh glove can be used for handling untamed rats.

To pick up an untamed mouse for examination in a research setting, transport the mouse to a rough surface or wire bar cage top by grabbing the middle of the tail to lift the entire mouse. Tug gently on the tail with one hand so that the mouse resists by clinging with its front legs, thus elongating the body. While maintaining traction on the tail, grasp the loose skin over the neck (just behind the ears) with the thumb and forefinger of the other hand, lift the mouse and press the tail to the palm of the same hand with the combined fourth and fifth fingers or tuck the tail between the fourth and fifth fingers of the same hand (Fig. 1.1). If not enough skin over the neck is grasped or if the skin over the shoulders is grasped instead, the mouse will be able to turn and bite the hand. If the skin is grasped too tightly (the eyes will bulge noticeably), the mouse will choke.

When picking up a rat by the tail, be very careful not to grasp the distal tail. Rats have a tendency to twist in mid air, which can result in the skin tearing off the restrained tail. If this happens, a tail amputation is advisable because gangrene is the usual sequela.* Instead, lift the rat near the base of the tail with the unprotected hand and transfer it to a rough or irregular surface as described for mice (in contrast to mice, rats can easily 'climb' their own tail up to your hand, so move quickly). Apply traction to the tail to elongate the body and lift the rat with the gloved hand by encircling and firmly embracing the body over the shoulder and neck region so that the thumb is pushing the near forelimb under the chin as a barrier to the head (and teeth) (Fig. 1.2). When properly restrained, the rat will not be able to bite the restraint glove,

---

*After anaesthetising the animal, use a rubber band pinched tightly around the proximal tail with forceps as a tourniquet, make an incision to create two opposing 1 cm long dorsal and ventral skin flaps, dissect proximally and use a surgical blade to sever cleanly between two tail vertebrae at least 1.5 cm proximal to the ends of the skin flaps, then use interrupted sutures to close the two 1 cm overhanging flaps.

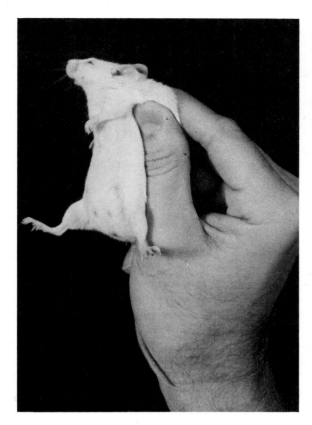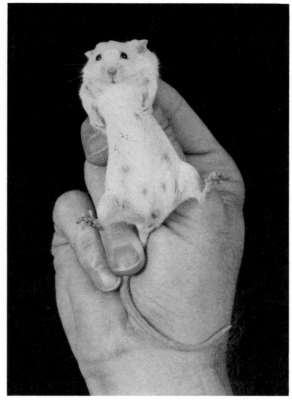

FIG. 1.1 Hand restraint for an untamed mouse. The skin over the neck and back is gathered from as far around the body as possible without including the forelimbs. This prevents the mouse from turning around and biting the thumb or fingers. The fourth and fifth fingers press the tail against the palm to immobilise the rear of the mouse. The middle finger helps to gather more skin over the back to further stabilise the skin between the thumb and index finger, further supporting the neck and middle section of the mouse.

which is desirable because the teeth can be damaged when the rat struggles and bites the glove at the same time. By maintaining slight traction on the tail, the rat can be comfortably controlled. If necessary, the hind feet can also be restrained by the hand holding the tail to increase control. **Do not grip the chest so tightly with the protectively gloved hand that respiration is hindered** (make sure rat is not gasping). Hypoxia, loss of consciousness and death can rapidly occur.

Injection

Rodent injections are usually limited to the intraperitoneal (IP) or subcutaneous (SC) routes.

Intramuscular (IM) injections should be avoided when possible in favour of the IP route because of the small muscle mass available. A 23 to 25 gauge long needle on a 1 ml syringe is satisfactory for injections. The nape of the neck is a good site for SC injections. The lower right quadrant of the abdomen is preferred for IP injections to avoid the caecum to the left. The needle is pointed cranially, angled at a 15–20° angle above the body, parallel to and to the right of the midline (the bladder must be avoided). To avoid visceral injections, it is a good policy to aspirate the syringe before injecting. A vacuum should be encountered. If blood or other liquids are aspirated, withdraw and reposition the nee-

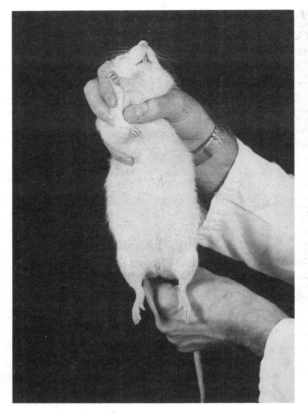 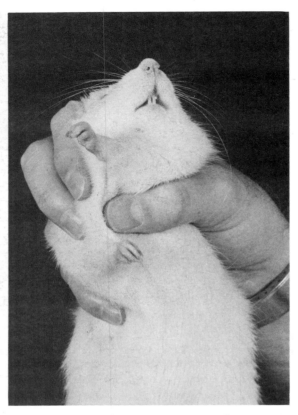

FIG. 1.2 Hand restraint for an untamed rat. (left) Overall view. One hand curls around the shoulder and neck area, and the other grabs the base of the tail. (right) Closeup of the shoulder and neck grip. The 'thumb pushes the near forelimb across the body under the chin. This prevents bites to the hand. The pointer and middle fingers force the far forelimb across and down under the end of the thumb.

dle. Before giving an IP injection to rats, some workers tilt the rat so that the head is lower than the abdomen in an attempt to slide the viscera cranially and away from the needle. However, the viscera are quite immobile because of the slight vacuum in the abdomen and this manipulation is of questionable value.

For intravenous (IV) injections, the lateral tail veins of both species are most accessible (the dorsal and ventral vessels are arteries, which usually give poor bleeding results). The process is greatly helped if the animals are placed under a heat lamp (not too close!) to dilate the tail veins prior to injection. Alternatively, the tails can be dipped in warm water for 1–2 min. If anaesthesia is not used, a restraint device is usually necessary because the tails are sensitive. Several types of clear plastic restraint devices which allow tail access are available commercially for rats (Fig. 1.3). A restraint tube allowing tail access fashioned from a 50 ml plastic centrifuge tube with a screw cap is useful for injecting mouse tail veins (Fig. 1.4).

Rats will take palatable liquids from a syringe, but if this fails or more careful oral dosing is required, ball-tipped gavage needles or flexible tubing can be used. A slightly curved 20 gauge gavage needle attached to a syringe can be used for rats and likewise a straight 22 gauge gavage needle for mice can be used. Care must be taken not to force the gavage needle because of the risk of oesophageal penetration and a poor prog-

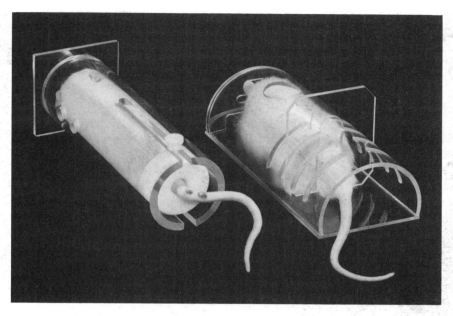

FIG. 1.3 Two types of commercial plexiglass rat restraint tubes. A doughnut-shaped disc moves along a groove to accommodate different body sizes in the left restrainer whereas a square-shaped plastic piece is inserted into slots along the top of the restrainer on the right to adjust for body size. Both models allow access to the tail and have holes and slots cut in the restraint tube to allow for injections. Note the marking at the base of the tail of the left rat made by a laboratory-type marker pen. This is a simple non-traumatic, temporary identification method.

nosis can result. Some people prefer flexible tubing that can be less damaging to the oesophageal mucosa. Mice and rats should not be dosed orally unless fully conscious to reduce the possibility of aspiration pneumonia, which

50 ml centrifuge tube

6 mm diameter hole cut in conical end of tube to allow protrusion of nose

Section of tube removed, then ends rejoined with nylon tape to give a total tube height of 7-8 cm

Nylon tape strips covering sharp edges of slot

7 mm wide vertical slot cut in tube that extends 5-8 mm above lid rim (tail comes out here for access)

Lid of centrifuge tube

FIG. 1.4 A mouse restrainer. A good mouse restraint tube can be made from a 50 ml polypropylene centrifuge tube and some nylon tape. The tube must be shortened and the ends rejoined as shown. The dimensions shown are adequate for a typical adult mouse.

usually has a poor prognosis. Total volumes should ideally be kept at about 1 ml in the rat and about 0.1 ml in the mouse.

Specimen Collection

Because rodents naturally urinate and defaecate when restrained in an unfamiliar environment, fresh urine and faecal samples can often be collected directly from the animal. If no urine or faeces are offered, some gentle prodding of the abdomen over the bladder with a finger may produce results.

The method of blood collection depends on the quantity of blood needed. The tip of the tail may be nicked to obtain a single drop of blood for a smear. However, several hundred microlitres of blood are frequently needed for serology and alternate methods are often required. To prevent hypovolaemic shock, a simple rule of thumb for all species is to limit blood collection at one time to 1% of body weight, which is converted to millilitres by assuming that 1 ml of blood weighs 1 g. Thus, the blood collection limits on a 25 g mouse and 250 g rat calculated by this method would be 0.25 and 2.5 ml, respectively.

Although some experienced workers can reliably bleed conscious rats via the jugular vein, it is probably easiest to obtain millilitre quantities of blood from the lateral tail veins. This can be a frustrating experience if the rat or tail are not warmed first to cause tail vasodilation. The best results are obtained under anaesthesia, but blood collection can be performed without anaesthesia using restraint devices. To obtain vasodilation, rats may be placed under a 100 W lightbulb while still in their cage (at least 12 cm away to prevent burns) for 5–10 min and their tails can be dipped in 40°C water for several minutes (or 50°C water for 10 s) just prior to bleeding. To prevent tail damage, it is prudent to check the temperature of the water with an ungloved hand if a thermometer is not available. A 1 or 3 ml syringe with a 21 or 23 gauge needle is inserted into a tail vein about 3 cm from the tip, with the needle nearly parallel to the vein. If the needle enters the vein properly, blood will appear in the needle hub. If blood enters the hub but does not flow into the syringe, better results can be obtained if the tail is gently massaged repeatedly over the lateral veins in one direction only from the base toward the tip. The application of some dilute dish soap to the tail helps the process by reducing friction, which reduces tail movement and prevents needle jarring. If blood flow begins and then stops, slightly withdrawing the needle, rotating the bevel, or gently directing the needle tip downward may solve the problem. If a haematoma appears at the injection site, try again in a new site in the opposite tail vein, or closer to the tail base in the same vein.

In contrast to the rat, the lateral tail veins of the mouse are not often useful for obtaining blood via venipuncture. Instead, dilated tail veins can be nicked with a lancet to produce blood droplets that can be collected with capillary tubes. A periorbital bleeding method also utilising a capillary tube has traditionally been used for mice, but this technique requires some practice to avoid eye injury and should be performed only on anaesthetised mice. After the mouse is grasped, bleeding is greatly facilitated if the eye is proptosed slightly out of the lids by the exertion of gentle downward pressure on the lower lid with one end of the capillary tube. The other (uncontaminated) end of the capillary tube is then placed into the medial canthus angled slightly rostral to the perpendicular of the plane formed by the face and rotated in place with gentle pressure until blood enters the tube. Although this method appears traumatic, in experienced hands it rarely causes permanent damage to the socket or globe.

Terminal blood collection is best performed by cardiac puncture (under anaesthesia) for both mice and rats. The animal is placed in a dorsal recumbency, then the needle is directed to the heart from a lateral approach through the left rib cage or from a ventral approach through the diaphragm (needle begins just to the left of the xiphoid process and is angled down and slightly to the left).

Diseases—An Introduction

Healthy mice and rats spend time each day keeping their coats clean and shiny. As they become ill, their coats become ruffled and unkempt and they lose weight (unthrifty). Their activity gradually decreases until they become reluctant to move and finally assume a characteristic posture — the back is hunched up, the fur is ruffled, the head is lowered and the eyes are closed or squinting. Respirations become more pronounced and rapid. This behaviour is a clear indicator of illness, but unfortunately does not reliably suggest a specific aetiology. However, based on historical data collected from thorough necropsies of animals obtained from commercial research suppliers in the early 1980s (Bhatt *et al.*, 1986) and the likelihood that a given agent will cause clinical signs, some predictions can be offered. In mice, *Mycoplasma pulmonis*, mouse hepatitis virus (MHV), or Sendai virus would most likely be encountered as the cause of illness. In rats, *M. pulmonis*, Sendai virus and sialodacryoadenitis virus (SDAV) would be the most likely cause of illness.

The use of antibiotics for treatment of bacterial diseases of rodents is problematic because most information on antibiotic selection and efficacy is based upon older accounts of a limited number of disease outbreaks and very few systematic studies are undertaken to evaluate the efficacy of newer drugs against rodent pathogens. However, it is clear that in some cases the use of antibiotics can suppress clinical signs, thus giving some benefit to individual animals. The potentially toxic (e.g. dihydrostreptomycin in gerbils) and gut flora-altering (e.g. penicillins in hamsters and guinea pigs) side effects of antibiotics are less of a concern in mice and rats when compared with other laboratory rodents.

For animals infected with viruses such as MHV and Sendai virus, supportive care is all that can be provided because effective antiviral agents have not been tested clinically. Fortunately animals infected with the common viruses (MHV, Sendai virus, SDAV) do well if they survive the acute phase.

Supportive care is recommended to help any sick animal through acute illness. The level of dehydration present should be assessed. If the skin on the scruff of the neck 'tents' when pinched and elevated with the fingers, IV fluids (0.9% saline, 5% dextrose) via an indwelling catheter in a tail vein may be needed to correct quickly the deficit fluid. Limiting the IV fluid rate to 10–20 ml/kg/h should help prevent pulmonary oedema (Muir and Hubbell, 1989).

Less severe dehydration can be treated with fluids by the SC or IP routes if the animals will not take fluids orally from a syringe. Individual preferences vary, but fruit-flavoured, sugared drinks are often accepted from a water bottle or syringe when water is not. Do not assume that a particular flavour used in a water bottle will appeal to all animals equally well. Liquid consumption should be monitored to make sure that an animal is not becoming dehydrated because the flavour is unpalatable. If the animal is not drinking, 40–80 ml of fluid per kg per day is required to maintain health (Waynforth and Flecknell, 1992). For a 25 g mouse, this would be 1–2 ml per day and for a 400 g rat, 16–32 ml per day. Fluids administered by the SC or IP route are best given in divided doses, perhaps 4 times during the day. Ideally, SC fluid injection volumes should be kept to about 0.5 ml per site on a mouse and about 5 ml per site on a rat to prevent pain from skin distension.

Additionally, animals should be kept warm and dry. A light bulb can be placed about 12 cm outside the cage at one end to allow the animal to move to its preferred temperature, but extreme caution must be used to prevent overheating. For instance, if an aquarium is used as a rodent cage, it is difficult to prevent overheating because ventilation is relatively poor. A sheltered area that allows the animals to escape the glare of the light and direct heat is a good idea when a warming light is used. If a suspended feeder is in use, some food should be placed in the cage so that the effort required to obtain food is minimised. The food should be replaced promptly if it gets wet or soiled.

Figure 1.5 found at the end of the chapter summarises the diseases discussed below.

Diseases of the Respiratory System

Bacterial Diseases

Mycoplasmosis

Agent. *M. pulmonis* is an important extracellular pathogen of mice and rats that colonises the respiratory epithelium. It is a bacterium in Class Mollicutes. The organism lacks a cell wall and with a diameter of as little as 0.3 μm, is very small for a bacterium. There is wide variability in pathogenicity between mycoplasma isolates (National Research Council, 1991).

Hosts. *M. pulmonis* can cause severe lesions in mice and rats. Rarely, hamsters, guinea pigs and rabbits can carry the organism, but do not develop lesions.

Clinical signs. Clinical signs may include respiratory distress, snuffling (rhinitis), nasal discharge and torticollis (secondary to otitis interna). Pulmonary abscesses are often present. Purulent endometritis and other genital infections have been described in highly susceptible rats such as the Lewis strain. However, it is important to remember that inapparent chronic infection is common.

Diagnosis. Diagnosis by culture of the respiratory tract in special medium is definitive, but ELISA testing of serum is much more cost-effective.

Treatment / control. Elimination of the organism from infected animals is not feasible, but tetracycline or tylosin may suppress clinical signs. Because disease is potentiated by high intracage ammonia levels, clinical signs (but not infection) may be prevented by proper cage sanitation. Concurrent respiratory infections such as Sendai virus (mice and rats) and sialodacryoadenitis virus (rats) also potentiate mycoplasma respiratory disease. In a colony setting, depopulation and restocking with uninfected animals is the best approach, but caesarian derivation of valuable strains is possible.

Streptococcus pneumoniae infection

Agent. *Streptococcus pneumoniae* is a Gram-positive lancet-shaped coccus that is often seen in pairs under the microscope (hence the earlier genus designation *Diplococcus*). The organism produces haemolysis on blood agar and can be differentiated from related streptococci by bile and ethylhydrocupreine (optochin) sensitivity (National Research Council, 1991).

Hosts. *S. pneumoniae* can cause severe respiratory infections in rats and guinea pigs, but only inapparent infections have been described in mice. Primates are also susceptible.

Clinical signs. Clinical signs include suppurative rhinitis, otitis media and interna and fibrinous lobar pneumonia, leading to septicaemia and death. Pleural and pericardial effusion may also be seen (even in the absence of gross pulmonary lesions). Torticollis or circling may be occasionally observed as sequelae of otitis interna.

Diagnosis. Diagnosis can be achieved by Gram-staining of effusion smears or contact impressions of affected organs as this will often reveal the Gram-positive diplococci. In the absence of typical gross or microscopic lesions, interpretation of positive cultures must be tempered by the fact that pneumococci can be commensals in the rat (and mouse) respiratory tract without any apparent adverse effect.

Treatment / control. Treatment with penicillin or another antibiotic indicated by antibiotic sensitivity testing may improve clinical signs, but elimination of pneumococci is not likely. Zoonotic infection is a possibility, but there is no current evidence that it is a reality.

CAR (cilia-associated respiratory) bacillus infection

Agent. This is an unusual bacterial pathogen that inserts itself onto the surface of ciliated respiratory epithelial cells. It is so elongated ($0.2 \ \mu$m $\times$ $6.0 \ \mu$m) that it can masquerade as a cilium on electron micrographs (National Research Council, 1991).

Hosts. It has been reported in laboratory mice, rats and rabbits, but its pathogenic potential as a potentiator of *M. pulmonis* respiratory disease has been demonstrated most clearly in rats. Recent reports suggest that bacilli from rats have characteristics different from those obtained from rabbits. Thus, CAR bacillus isolates may eventually be differentiated into more than one species.

Clinical signs. Clinical signs in rats are usually identical to those of severe *M. pulmonis* respiratory infections. The severity of natural uncomplicated infections is unclear. Descriptions of clinical disease in mice or other rodents are very sparse.

Diagnosis. Although it is now possible to culture the organism in artificial media or a cell line in some laboratories (Cundiff *et al.*, 1994; Schoeb *et al.*, 1993), serological testing is widely available and represents an economical approach to screening. Confirmation of the organisms on respiratory tissue sections by silver stain would be important to verify a serological diagnosis.

Treatment / control. There is no known treatment, but given the apparent common clinical association with *M. pulmonis* infection, therapy aimed at suppressing the clinical signs of *M. pulmonis* would probably be helpful. Control by caesarian derivation appears to be effective in breeding colonies.

Corynebacterium kutscheri *infection*

Agent. *C. kutscheri* is a Gram-positive diphtheroid bacillus.

Hosts. Mice and rats are most often infected. Rarely, guinea pigs may be infected.

Clinical signs. *C. kutscheri* usually exists in mice and rats as a subclinical infection. In active infections in rats, respiratory distress (dyspnoea, weight loss, anorexia, hunched posture) related to pulmonary lesions (necropurulent parenchymal lesions) is more typical, whereas in mice general malaise secondary to necropurulent lesions of multiple abdominal organs is more common. Lesions in the lungs may become granulomatous over time, which led some workers to refer to *C. kutscheri* infections as 'pseudotuberculosis' (National Research Council, 1991).

Diagnosis. Diagnosis is primarily by culture of affected organs and evaluation of microscopic lesions, but the bacilli may sometimes be presumptively identified by their tendency to assume a characteristic 'Chinese letter' arrangement in Gram- or silver-stained tissue smears. Greyish to yellow dome-shaped non-haemolytic colonies develop on blood agar, but no growth is seen on MacConkey's agar.

Treatment / control. Tetracycline, chlortetracycline, chloramphenicol and other antibiotics may be effective in limiting clinical signs if treatment is begun early enough, but elimination of the organism is unlikely. Chronic carriage and shedding is a problem.

Viral Diseases

Sendai virus (SV) infection

Agent. Sendai virus is an RNA virus in the family Paramyxovirus. All known strains are antigenically very similar.

Hosts. Mice and rats are the main hosts. Hamsters can be infected, but are resistant to disease.

Clinical signs. In naive animals, respiratory distress, prolonged gestation, neonatal death and poor growth may be seen. In enzootically infected colonies, neonates are passively protected by maternal antibodies until mild subclinical infections occur at 1–2 months of age. Although some mouse strains (e.g. 129, DBA) are very sensitive to Sendai virus infection alone, more severe clinical signs including death, are usually the result of concurrent mycoplasma or CAR bacillus respiratory infections. There is no carrier state in immunocompetent animals that survive the initial episode.

Diagnosis. SV infection is difficult to diagnose based on clinical signs alone. Serology is usually reliable and observation of characteristic microscopic respiratory lesions is helpful. ELISA serum testing and lung histopathology are used in a laboratory setting.

Treatment / control. There is no specific treatment, but supportive treatment may help. Adult rodents clear the infection in about a week, but in a breeding colony an enzootic infection can be established because of the continuing presence of susceptible neonates. To control established infections, pups should be euthanased and all breeding should cease for 6–8 weeks to allow the adults to clear the infection completely. Adults usually completely recover if they survive acute infection unless other complicating infections are present. SV is one of the most highly contagious infections of mice and rats (National Research Council, 1991).

Diseases of the Digestive System

Bacterial Diseases

Citrobacteriosis

Agent. *Citrobacter freundii* is a Gram-negative facultative anaerobic rod measuring 1 μm wide by 2–6 μm long. The biotype (4280) of *C. freundii* known to cause disease is positive for ornithine decarboxylase, ferments rhamnose, produces hydrogen sulphide and reduces nitrate (in contrast with non-pathogenic biotypes that do not). The designation 4280 is a numerical key derived from biochemical assay results used for identification purposes in a commercial kit.

Hosts. Only mice are known to be affected.

Clinical signs. This organism initiates a unique colonic mucosal hyperplasia that results in diarrhoea and a prolapsed rectum. Affected mice will appear sick and high mortality may result. The colon and caecum may be grossly thickened on necropsy. The disease is self limiting in adults in 4–6 weeks, but may persist longer in younger mice.

Diagnosis. Diagnosis is based on isolation of the pathogenic biotype from culture of the colon and observation of the characteristic gross and microscopic lesions.

Treatment / control. Tetracycline or neomycin in the drinking water may control symptoms. Depopulation and restocking with uninfected animals is recommended in a colony setting.

Tyzzer's disease

Agent. Tyzzer's disease is caused by a fastidious bacterium now identified as *Clostridium piliforme* (formerly *Bacillus piliformis*). The vegetative form is an obligate intracellular pathogen that quickly loses viability after the host's death. However, the spores are very stable and can survive at room temperature for a year or more. The spores are resistant to formaldehyde, organic iodine,

benzalkonium chloride, ethanol and phenolic compounds. High heat (70°C for 30 min, 80°C for 15 min) and 0.3% sodium hypochlorite (dilute bleach) for 5 min will inactivate the spores (National Research Council, 1991).

Hosts. This bacterial pathogen affects a variety of species including mice, rats, hamsters, gerbils (most susceptible), guinea pigs, gerbils, rabbits, cats, dogs and monkeys. Of the rodents, the gerbil is considered most susceptible.

Clinical signs. Clinical signs are mild to severe and may include diarrhoea, but are non-specific (typical sick mouse or rat). Gross lesions, when present, may range from multiple pale foci in the liver to a dilated ileum and caecum to myocardial inflammation.

Diagnosis. Diagnosis is by histopathology (silver stain of organisms in characteristic lesions) or by serology.

Treatment / control. Typically, stress (inadequate cage sanitation, hot/cold environment, overcrowding) contributes to disease expression. Control is very difficult because spores shed in faeces can persist for a year or more. Repopulation after a thorough room and cage cleaning is best in large populations. Oral tetracycline may prevent mortality, but will not eliminate the chronic infection. Supportive therapy may be needed during the early infection phase.

Viral Diseases

Sialodacryoadenitis virus (SDAV)

Agent. This is a rat coronavirus pathogen that shares antigenic cross reactivity with mouse hepatitis virus (MHV), a coronavirus pathogen of mice. Earlier, some rat coronaviruses noted to cause mild respiratory lesions were termed rat coronavirus (RCV) isolates in contrast with the SDAV isolates that caused the classic signs described below, but with the realisation that SDAV and RCV isolates cause similar typically mild respiratory lesions in adults, many workers now consider RCV isolates to be variants of SDAV.

Host. Only rats are known to be naturally infected.

Clinical signs. As with Sendai virus infections (and MHV infections of mice below), clinical signs depend on the immune status of the animal at the time of infection. In enzootically infected breeding colonies neonates are protected by maternal antibodies until they are older when they typically exhibit only mild conjunctivitis (some blinking may be observed). In naive rats, high morbidity and low mortality is observed. Classic clinical signs include sneezing, grossly swollen necks (due to inflammation and swelling of salivary glands, lacrimal glands and lymph nodes), porphyrin staining around eyelids (Harderian hypersecretion), suborbital swelling (inflamed Harderian and intraorbital lacrimal glands) and keratitis and corneal ulcers (due to loss of tears). Occasionally an animal will have permanent eye damage (megaloglobus, chronic keratitis), but complete recovery in 1–2 weeks is typical. There is no carrier state in rats that survive the initial episode. Weanlings can be more severely affected and deaths might be expected in such populations. There is evidence that SDAV can exacerbate *M. pulmonis* infections (National Research Council, 1991).

Diagnosis. Diagnosis can be made with some confidence if the classic swollen neck is observed. Serology is very helpful, but remember that in the absence of a classic presentation of a swollen cervical area or corroborating microscopic lesions, a positive serological test may simply indicate previous exposure. The appearance of typical lesions in the salivary and lacrimal glands is very helpful. While the submaxillary (mixed serous–mucous) and parotid (serous) salivary glands are often severely affected, the mucous sublingual salivary gland is paradoxically spared from damage.

Treatment / control. Treatment is supportive. Adults shed virus for only about a week and usually show a complete clinical recovery within 1–2 weeks. To control established infections, any pups should be euthanased and all breeding should cease for 6–8 weeks to allow the adults to clear the infection completely.

Mouse hepatitis virus (MHV)

Agent. MHV is a coronavirus pathogen of mice. The name MHV is misleading because the liver is only one of several organs affected and liver lesions do not predominate in all virus strains. There is significant variability in the pathogenicity of different virus strains and in the susceptibility of different mouse strains.

Host. Only mice are known to be naturally infected.

Clinical signs. As in Sendai virus (mice and rats) and SDAV infections (rats only), clinical signs depend on the immune status of the mice when infected. In enzootically infected colonies, clinical signs are usually mild because neonates are protected by maternal antibodies when they would be most susceptible to infection. In naive mice, clinical signs are usually non-specific (ruffling, hunched posture, photophobia). Naive immunocompetent adults usually exhibit mild signs and clear the virus in 7–10 days. In naive neonates, infections are more severe and can result in diarrhoea and death. There is no carrier state in immunocompetent adults (National Research Council, 1991).

MHV infections tend to exhibit one of two disease patterns depending on the tissue tropisms of the virus strain. In the respiratory disease pattern, initial infection of the nasal passages progresses to respiratory tract infection and vascular dissemination to internal organs such as lymph nodes, thymus, liver, bone marrow and spleen. Intestinal tract involvement is minimal. In the enteric pattern, infection is restricted to the nasal passages and intestines, with the liver and other abdominal organs being variably infected. The lungs are usually not involved. Despite the existence of these two disease patterns, differences in clinical signs are not significant.

Diagnosis. Diagnosis is based upon serology and histopathology.

Treatment / control. Treatment is supportive. MHV is widely distributed in conventional research colonies and is likely to be present in many pet breeding colonies where enzootic infections are easily established. In such cases the infection can be eradicated by euthanasing susceptible pups and stopping all breeding for 6–8 weeks to allow the adults to clear the infection completely (as in Sendai and SDAV infections).

Endoparasites

There have been numerous intestinal parasites identified in mice and rats, but few would be expected to cause clinical problems in immunocompetent adult mice or rats (National Research Council, 1991). Only two are discussed here. *Hymenolepis* tapeworm infections are discussed because of their zoonotic potential and pinworm infections are discussed because they are very common and can cause clinical signs in some rodents.

Hymenolepis *tapeworm infections*

Agents / hosts. *Hymenolepis nana* (dwarf tapeworm) and *Hymenolepis diminuta* (rat tapeworm) can infect mice, rats and other rodents. Adults attach to the mucosa of the small intestine and shed eggs in the faeces. *H. diminuta* has a 3–4 week indirect life cycle utilising flea or beetle intermediaries and is easily eliminated by vector control and regular bedding changes to remove eggs before they become patent. In addition to the indirect route, *H. nana* can also utilise a direct infection cycle without intermediates as well as internal autoinfection without external egg passage. This makes control of *H. nana* more difficult.

Clinical signs. Infections are rarely pathogenic in adults, but heavy infections in young may cause weight loss, intestinal obstruction and even death.

Diagnosis. Diagnosis is by identification of the egg in faecal floats (three pairs of hooks in the 40–60 μm × 30–55 μm *H. nana* egg or in the larger 60–90 μm × 50–80 μm *H. diminuta* egg) or by identification of adult or cysticercal stages by histopathology.

Treatment / control. Niclosamide, praziquantel and thiabendazole have been recommended as treatment for either cestode. Proper sanitation is critical to controlling egg dispersion until adults and larvae are eliminated. Although mostly a potential problem for children in developing countries, both cestodes can infect humans and should be treated aggressively as soon as the diagnosis is made.

Pinworm infections

Agents / hosts. *Syphacia obvelata* and *Syphacia muris* are the common pinworms of mice and rats, respectively (some crossover does occur). Gravid females migrate out of the bowel and lay eggs on the perineal skin; these are then ingested to continue the direct life cycle.

Clinical signs. Both pinworms are highly infectious and can compromise health, but clinical signs (diarrhoea, rectal prolapse, unthriftiness) will be infrequent except in younger animals with very high worm burdens.

Diagnosis. Antemortem diagnosis is by identification of the ova on adhesive tape impressions of the anal area or in faecal samples. The eggs of both species are somewhat banana-shaped, being about 130 μm × 40 μm (*S. obvelata*) or 75 μm × 30 μm (*S. muris*).

Treatment / control. Ivermectin has proved to be an effective treatment. Three oral doses at 2 mg/kg (in oil or propylene glycol) spaced 1 week apart have been effective for *S. muris* infections in rats (Huerkamp, 1993). Two doses, as detailed above, 10 days apart are reportedly effective in eliminating *S. obvelata* in mice (Flynn *et al.*,

1989). Alternatively, 2 μg/ml ivermectin in the water bottle for 21 days has been used to eradicate *S. muris* from rats (Diggs *et al.*, 1990). Some authors have expressed concern about the potentially toxic effects of ivermectin (particularly in breeding colonies) and have recommended fenbendazole as a safer alternative (150 mg/kg formulated in the feed; two 1-week feeding periods were separated by a week of feeding with normal chow (Coghlan *et al.*, 1993)). Accumulating evidence suggests that C57BL/6 mice may be hypersensitive to ivermectin, so other agents should probably be used in this strain. Pinworm eggs are so light that they easily float in the air from room to room, making control very difficult. Infected animals must be treated at the same time as rigorous sanitation procedures are followed to eliminate infections in multiroom housing environments.

Non-Infectious Diseases

Malocclusion

Aetiology. Accidental trauma, genetic, or developmental problems can result in misaligned incisor roots. Also, the traumatic permanent loss of a tooth (via root damage) prevents the natural grinding action of opposing incisors and results in tooth overgrowth.

Clinical signs. If malocclusion is present, the lower incisors will often grow until they curve back and pierce the soft palate, ultimately resulting in mouth trauma and starvation. Always check for malocclusion carefully during the physical examination.

Treatment. A dedicated pair of guillotine-style dog toenail clippers can be used to trim the teeth on a weekly or biweekly basis to prevent oral trauma and starvation. Protective goggles should be worn. Usually, this is a procedure that does not require general anaesthesia, but care must be taken not to twist the teeth during clipping, or additional tooth damage may occur. The hemi-mandibular joint is flexible enough to allow the lower incisors to bend apart when manipulated in an anaesthetised animal. This is normal and should not be mistaken for osteomalacia.

Diseases of the Genitourinary System

Bacterial Infections

Leptospirosis

Agents. Members of the genus *Leptospira* are Gram-negative, motile, corkscrew-shaped rods about 0.1 μm $\times$ 6–12 μm long. Many serovars of pathogenic *Leptospira interrogans* have been isolated from animals. Although many species can infect mice and rats, most commonly, mice are infected with *L. interrogans* serovar *ballum* (Foster *et al.*, 1982) and rats are infected with *L. interrogans* serovar *icterohemorrhagiae* (Baker *et al.*, 1979).

Hosts. Wild mice are considered the natural reservoir of *L. ballum*. Many mammals and reptiles can be infected with leptospires, which colonise renal tissue and are shed in the urine. Hamsters, young guinea pigs and gerbils are more susceptible to infection than mice or rats. Humans are also susceptible.

Clinical signs. Rodents are unusual in that they can harbour lifelong patent leptospire infections without any clinical signs. In humans, the disease varies from inapparent infections to serious complications leading to death. Human infections can result in sudden illness characterised by weakness, headache, myalgia, malaise, fever and chills. Conjunctivitis and rash often follow, as does a painful orchitis in men. Chronic weight loss and malaise can occur if proper treatment is not obtained.

Diagnosis. Diagnosis is primarily by culture of kidneys or urine in special media or by serology (usually provided by specialised laboratories). In some cases, inoculation of 3–4-week-old hamsters with fresh kidney tissue from suspected cases is performed to detect low levels of infection. The organisms can sometimes be identified in smears of infected tissue or in urine by dark-field illumination or phase-contrast microscopy.

Treatment / control. Because of the potentially serious zoonotic hazard, euthanasia of infected animals is indicated. Infection is transmitted through secretions from the nose, mouth and eyes of infected rodents to humans through abrasions or by aerosols. It is imperative that contact between wild and pet or research animals is prevented. There are intermittent reports of zoonotic infections acquired through contact with urine from both research and pet mice and rats. A high index of suspicion should be maintained whenever members of a pet owner's family report persistent non-specific malaise, weight loss, or 'flu-like symptoms. Physicians can miss a diagnosis of leptospirosis because it is uncommon. The same is true of lymphocytic choriomeningitis (LCMV, see below).

M. pulmonis *endometritis and pyometra*

Agent. *M. pulmonis* has been described earlier (see *Diseases of the Respiratory System* above).

Host. Although several strains of rat may have natural *M. pulmonis* infections of the genital tract, only LEW rats are reported to have serious reproductive tract disease. The LEW rat is also very susceptible to respiratory mycoplasmosis.

Clinical signs. Clinical signs are non-specific, but reduced reproductive function would be expected.

Diagnosis. Antemortem diagnosis is difficult, but radiographs might be of some use. Purulent endometritis, pyometra, salpingitis, or perioophoritis might be seen on necropsy. Culture of the affected reproductive tissue would be definitive.

Treatment / control. For control and treatment of infections see the discussion of *M. pulmonis*

in the section entitled *Diseases of the Respiratory System*.

Preputial gland abscesses

Agents. A variety of bacterial pathogens, including *Staphylococcus aureus* and *Pasteurella pneumotropica,* can infect the preputial glands.

Hosts. Both mice and rats can be affected. Nude mice are predisposed to this problem.

Clinical signs. Such abscesses usually present as firm bilateral spherical swellings around the penis. In advanced cases, ulceration of overlying skin may be seen.

Diagnosis. The gross appearance is usually adequate to make the diagnosis. However, rare preputial neoplasms can mimic abscesses (this is more likely if a unilateral presentation is seen). Evaluation of a smear made from a fine needle aspirate will allow differentiation between the two.

Treatment / control. Lancing the abscess(es) under anaesthesia to allow drainage is often all that is required, but an antibacterial ointment may promote healing. If found, preputial gland neoplasms should be removed surgically.

Parasitic Infections

Trichosomoides crassicauda

Agent. The 9–10 mm long female nematode lives in the urinary bladder, anchored at one end to the transitional epithelium. The much smaller male resides permanently within the reproductive tract of the female. Eggs are passed out through the urine.

Host. Only the rat is infected.

Clinical signs. Although most infections are subclinical, irritation of the bladder can result in the presence of urinary leucocytes, calculi or even tumours. Eosinophilia is also seen sometimes. Dysuria and unthriftiness may be seen occasionally in rats with severe burdens of calculi or tumour tissue.

Diagnosis. Bladder stones may be palpable, but antemortem diagnosis is most likely by identification of the characteristic heavy-walled, double-plugged oval 60 μm $\times$ 30μm egg in the urine. The female can be identified in the bladder at necropsy.

Treatment. A single 3 mg/kg oral dose of ivermectin in propylene glycol is reported to be effective (Summa *et al.*, 1992). Ivermectin treatment as described above for pinworms might also be effective.

Diseases of the Nervous System

Other than torticollis and circling secondary to otitis interna caused (most commonly) by *M. pulmonis* or *S. pneumoniae*, specific dysfunction of the nervous system in mice and rats is rarely observed. Murine encephalomyelitis virus (MEV) infects both mice and rats and can cause poliomyelitis and demyelination leading to clinical signs of flaccid paralysis of the rear legs. This is extremely rare, however, occurring only in about one in several thousand infected animals. Rats may be infected with the microsporidian protozoan *Encephalitozoon cuniculi*, which can cause brain and kidney lesions more commonly in rabbits, but clinical signs in rabbits or rats are very rare. Diagnosis of both MEV and *E. cuniculi* is based on characteristic histopathology and serological testing. There is no treatment for MEV or *E. cuniculi* and no known zoonotic potential.

Although rabies is extremely rare in wild mice or rats and non-existent in research or commercial facilities (except in experimental studies of the virus), clients may wonder about the likelihood of rodent bites transmitting the disease to humans. Because all warm-blooded animals are potentially infected by rabies virus, mice and rats must be considered a possible source of the virus. However, mice and rats are not a significant rabies reservoir in most parts of the world and there are very few reports of rodent to human rabies transmission over the past 40 years (Baker *et al.*, 1979; Foster *et al.*, 1982). In experimentally infected mice, flaccid paralysis and sometimes convulsions occur 7–24 days after inoculation. Death follows about 24 h later (Foster *et al.*, 1982).

Although local or federal health officials and physicians should be consulted for current policies, human anti-rabies prophylaxis is not usually warranted for bites by pets or research rodents. In areas where the rodent population is known to harbour rabies, or if a wild rodent exhibits uncharacteristically aggressive behaviour (wild rodents fear humans unless they have been fed), human anti-rabies prophylaxis might be considered when a bite occurs. An exceptional circumstance that would probably warrant prophylaxis would be if a pet mouse or rat survived the bite of a rabid carnivore, then bit a human (Bhatt *et al.*, 1986). As is the practice with other animals suspected of rabies infection, the head of the rodent would be needed for analysis by the responsible government laboratory. There are no vaccines commonly used to immunise rodents against rabies. But given the susceptibility of mice to the virus, only a killed vaccine would be indicated in those exceptional cases when immunisation was indicated.

Diseases of the Integument and Musculoskeletal System

Fungal Diseases

Dermatophytosis

Agents. Several species of fungi in the genera *Trychophyton* (including *mentagrophytes*) and *Microsporum* (including *gypseum*) can cause dermal lesions.

Hosts. Dermatophytes have a very wide host range, including rodents, rabbits, carnivores and people.

Clinical signs. Mice and rats can carry inapparent, chronic infections. When they occur, lesions consist of small to confluent scaly areas of alopecia.

Diagnosis. Differentiation of skin lesions from mites is by identification of mycelia or arthrospores in skin scrapings from the periphery of the lesion digested with 10% potassium hydroxide. Wood's lamp fluorescence of the lesion may also be helpful. Culture of the organisms on Sabouraud's or equivalent media assists diagnosis. Hair brushings from suspected asymptomatic carriers may also be examined and cultured.

Treatment / control. The actual incidence in research settings is very low and the incidence in pets is probably low as well. Inapparent infections are not likely to be investigated unless a diagnosis of ringworm is made in an exposed human. Prolonged treatment (30–60 days) with griseofulvin at 25 mg/kg PO may cure the infection, but periodic follow-up skin scrapings to evaluate therapy efficacy are advisable. Dermatophytes are not usually important pathogens of mice and rats, but the zoonotic potential of these pathogens must be appreciated.

Parasitic Diseases

Mites

Agents. A large number of mites have been recovered from wild rodents, but infections in laboratory animals are becoming very rare. The prevalence in the pet population is unknown. Of the many mites described, only the mouse fur mites *Myobia musculi* (more pathogenic) and *Mycoptes musculinus* have much pathogenic potential. Rats have similar, though generally fewer pathogenic mites (e.g. *Radfordia ensifera*). *Liponyssus* (formerly *Ornithonyssus*) *bacoti*, the tropical rat mite, has zoonotic potential. All are arthropods in the order Acarina.

Hosts. *M. musculi* and *M. musculinus* are found primarily on mice, rarely on other rodents. *Radfordia ensifera* is found primarily on rats, rarely on other rodents. *Liponyssus bacoti* infects both mice and rats.

Clinical signs. Ulcerative skin lesions on the dorsum of mice may be produced by the fur mite *M. musculi* (more pathogenic) or *M. musculinus*. Similar but milder lesions may be caused by *R. ensifera* infection of rats. *L. bacoti*, the tropical rat mite, can cause general unthriftiness and anaemia if infections are allowed to continue unchecked. It will cause a papular rash on humans. C57BL/6 mice can develop allergic sensitivities to mites that result in more severe lesions than normal.

Diagnosis. Diagnosis is by identification of parasites in skin scrapings or pelt brushings or by examination of the pelt with a magnifying glass. At necropsy, a pelt placed in a Petri dish in the refrigerator will allow identification of mites as they abandon the cooling pelt. Rarely, *Sarcoptes scabiei* may also be found on mice and rats and can also cause zoonotic infections.

Treatment / control. Control and eventual elimination is possible by dusting the animal, cage and (in the case of *Liponyssus* infestation) surrounding areas with pyrethrin or carbaryl weekly for several weeks (periodic rechecks would be advisable). Ivermectin is reportedly effective for fur mite infestations (see *Pinworm infections* above), or place a drop of 1% ivermectin diluted 1:100 in 1:1 propylene glycol/water, 3 treatments 1 week apart, and might be used in conjunction with light dusting of the environment for a more rapid cure. The toe nails should be kept short to prevent secondary self trauma of pruritic lesions.

Lice

Agents. *Polyplax serrata* and *Polyplax spinulosa* in the order Anoplura are the only lice likely to be encountered in mice and rats. These lice are known vectors of *Encephalitozoon cuniculi*, *Eperythrozoon coccoides* and *Haemobartonella muris*.

Hosts. Mice are infested with *P. serrata* and rats are infested with *P. spinulosa*.

Clinical signs. Heavy infestations of these blood sucking lice can lead to unthriftiness, restlessness and dermal pruritus.

Diagnosis. Diagnosis is as described above for mites.

Treatment / control. Treatment is as for mites. Lice and mites should not be tolerated in research animals or pets. In a research setting, depopulation and restocking with uninfected animals is usually the most effective action.

Fleas

Agents. Rodent fleas of the genera *Xenopsylla* and *Nosopsylla* as well as others are important because they are the vectors of serious zoonotic infections such as *Yersinia pestis* (plague) and *Rickettsia typhus* (scrub typhus). They also act as an intermediate host for *Hymenolepis* tapeworms. Fleas are insects in the order Siphonaptera (National Research Council, 1991).

Hosts. Mice and rats can be infested by a wide variety of fleas, but such infestations are very rare in modern laboratory settings. Wild rodent populations are always a potential source of infestation for laboratory and pet rodents alike.

Clinical signs. Clinical signs in rodents are poorly documented, but presumably severe infections could produce pruritic lesions.

Diagnosis. Diagnosis is by visualisation of fleas on affected mice or rats.

Treatment / control. Standard flea control measures such as carbaryl dusting or pyrethrin sprays should be effective in eradicating rodent fleas from pets (Fox *et al.*, 1984).

Non-Infectious Diseases

Ringtail

Relative humidity levels below 40% can result in annular constrictions on the tails of rats that can progress to necrosis and tail sloughing in neonates. Treatment is palliative. The condition is prevented by raising the relative humidity to 40–70%, preferably to at least 50%. The condition has also been reported rarely in mice.

Foot lesions

Plantar foot lesions are sometimes seen on mice or rats housed on wire floors. Treatment with topical antibiotic salves and removal of affected animals to shoebox-style cages with soft bedding helps. This condition is controlled by improving cage sanitation (reducing faecal bacteria counts) and discontinuing the use of floors with rough or sharp surfaces.

Barbering

Dominant male and female mice in groups will sometimes chew off sharply delineated patches of facial and body hair from less dominant mice. The hairs are 'barbered' so close that the skin looks clean shaven. Typically, the dominant mouse will be the only one in the group not barbered. A similar condition (muzzle alopecia) is sometimes seen in mice that have worn the hair off both sides of their muzzle while eating between cage bars. In both conditions the skin has a normal appearance (although the mouse may not) and neither condition usually causes any problems. Although less common, rats will also barber guinea pigs too. A skin scraping will be negative for dermatophytes or parasites.

Bite wounds

In contrast to the benign practice of barbering, dominant mice will sometimes repeatedly bite their cagemates. Small scabs (and focal alopecia) will appear on the tail and dorsum of subordinates (sometimes the perianal area is also involved) and periodic squealing will be heard as attacks occur. Subordinates lose weight because they are constantly harassed and may die of their wounds. The only control measure is to remove the dominant mouse from the group. Once the offender is removed, the subordinates usually quickly recover body weight and heal. Males tend to be more prone to biting and some strains (e.g. C57BL/6, BALB/c) are extremely aggressive.

Systemic Diseases

Bacterial Diseases

Salmonellosis

Agent. *Salmonella enteritidis* is a Gram-negative, non-spore-forming rod about 1 μm wide $\times$ 3 μm long. Currently all salmonella isolates are considered to be *S. typhi* (human infections only), *S. choleraesuis* (usually swine) or *S. enteritidis* (many animals, see below). Most isolates previously identified as separate species (e.g. *S. typhimurium*, *S. amsterdam*, *S. newport*, *S. dublin*) are now considered to be one of more than 1000 serotypes of *S. enteritidis* and are properly written, for example, as *S. enteritidis* serotype typhimurium or *S. enteritidis* serotype amsterdam. However, in the literature the old method (i.e. *S. typhimurium*) is often still employed for convenience. Rodents are usually only susceptible to the *S. enteritidis* serotypes (National Research Council, 1991).

Hosts. *S. enteritidis* is a serious pathogen of mice, rats and most other rodents and mammals. It also infects poultry and reptiles (there were so many cases of human salmonellosis cases attributed to small pet turtles that interstate shipments were banned over 20 years ago in the US). Experimental *S. enteritidis* serotype typhimurium infections of mice are an important model of human *S. typhi* (typhoid fever) infections.

Clinical signs. Clinical signs in rodents range from asymptomatic to nonspecific (ruffled fur, hunched posture) to acute death. Diarrhoea is seen occasionally. Asymptomatic chronic shedders are not uncommon and culture is not always effective in identifying such shedders because shedding varies over time. Multifocal pale hepatic lesions and splenomegaly are typical but variable, depending on the stage and severity of disease. Ulcerative caecitis is more common in the rat. In humans, infections can range from diarrhoea and other gastrointestinal symptoms to full blown systemic disease characterised by fever, chills, weakness and even death.

Diagnosis. Diagnosis is by culture of bacteria from affected organs or faeces using standard media, and by histopathology.

Treatment / control. Because of the clear zoonotic potential, depopulation rather than treatment is used to control infections. Prevention of contact with wild rodents is critical because they can be salmonella carriers.

Streptobacillosis

Agent. *Streptobacillus moniliformis* is a large (0.4 μm $\times$ 3 μm) Gram-negative bacillus that is an oral cavity commensal of wild and laboratory rats. It is spherical or club-shaped. The taxonomy is problematic and numerous other names have been proposed periodically (*Streptothrix muris ratti*, *Nocardia muris*, *Actinomyces muris*, *Haverhilia multiformis*, *Asterococcus muris*).

Hosts. The rat is the natural host. Mice, guinea pigs and humans can be infected by exposure to, or bites from, rats.

Clinical signs. In its role as a commensal, it causes no clinical signs in rats. Infections in mice are septicaemic with internal organ involvement and high mortality. Classical signs in mice that survive acute infection include chronic arthritis, limb deformity and even limb amputation ('ectromelia', see mousepox infection below). *S. moniliformis* (and another commensal, *Spirillum minus*) cause rat bite fever, a potentially serious infection of humans transmitted by the bite of a rat (or rarely, a mouse) and characterised by regional lymphadenopathy, macular rash on extremities, fever, malaise, chills and myalgia.

Diagnosis. Diagnosis is by culture of joint fluid, blood, or affected organs.

Treatment / control. Timely antibiotic therapy in humans is essential—penicillins and less often tetracyclines and streptomycin have been the antibiotics of choice in humans (Foster *et al.*, 1982). Infected rodents are euthanased because of the zoonotic potential. The disease is rare in modern research rodents, but the prevalence in pets is unknown. Exposure of pet and laboratory rodents (and humans) to wild rats should be prevented.

Viral Diseases

Lymphocytic choriomeningitis virus (LCMV) infection

Agent. LCMV is an RNA virus in the family Arenavirus. Virus particles bud from the plasma membrane and can form large intracytoplasmic inclusions.

Hosts. Wild mice are the principal reservoir. Laboratory mice and hamsters serve as the most important source of infection in research settings (as are infected transplantable tumours, cell lines and other biological materials). Other rodents, rabbits, primates and humans are also susceptible, but are not known to transmit the virus. Recent zoonotic infections in laboratory settings have been caused by hamsters.

Clinical signs. Natural infections of both mice and hamsters can be subclinical, resulting in asymptomatic chronic shedding in urine, saliva and milk. In mice, neonatal stunting may occur and immune complex deposition in the kidneys of 7–10-month-old adults can result in renal failure and a typical sick mouse. In humans, 'flu-like symptoms (fever, headache, myalgia, vomiting, sore throat, photophobia) are most common, but rash, diarrhoea, cough, lymphadenopathy, orchitis, delirium, or amnesia can also be seen. Deaths have occurred (National Research Council, 1991).

Diagnosis. Diagnosis is principally by serology.

Treatment / control. Because of the zoonotic potential, infected animals are euthanased. Prevention of contact with wild mice is critical because they are frequent carriers of LCMV. Vet-erinarians should maintain a high index of suspicion when members of the pet owner's family report severe 'flu-like symptoms.

Hantavirus infection

Agent. Hantaviruses form the relatively new genus Hantavirus in the family Bunyaviridae. The prototype virus is Hantaan virus, named after the Hantaan river in Korea.

Hosts. Small mammals, particularly rodents, are the reservoir for hantavirus infections. Humans can be infected. The known rodent hosts and human disease syndromes associated with hantaviruses (if any) are as follows: field mice (*Apodemus* sp.) in Korea (Korean haemorrhagic fever, KHF) and China (epidemic haemorrhagic fever, EHF); bank voles (*Clethrionymus* sp.) in Scandinavia (nephropathica epidemicus, NE); the meadow vole (*Microtus pennsylvanicus*) in the Eastern US (no known disease); deer mice (*Peromyscus maniculatus*) in the Western US (hantavirus pulmonary syndrome, HPS); and wild and laboratory Norwegian rats (*Rattus norvegicus*) in Korea, China, the former Soviet Union, Japan, Scandinavia, UK, France, The Netherlands and Belgium (various syndromes in animal caretakers and laboratory research personnel).

Clinical signs. Infections in rodents can be persistent and are usually asymptomatic. Aerosol transmission of the virus can occur as virus is shed from lungs, urine, saliva and faeces. Bites can also be a source of zoonotic infections. In laboratory settings, rats and humans have been infected by transplantable tumours and cell lines. When such materials are obtained from areas with endemic hantavirus infections, they should be screened. One method is to use an antibody production test. A susceptible species (usually a mouse) is injected by one or more routes with a suspension of test cells over a period of several weeks. The test animals are then bled and the serum used to check for antibodies against a single pathogen or an entire range of pathogens by serology (Foster *et al.*, 1983; National Research Council, 1991).

In humans, symptoms range from mild to moderate in the NE syndrome (acute onset of fever, headache, nausea, vomiting, followed by proteinuria, oliguria, haematuria, thrombocytopenia, then by polyuria and recovery in about 3 weeks) to more severe in the KHF syndrome (fever, headache, myalgia, haemorrhages (cutaneous petechiae, haemoptysis, haematuria, haematemesis, melaena) and proteinuria). Up to 20% of patients with KHF develop shock, significant haemorrhages and renal failure and up to half of these patients may die (National Research Council, 1991). Recent human infections in the US have primarily affected the lungs (HPS). These patients have developed fever, myalgia, hypotension and pulmonary dysfunction (acute adult respiratory distress syndrome or bilateral pulmonary infiltrates). Gastrointestinal symptoms have also occurred and haemoconcentration and thrombocytopenia are common. Mortality has been over 60% (Rand, 1994).

Treatment / control. Infected animals should be euthanased because of the severe zoonotic threat. A significant number of transplantable plasmacytomas derived from LOU strain rats in Belgium were found to be contaminated with hantavirus and such material may yet exist in research freezers around the world. Researchers should always screen transplantable tumours and cell lines from areas with endemic hantavirus infections before use. Infected pet mice and rats have not been implicated in zoonotic infections so far, but practitioners should be alert to the possibility. Exposure of pets and research animals to wild rodents should be strictly prevented.

Mousepox, rat poxvirus

Agents. Poxviruses are large DNA viruses with a characteristic dumbbell-shaped nucleus.

Hosts. The mousepox disease virus is called 'ectromelia virus' because of the classic early observations of the necrotic amputations (ectromelia) in naturally infected mice. Rats will seroconvert when experimentally infected, but

quickly clear the virus and do not get lesions. Poxviruses in rats from the former Soviet bloc countries have been reported sporadically, important principally because of the severe zoonotic infections that resulted.

Clinical signs. Ectromelia virus is an important pathogen of laboratory mice that causes highly variable clinical manifestations. Depending on the mouse strain, virus strain and previous exposure history of the mouse, explosive epizootics to silent enzootics may occur. Classic clinical signs include cutaneous papules, erosions, or crusts on the face and extremities and necrotic amputations of the feet or tail. Little is known about rat poxviral infections, but the symptomatology is apparently similar to that described above for ectromelia virus infection in mice. Ectromelia virus has no known zoonotic potential. It was probably a major contaminant of a 'murine typhus rickettsia' vaccine given to hundreds of thousands of people in the 1930s and 1940s. No significant reactions were reported in that population (Foster *et al.*, 1982). In contrast, there have been reports of zoonotic poxviral infections contracted from rats in the former Soviet bloc countries. Human symptoms include headaches, fatigue, cough and diarrhoea; some patients also had a rash on the head, shoulders, knees and hands.

Diagnosis. Diagnosis is based on typical lesions, histopathology and serology.

Treatment / control. There is no treatment and depopulation is usually the course of action in a research setting. Until more information is available, great caution should be exercised when obtaining rats and transplantable tumours or cell lines from the former Soviet bloc nations.

Diseases of the Haematopoietic System

Few specific diseases of this system are likely to result in clinical problems. *Haemobartonella muris* (rats) and *Eperythrozoon coccoides* (mice) are rickettsial pathogens transmitted by *Polyplax* lice. *H. muris* can cause anaemia and weight loss, but both agents usually cause subclinical infections. They can be identified, by Giemsa staining of blood smears, as coccoid or rod-shaped forms in or on erythrocytes. Diagnosis is likely to be accidental. There is no treatment. Control is by vector elimination.

Diseases of Aged Mice and Rats

Mice

Neoplastic lesions

Because of the importance of environmental and genetic factors, different strains of mice have very different prevalences of tumours. The most common tumours that would easily be recognised are mammary neoplasms (adenocarcinomas and carcinomas). They present as growing rounded masses under the skin of the neck, flank, inguinal or axillary region (remember the wide distribution of mammary tissue in rodents). They can be differentiated from other tumours and abscesses by cytology of fine needle aspirates. Mammary tumours will metastasise eventually (often to lung), but surgical removal will maintain the quality of life as long as possible.

Some mice are infected by any of a number of mouse mammary tumour viruses (MMTV), retroviruses which can exist as proviruses in the DNA of the mouse. Infection with MMTV predisposes mice to the development of mammary adenocarcinomas. Mice certified free of MMTV are readily available from commercial sources.

Other fairly common tumours of aged mice are lymphocytic leukaemias, alveologenic carcinomas, hepatic carcinomas, testicular interstitial cell tumours and ovarian tumours, depending on the mouse strain (Foster *et al.*, 1982). When possible (e.g. testicular tumour), surgical removal is helpful in increasing the quality of life and lifespan.

Non-neoplastic lesions

Amyloidosis is common in aged mice of some strains, particularly C57BL/6. Amyloid deposits are found in the intestines, spleen, liver, lung, thyroid and mesenteric lymph nodes. Mice will become ill as vital organ functions decrease and there is no treatment (Foster *et al.*, 1982).

Mice of some strains (CBA, DBA, others) are prone to dystrophic calcification of internal organs. Often such calcification is noted as an incidental finding in heart muscle, intestinal smooth muscle, brain and renal tubules. Rarely are such lesions associated with disease.

Atrial thromboses are found in aged mice of some strains such as RFM and the thrombus can be large enough to restrict blood flow significantly. Pulmonary congestion, hydrothorax, ascites, subcutaneous oedema and an enlarged heart (as well as unthriftiness) can result. Diagnosis is very difficult and there is no known treatment.

Glomerulonephritis of autoimmune (e.g. NZB strain) or unknown cause (in contrast to renal dysfunction caused by amyloidosis) is also diagnosed in aged mice. Descriptions of clinical signs are sparse, but would presumably be those of renal failure. Treatment would be difficult, but the feeding of a palatable low-protein diet might stabilise renal function.

Osteoarthrosis is common in aged mice and can make locomotion difficult. Palliative treatment might consist of acetaminophen or aspirin in the drinking water to alleviate acute episodes of discomfort.

Rats

Neoplastic lesions

A variety of tumours has been described, but generalisations are extremely difficult to make because of the varied genetic and environmental background of the animals and the wide differences in methods of detection (Baker *et al.*, 1979).

As opposed to the mammary adenocarcinomas and carcinomas usually seen in mice, fibroadenomas are the more common mammary tumour in female rats (males may also rarely develop mammary tumours). Mammary fibroadenomas can continue to grow until they approach 40–50% of the total body weight of the rat and make locomotion almost impossible. As in the mouse, surgical removal is the treatment of choice for maintaining quality of life. Because they tend to be less invasive, if caught early enough, a complete cure is possible.

The F344 (Fisher) rat is susceptible to a mononuclear cell leukaemia that has been variously described as monocytic, myelomonocytic, or unclassified. It can affect up to 25% of F344 rats as they age. Splenomegaly is consistent and may be picked up on physical examination or radiographs. Hepatomegaly and lymphadenopathy can also be noted on occasion. During the early stages of the disease, atypical mononuclear cells may be spotted in blood smears. As the disease progresses, a leucocytosis (up to 180,000/μl) consisting of up to 90% leukaemic cells can occur. A haemolytic anaemia may also occur. On staining with Wright–Giemsa stain, the leukaemic cells appear as large mononuclear cells with oval or slightly lobulated nuclei containing one to two nucleoli and abundant blue cytoplasm with azurophilic granules. There is no treatment. Leukaemias in other rat strains are not as common.

Non-neoplastic

Chronic renal disease is a significant cause of morbidity and mortality in aged rats. Rats fed refined diets tend to develop lesions and die from renal failure earlier than rats fed diets containing at least some natural ingredients, although the aetiology remains obscure. End stage kidneys are yellowish and bilaterally enlarged, have roughened nodular to granular surfaces, are often pitted and can contain multiple cortical cysts up to 3 mm in diameter. At 12–14 months of age, up to half of some rat strains will have a proteinuria of > 20 mg/dl (young rats have protein values of < 5 mg/dl) (Baker *et al.*, 1979). Glomerulosclerosis and interstitial fibrosis develop progressively. Clinical signs include polydypsia, hydrothorax, fibrous osteo-

dystrophy and ascites. Elevated BUN and creatinine, hypercholesterolaemia and hypertension are also seen. These complications are usually most significant in rats at least 2 years old. By the time clinical signs are noted, kidney damage is already present and treatment is rarely attempted in a laboratory setting. However, the use of a palatable low protein feed might stabilise renal function and maintain quality of life.

Some rat strains develop myocardial degeneration and fibrosis of unknown aetiology as an ageing lesion. Clinical signs of cardiac insufficiency are rare and a diagnosis is usually made incidentally after the death of the animal.

Spinal nerve root degeneration (radiculoneuropathy) is found in some rats at around 2 years of age. Myelin sheath swelling and nerve degeneration are seen in the cauda equina, ventral spinal roots and white matter of the spinal cord. Some consider the hind limb skeletal muscle degeneration often seen to be a separate syndrome, but the onset of muscle degeneration often coincides with nerve lesions. Clinical signs are posterior paresis, paralysis and motor disturbances (gait and movement abnormalities). The aetiology is unknown and there is no treatment. Euthanasia should be considered when it is difficult for the animal to reach food and water, or when skin lesions caused by contact with urine and faeces become a chronic problem unresponsive to topical therapy.

Polyarteritis nodosus is an inflammatory condition of blood vessels of unknown aetiology. Blood vessels become infiltrated by neutrophils and mononuclear cells, mural thrombi form and there is intimal proliferation. This leads to reduced blood flow, aneurysms and degeneration. Pancreatic, mesenteric, spermatic, hepatic, coronary, ovarian, uterine, cerebral, adrenal and other arteries are commonly affected. Affected arteries are enlarged, nodular, hard and have outpouchings (aneurysms). Clinical signs are non-specific and there is no treatment. Mortality can be caused by myocardial infarction, catastrophic blood loss from aneurysm rupture, or other sequelae secondary to the distribution of affected vessels in vital organs.

References

Baker, H. L., Lindsey, J. R. and Weisbroth, S. H. (eds) (1979) *The Laboratory Rat, Vol. 1, Biology and Diseases*. Academic Press.

Bhatt, P. N., Jacoby, R. O. and Morse III, A. E. (eds) (1986) *New, Viral and Mycoplasmal Infections of Laboratory Rodents (Effects on Biomedical Research)*. Academic Press.

Coghlan, L. G., Lee, D. R., Psencik, B. and Weiss, D. (1993) Practical and effective eradication of pinworms (*Syphacia muris*) in rats by use of fenbendazole. *Laboratory Animal Science* **43**, 481–487.

Cundiff, D. D., Besch-Williford, C. L., Hook Jr, R. R., Franklin, C. L. and Riley, L. K. (1994) Characterisation of cilia-associated respiratory bacillus isolates from rats and rabbits. *Laboratory and Animal Science* **44**, 305–312.

Diggs, H. E., Feller, D. J., Crabbe, J. C., Merrill, C. and Farrell, E. (1990) Effect of chronic ivermectin treatment on GABA receptor function in ethanol withdrawal-seizure prone and resistant mice. *Laboratory and Animal Science* **23, 40**, 68–71.

Flynn, B. M., Brown, P. A., Eckstein, J. M. and Strong, D. (1989) Treatment of *Syphacia obvelata* in mice using ivermectin. *Laboratory and Animal Science* **39**, 461–463.

Foster, H. L., Small, J. D. and Fox, J. G. (eds) (1981) *The Mouse in Biomedical Research Vol. 1, History, Genetics and Wild Mice*. Academic Press.

Foster, H. L., Small, J. D. and Fox, J. G. (eds) (1982a) *The Mouse in Biomedical Research, Vol. 2, Diseases*. Academic Press.

Foster, H. L., Small, J. D. and Fox, J. G. (eds) (1982b) *The Mouse in Biomedical Research, Vol. 4, Experimental Biology*. Academic Press.

Foster, H. L., Small, J. D. and Fox, J. G. (eds) (1983) *The Mouse in Biomedical Research, Vol. 3, Normative Biology, Immunology and Husbandry*. Academic Press.

Fox, J. G., Cohen, B. J. and Loew, F. M. (eds) (1984) *Laboratory Animal Medicine*. Academic Press.

Guide for Care and Use of Laboratory Animals (1985) US Department of Health and Human Services. National Institutes of Health Publication 86–23.

Harkness, J. E. and Wagner, J. E. (eds) *The Biology and Medicine of Rabbits and Rodents*, 3rd edn. Lea and Febiger, Philadelphia.

Huerkamp, M. J. (1993) Eradication of pinworms from rats kept in ventilated cages. *Laboratory and Animal Science* **43**, 86–90.

Muir, W. W. and Hubbell, J. A. E. (eds) (1989) *Handbook of Veterinary Anesthesia*. C. V. Mosby.

Rand, M. S. (1994) Hantavirus: An overview and update. *Laboratory Animal Science* **44**, 301–304.

Rugh, R. (1990) *The Mouse. Its Reproduction and Development*. Oxford University Press.

Schoeb, T. R., Dybvig, K., Davidson, M. K. *et al.* (1993) Cultivation of cilia-associated respiratory bacillus in artificial medium and determination of the 16S rRNA gene sequence. *Journal of Clinical Microbiology* **31**, 2751–2757.

Summa, M. E. L., Ebisui, L., Osaka, J. T. and de Tolosa, E. M. C. (1992) Efficacy of oral ivermectin against *Trichosomoides crassicauda* in naturally infected laboratory rats. *Laboratory Animal Science* **42**, 620–622.

Veterinary Clinics of North America Small Animal Practice (1994) *Exotic Pet Medicine II*, Vol. 24, pp. 89–102.

Waynforth, H. B. and Flecknell, P. A. (1992) *Experimental and Surgical Technique in the Rat*, 2nd edn. Academic Press.

White, W. (1994) Seminar on rodent behaviour presented at Southeastern AALAS meeting in Augusta, Georgia, US on August 19, 1994.

Further reading

Baker, H. L., Lindsey, J. R. and Weisbroth, S. H. (eds) (1979–1980) *The Laboratory Rat*, Vols 1 and 2, Academic Press.

Bhatt, P. N., Jacoby, R. O. and Morse III, H. C. (eds) (1986) *Viral and Mycoplasmal Infections of Laboratory Rodents (Effects on Biomedical Research)*. Academic Press.

Flynn, R. J. (1972) *Parasites of Laboratory Animals*. Iowa State University Press, Ames, Iowa.

Foster, H. L., Small, J. D. and Fox, J. G. (eds) (1979–1982) *The Mouse in Biomedical Research*, Vols 1–4, Academic Press.

Fox, J. G., Cohen, B. J. and Loew, F. M. (eds) *Laboratory Animal Medicine*. Academic Press.

Harkness, H. E. and Wagner, J. E. (1989) *The Biology and Medicine of Rabbits and Rodents*, 3rd edn. Lea and Febiger, Philadelphia.

Laber-Laird, K. and Proctor, M. (1993) An example of a rodent health monitoring program. *Laboratory Animal* **22**(8), 24–32.

National Research Council (1991) *Infectious Diseases of Mice and Rats*. National Academy Press, Washington, DC.

30   M. T. Fallon

National Research Council (1992) *Recognition and Alleviation of Pain and Distress in Laboratory Animals*. National Academy Press, Washington, DC.

Owen, D. (1972) *Common parasites of laboratory rodents and lagomorphs*. MRC Laboratory Animals Centre Handbook No. 1, Medical Research Council, London.

Waynforth, H. B. and Flecknell, P. A. (1992) *Experimental and Surgical Technique in the Rat*, 2nd edn. Academic Press.

(*Data Tables follow*).

Data Tables

COMMON DISEASES—RATS AND MICE					
Disease/agent	Animals(s) affected	Clinical signs	Diagnosis	Treatment and control	Comments
Respiratory system					
Respiratory mycoplasmosis (*M. pulmonis*)	Rat, mouse	Respiratory distress Nasal discharge Torticollis from otitis interna	Culture Serology Histopathology of lung, ear	Tetracyline may control symptoms	Persistent infection the norm. Treatment unlikely to eliminate infection
Sendai virus	Mouse, rat	Respiratory distress	Serology Histopathology of lung	Supportive therapy	Virus clears within about a week from adults, which usually recover completely. Exacerbates *M. pulmonis* infection
Cilia-associated respiratory (CAR) bacillus	Rat, mouse (rabbit also, but no clinical signs)	Respiratory distress Pathogenicity without *M. pulmonis* coinfection unclear	Serology Special histopathology stains	Supportive; tetracycline may control concurrent mycoplasma infections	Persistent infection the norm
Corynebacterium kutscheri	Rat (primarily res-piratory), Mouse (systemic)	Respiratory distress (rat) General unthrifti-ness (mouse)	Culture Histopathology	Tetracycline or chloramphenicol may control symptoms	Persistent infection likely. Treatment unlikely to eliminate infection
Gastrointestinal system					
Sialodacryo-adenitis virus (SDAV)	Rat	Swollen cervical region Photophobia Porphyrin staining of face	Serology Typical histopathology of salivary and other glands in head	Supportive therapy	Virus clears in about a week from adults, who usually completely recover. Exacerbates *M. pulmonis* infection
Mouse hepatitis virus (MHV)	Mouse	Weight loss Dehydration	Serology Typical histopathology	Supportive therapy	Virus clears in about a week from adults, who usually completely recover
Mouse rotavirus and rat rotavirus-like agent	Mouse, rat	Diarrhoea in suckling animals	Serology Histopathology	Supportive therapy; fluids may prevent dehydration	Not a problem in adults, who may have positive serology from earlier infections

Fig. 1.5—continued

COMMON DISEASES—RATS AND MICE					
Disease agent	Animals(s) affected	Clinical signs	Diagnosis	Treatment and control	Comments
Tyzzer's disease (*Clostridium piliforme* infection)	Mouse and rat, sucklings most affected	Diarrhoea Weight loss	Serology Histopathology	Oxytetracyline, tetracyline may suppress clinical signs	Persistent infections common. Spores difficult to eradicate
Citrobacteriosis (*Citrobacter freundii* biotype 4280 infection)	Mouse	Weight loss Dehydration Colon enlargement is the striking gross finding, rectal prolapse may be seen	Culture Histopathology	Tetracycline or neomycin may suppress infection	Recovery will be gradual as gut returns to normal over several weeks
Cestodiasis (Dwarf tapeworm, *Hymenolepis nana* and rat tapeworm, *Hymenolepis diminuta*)	Mouse, rat, (younger animals usually affected)	Weight loss Intestinal obstruction	Ova can be identified in faecal floats; adult or cysticercal stages by histopathology	Vector control, proper bedding changes, treat with niclosamide, praziquantel, or thiabendazole	Zoonotic threat, particularly in children
Pinworm infection (*Syphacia obvelata*, mouse, *Syphacia muris* rat)	Mouse, rat (crossover occurs, younger animals usually affected)	Diarrhoea Rectal prolapse Unthriftiness	Ova identified on cellophane tape impressions of the anal area or in faecal samples	Ivermectin is effective treatment	Control very difficult because eggs float in air and spread infection. Not zoonotic
Malocclusion (incisor overgrowth)	Mouse, rat (other rodent and rabbits)	Weight loss, soft palate trauma, presence of crumbled but uneaten food in pan	Examination of incisors	Clip overgrown incisors even with other paired tooth every 1–2 weeks; provide soft food during healing	
Genitourinary system					
Leptospirosis (*Leptospira* spp. infection)	Mouse, rat, many mammals and reptiles	Usually infections are asymptomatic	Culture of kidneys or urine (special media required), or by serology	Prevent contact with wild rodents	Euthanasia indicated if infections detected because of zoonotic infections. Listen when family members report severe 'flu-like symptoms

Fig. 1.5—continued

COMMON DISEASES—RATS AND MICE					
Disease agent	Animals(s) affected	Clinical signs	Diagnosis	Treatment and control	Comments
M. pulmonis endometritis and pyometra	LEW strain rats	Unthriftiness Sterility	Culture of affected tissue Serology	Treat with tetracyline	Treatment unlikely to eliminate infection
Preputial gland abscesses (*Staphylococcus aureus, Pasteurella pneumotropica* and other bacteria)	Mouse (nude mice are predisposed), rat	Swellings around the penis	Fine needle aspirate will differentiate abscess from neoplasm	Lance abscesses, apply antibacterial salve until healed	Check cytology to rule out preputial gland neoplasms
Urinary bladder nematodiasis *Trichosomoides crassicauda*	Rat	Dysuria Unthriftiness; bladder calculi may be palpable	Ova present in urine; female can be observed in bladder postmortem	Ivermectin will eliminate parasite	Male residues completely within reproductive tract of female
Nervous system					
Otitis interna (*M. pulmonis* infection most common)	Rat, mouse	Torticollis, circling	Serology Postmortem culture Histopathology	Tetraycline Penicillin, others	Torticollis rarely responds to antibiotic treatment. Euthanasia usually indicated due to inability to eat or drink
Mouse encephalomyelitis virus	Mouse	Flaccid paralysis of rear limbs	Serology Histopathology	Supportive therapy	Euthanasia if mobility severely affected Other clinical signs are rare
Integument and musculoskeletal system					
Mammary tumours	Fibroadenomas common in rats, adenocarcinomas more common in mice	Small to large movable tumours on ventrum or higher on body	Cytology of fine needle aspirate	Surgical removal	Goal is to maintain quality of life; depending on size and grade, tumour may return

Fig. 1.5—continued

COMMON DISEASES—RATS AND MICE					
Disease agent	Animals(s) affected	Clinical signs	Diagnosis	Treatment and control	Comments
Ringtail	Rat, rarely mouse	Annular constrictions in tail and, rarely, gangrene of distal limbs	Examination of tail and limbs	Increase humidity to 50%; treat tail topically, amputate if necessary	Euthanase if limb loss interferes with quality of life
Pododermatitis	Rat, other large rodents, rabbit	Acute or chronic inflammation of plantar surface of foot; granulation tissue may be present	Examination of feet (usually rear ones involved)	Transfer animal to soft bedding from wire floors, clean wire floors more often, remove sharp edges; treat topically	Many times lesions do not respond to treatment. Prevention is very important
Barbering	Mouse, sometimes rat	Hair patches on lower ranking animal chewed down to bare skin (but usually no lesions on skin)	Bare skin present around muzzle, face, or neck area; use skin scrape to rule out ecto-parasites, fungi	None usually needed; animals may be separated	Highest ranking animal usually has no hair loss
Bite wounds	Mouse, rarely rat	Small lacerations and crusty lesions on the tail and rump (around head area in rats); periodic squeals of pain will be heard in cage; Weight loss	Pattern of wounds and observation of aggressive behaviour in cage; skin scrapes can be used to rule out ecto-parasites, fungii	Remove dominant mouse or separate mice into individual cages; lesions can be treated topically	C57BL/6 and BALB/C mouse strains are usually more aggressive than others
Dermatophytosis (*Trichophyton* spp. and *Microsporum* spp.)	Most mammals	Small areas of alopecia and scaly skin (lesions may be very mild)	Wood's lamp examination; identification of pathogen in skin scrapes taken from periphery of lesion, culture on specific media	Griseofulvin therapy for 30–60 days	Data on treatment success rate are lacking Zoonotic potential must be considered during treatment and follow-up

Fig. 1.5—continued

COMMON DISEASES—RATS AND MICE					
Disease agent	Animals(s) affected	Clinical signs	Diagnosis	Treatment and control	Comments
Acariasis (*Myobia musculi, Mycoptes musculinus,* mouse, *Sarcoptes scabiei* in mouse or rat; other mites also)	Mouse, similar though fewer fur mites in rats	Ulcerative skin lesions on dorsum produced by mites and scratching, pathogenic	Identification of mites on pelt with magnifying glass or in skin scraping	Ivermectin will eliminate mites from animal Carbaryl dust may be used on cages and environment	*S. scabiei* and *Liponyssus bacoti* have zoonotic potential, but are rare
Peliosis (*Polyplax serrata,* mouse, *Polyplax spinulosa,* rat)	Mouse, rat	Dermatitis Anaemia Weight loss	Identification of lice on pelt with magnifying glass or in skin scraping	Ivermectin therapy or carbaryl dusting of animal	Vectors for *Encephalitozoon cuniculi, Eperythrozoon coccoides* and *Haemobartonella muris,* among others
Fleas	Mouse, rat (rare in both)	Dermatitis	Idenfitication of fleas on pelt	Carbaryl dust or pyrethrin spray	Elimination is important because fleas are vectors for zoonotic diseases
Systemic diseases					
Salmonellosis (*Salmonella enteritidis* infection)	Most mammals	Possibly diarrhoea Dehydration asymptomatic shedders common	Culture of faeces	None; prevent exposure to wild rodents	Zoonotic hazard indicates euthanasia
Lymphocytic choriomeningitis	Wild rodents are reservoir Mouse, hamster most suscep-tible	Usually infections are asymptomatic; virus shed in urine, saliva milk	Serology	None; prevent exposure to wild rodents; screen transplantable tumours and cell lines	Zoonotic hazard indicates euthanasia. Hamsters have been the source of most recent zoonotic infections Listen when family members report severe 'flu-like symptoms
Hantavirus infection	Wild mice, voles, other rodents; lab rats	Usually infections are asymptomatic; virus shed by aerosol and (less commonly) bites	Serology	None; prevent exposure to wild rodents; screen transplantable tumours and cell lines	Zoonotic hazard indicates euthanasia.

Fig. 1.5—continued

COMMON DISEASES—RATS AND MICE					
Disease agent	Animals(s) affected	Clinical signs	Diagnosis	Treatment and control	Comments
Streptobacillosis (*Streptobacillus moniliformis*)	Mouse, oral cavity commensal in wild and lab rats	Mice that survive acute infection get chronic arthritis and limb deformity; no lesions in rats	Culture; rule out mousepox in mice when limb deformity is observed	None; infected stock are usually euthanased	*S. moniliformis* (and *Spirillum minus*) are the agents of rat bite fever in humans
Mousepox/ ectromelia (mousepox virus)	Mouse	Cutaneous papules, erosions, or crusts on the face and extremities, and necrotic amputations of the feet or tail; asymptomatic infection also common	Serology Histopathology; a vaccine has been used in the past to protect mice from disease in some facilities	None; in research setting, euthanasia is usually recommended to control spread; screen transplantable tumours and cell lines	Mice can recover, but can shed virus chronically
Poxviral infection in rats	Rat	Similar to skin lesion in mousepox infection of mice	Difficult at this time, histopathology would be helpful; rats from former Soviet republics and Eastern Europe have been the source	None	Serious zoonotic infections have been reported

Fig. 1.5 Common diseases—rats and mice.

PHYSIOLOGICAL DATA—RATS AND MICE		
	Mice	Rats
Adult weight	18–40 g	250–1000 g+
Life span	1–3 years	2–3 years
Water consumption (per day)	15 ml/100 g b.w.	8–11 ml/100 g b.w.
Food consumption (per day)	15 g/100 g b.w.	5 g/100 g b.w.
Heart rate	300–600+/min	300–500/min
Respiratory rate	150–170/min	80–90/min
Tidal volume (ml)	0.09–0.38	1.5
Urine output	0.5–1.0 ml/day	5.5 ml/100 g b.w./day

As will be clear from some of the normal values given, tremendous variation in some parameters will be observed depending on the strain of mouse or rat tested, age, sex, diet, and a host of other environmental and procedural factors. Data taken from Fox *et al.* (1984) and Harkness and Wagner (1989).

Fig. 1.6 Physiological data—rats and mice.

HAEMATOLOGICAL VALUES—RATS AND MICE		
	Mice	Rats
Blood volume	5–6 ml/100 g b.w.	6 ml/100 g b.w.
PCV %	42–44	39–55
RBC x 10^6/mm^3	8.7–12.5	6–10
Haemoglobin g/dl	10.2–16.2	11–19.5
Reticulocytes per 1000 RBCs	0–3	0–3
Total WBC x 10^3/ml	5–12	6–15
Neutrophils %	7–40	9–34
Eosinophils %	0–4	0–6
Lymphocytes %	55–95	65–85
Basophils %	0–1.5	0–1.5
Monocytes %	0.1–3.5	0–5
Platelets x 10^3/mm^3	100–1000	500–1300
PTTs	55–100	17–25
Data taken from Fox *et al.* (1984), Harkness and Wagner (1989) and Baker *et al.* (1979).		

FIG. 1.7 Haematological values—rats and mice.

CLINICAL CHEMISTRY VALUES—RATS AND MICE		
	Mice	Rats
Calcium (mg/dl)	3.2–10	5.3–13.0
Phosphorus (mg/dl)	2.3–9.2	5.3–8.3
Sodium (mEq/l)	132–162	140–150
Chloride (mEq/l)	92–106 .	100–113
Potassium (mEq/l)	5.0–7.6	4.3–5.6
Glucose (mg/dl)	60–228	50–135
BUN (mg/dl)	17–28	6–23
Creatinine (mg/dl)	0.3–1.0	0.2–0.8
Total bilirubin (mg/dl)	0.1–0.9	0.2–0.55
Total protein (g/dl)	3.5–7.2	5.6–7.6
Albumin (g/dl)	2.5–4.8	3.8–4.8
Globulin (g/ml)	0.6	1.8–3.0
Cholesterol (mg/dl)	26–82	40–130
Alkaline phosphatase (IU/l)	47–85	16–90
AST/SGOT (IU/l)	74–232	
ALT/SGPT (IU/l)	26–54	20–90
Data taken from Harkness and Wagner (1989), Baker *et al.* (1979), Foster *et al.* (1983) and Fox *et al.* (1984).		

FIG. 1.8 Clinical chemistry values—rats and mice.

REPRODUCTIVE DATA—RATA AND MICE		
	Mice	Rats
Puberty	5–8 weeks	6–8 weeks
Oestrous cycle	Polyoestrous	Polyoestrous
Duration of oestrous cycle	4–5 days	4–5 days
Gestation	19–21 days	21–23 days
Average litter size	4–12 pups	8–14 pups
Birth weight	1.0–1.5 g	5–6 g
Eyes open	12–13 days	10–12 days
Weaning age	3–4 weeks	3–4 weeks
Postpartum oestrus	within 24 h (fertile)	within 24 h (fertile)
Mammae	5 pairs	6 pairs
Data taken from Fox *et al.* (1984) and Harkness and Wagner (1989).		

FIG. 1.9 Reproductive data—rats and mice.

2

Gerbils

KATHY LABER-LAIRD

Introduction

Gerbils are rodents whose native habitat includes China, Mongolia, India and Africa. They are the most common and widely distributed mammal in South Africa. There are 12 genera in the subfamily Gerbillinae, but only one species, *Meriones unguiculatus*, is typically available in North America and Europe. Tracing the family line of the American-raised Mongolian gerbil is an easy task. They were derived solely from 11 pairs of animals that Dr V. Schwentker imported from the Kitasato Institute, Japan, in 1954 (Norris, 1987).

Due to their relatively recent introduction into the US when compared with other rodents and their limited regional availability, gerbils have not received the 'pet-press' that other rodent species enjoy. Gerbils, however, can easily be described as the ideal pet rodent. They have no unusual dietary requirements and they require little in the way of maintenance. They possess a curious disposition and are active, interesting animals to observe. They have an attractive appearance and are easy to handle. A practitioner dealing with gerbils not only has to have knowledge about their diseases and treatments but also about husbandry requirements, biology and behaviour as these variables can strongly affect the health and well-being of the animal.

Unique Biology

The typical adult Mongolian gerbil is agouti, having a slightly lighter coat colour ventrally. The skin is darkly pigmented. Other coat colours that have resulted from genetic mutations and have been perpetuated include black, piebald, dove and cinnamon. Hairless and albino gerbils have also been produced. Unlike rats and mice, gerbils have fully furred tails, ears and foot pads.

The average lifespan for females and males is 2.7–3.2 years and 2.1–2.9 years, respectively. The male weighs approximately 5% more than the female. Both sexes continue to grow up to 18 months of age, but attain 70% of their mature body weight by 90 days of age. Body weights of adults can vary considerably depending on the animal's diet. Ranges are between 50 and 90 g with males being larger than the females (Robinson, 1979).

The haemogram of the gerbil is unique due to the presence of a large number of basophilic stippled and polychromatophilic red blood cells. The high number of polychromatic cells or reticulocytes corresponds to the animals' short erythrocyte lifespan (Dillon and Glomski, 1975). The basophilic stippled cells have been labelled both as cells containing precipitated cytoplasmic ribonucleoprotein or *Haemobartonella*-infected red blood cells (Najarian, 1961). Since the cell type has been found in gerbils from multiple sources at multiple time points and has never been associated with any pathology, it is more likely to be a physiological rather than an infectious condition. The gerbil exhibits significant sex-linked differences in packed cell volume, haemoglobin levels, white blood cell and lymphocyte counts. Gerbils are also very sensitive to dietary cholesterol. It is not unusual to have lipaemic serum in animals consuming a diet heavy in seeds (Ruhren, 1965). Normal physiological, haematological and clinical chemistry values are listed in Figs 2.9–2.11 found at the end of the chapter.

Both male and female gerbils have a unique glandular structure appearing as an oval hairless tan-coloured region located in the mid-ventral abdominal region. This ventral scent gland releases a secretion which allows the animals to mark and then identify territory. The gland is typically larger in males since they mark more frequently than females. Females mark predominantly during pregnancy and lactation (Wallace *et al.*, 1973). Other unique features specific to glandular structures include the adrenals which are very large relative to other rodents (three times the size of those in the rat) and which produce 19α-hydroxycorticosterone rather than corticosterone (Holmes, 1985). The gerbil's thymus, located in the thorax, persists into adulthood.

The Mongolian gerbil's natural habitat has wide temperature fluctuations; consequently the gerbil has the ability to adapt to wide ranges of temperatures. It is reported that they can tolerate temperatures ranging from greater than 38°C (100°F) to below freezing with no adverse physiological effects (Robinson, 1959). Thermoregulation in the gerbil is governed by the secretions of the Harderian gland (located behind the eye at the medial canthus). The gland also has chemosignalling functions as the secretions can stimulate proceptive behaviour in oestrous females (Holmes, 1985). The gland is prompted to secrete when the gerbil blinks its eyes. The secretions, composed of protoporphyrin pigments and fatty acids, are carried through the lacrimal canal and out through the nares. The secretions are mixed with saliva and groomed over the entire body. Grooming is evoked by thermogenic events, such as when the animal has a change in body temperature caused by ambient temperature changes or by environmental stimuli. If the animal needs to increase its body temperature, the lipids and pigments from the Harderian gland are groomed over the body to insulate and increase radiant absorption. If the animal needs to decrease its body temperature, the Harderian gland secretions decrease and the animal sandbathes and grooms predominantly with saliva which removes lipids from the coat and allows evaporative cooling (Thiessen, 1988).

Because the evolution of the gerbil has been influenced by desert ecology, the gerbil's kidneys have a tremendous concentrating ability. In the wild, gerbils need not consume water, but instead receive their fluid requirements solely from food sources. They secrete only drops of urine each day and the water content of the faeces is minimal; subsequently the odour associated with these animals is also minimal.

Behaviour

Gerbils are curious, pleasant animals that can make excellent pets once an understanding of their behavioural characteristics has been achieved. In the wild, they live in groups or social units composed of 2–17 males and females. The group occupies a territory as defined by clusterings of burrows and areas of activity. The size of the territory correlates with the size of the group. The group acts cooperatively to defend the territory from other gerbil groups. The Mongolian gerbil's natural habitat is one of extremes, with distinct seasonal variability in food supply. In the summer months, leaves and stems are plentiful. However, in the winter, the gerbil has to depend on the hoard of seeds that has been gathered and stored within the burrows. All ages and sexes participate in the gathering of food. The group efforts to defend this territory allow careful preservation of the food supply (Agren *et al.*, 1989). Within the established group no fighting occurs. However, there can be significant aggression and trauma, particularly involving females, when new adult animals enter the territory. In a captive environment, the best way to avoid this situation is to introduce new animals with established groups into a clean cage, however, fighting may still occur.

Within the group, there is a social hierarchy which dictates defined duties. Males are dominant and bigger animals rule the smaller. Physical evidence of dominance may be observed by barbered tails (hair removal from the subordinate animal by the dominant) especially in crowded conditions. Males tend to be more active than females and if given the opportunity will range to the limits of any given territory.

Males are responsible for defining the borders of the territory, then identifying them by marking with the ventral scent gland. Females have the responsibility for initiating copulation. Although it has been documented that gerbils form monogamous pairs in caged environments, in the wild there is evidence suggesting that only some gerbils appear to form monogamous mating pairs for life while others do not (Agren *et al.*, 1989).

Additional group activities include grooming, playing and sleeping. Gerbils occupy several hours a day using their teeth and tongues to groom themselves and other group members. Pups are particularly playful animals with behaviour which includes chasing or 'wrestling' with each other. Adults spend a great deal of time scratching at surfaces, digging, hoarding food and if given the opportunity, burrowing or nest building.

Gerbils use a variety of means to communicate. When gerbils are excited, mating, or feel threatened, they 'foot stomp'. This is an action where both rear paws are elevated and rapidly thumped against the ground. Pregnant animals tend to foot stomp in response to any disturbance. A gerbil exposed to danger on the surface of the burrow system thumps the hard, packed desert soil which reverberates the message to the other animals in the area. Adult gerbils rarely make audible noises, but occasionally squeals can be heard from adolescent animals or from adults if courting or fighting. Urine odours allow the gerbil to distinguish male from female as well as to discriminate between familiar and unfamiliar gerbils. Recognition of familiar odours will promote affiliative behaviour, while unfamiliar odours promote aggression (Brown *et al.*, 1988). If a particular animal in the group is stressed, caused by predator exposure for example, a body odour is produced which causes other members of the group to avoid that animal. This is thought to be a survival mechanism in the wild (Cocke and Thiessen, 1986).

Unlike other rodent species, gerbils are not specifically nocturnal. In the wild, they are diurnal with a crepuscular tendency. In captivity, it has been observed that they are active over 24 h with a slight increase in activity during the night.

Reproduction

Mating

Males become sexually mature between 70 and 84 days with testes descending around 30 days of age. As is typical of all rodents, the testicles can be retracted into the abdominal cavity throughout life. Females become sexually mature between 86 and 109 days. Early maturing females reproduce when younger and throughout their breeding lives will have more young per litter, but with reduced maternal behaviour (Clark *et al.*, 1986). Females tend to discontinue breeding by approximately 18 months of age while spermatogenesis ends by 24 months (Wagner and Farrar, 1987).

Sexual receptivity occurs in the gerbil at three distinct time points:

1. Every 4–6 days during the oestrous cycle which occurs throughout the year with the exception of a slight winter breeding depression.
2. Within 24 h postpartum.
3. Postweaning.

While lactating, the female will not mate as the vaginal opening decreases with the formation of a membrane.

Cytological detection of oestrus from vaginal smears is not as obvious in gerbils as it is in rats and mice. The recommended way to mate gerbils is to allow them to form male/female pairs before sexual maturity (by 10 weeks). A breeding trio of one male and two females also allows for successful matings. If it becomes necessary to introduce a male to a mature female, suggested approaches include anaesthetising both sexes and allowing them to recover in a clean cage, or introducing the female housed in a smaller cage into the male's larger cage for 24 h prior to housing them openly together. In a typical cycle of 12 h light–12 h dark, mating will occur in the late afternoon. The number of intromissions preceding ejaculation can be very high with the period of time required being up to 6 h. Copulation plugs are formed but are difficult to find because they are small and formed deep within the vagina. If the gerbil becomes pregnant, the vaginal smear will be dominated by leucocytes, with blood evident from day 12 onwards (Norris and Adams, 1981).

The housing environment has a significant impact on breeding success. Females housed together have a low incidence of oestrus; however, if a male is introduced into the cage, the females will start to cycle. This phenomenon is referred to as the Bruce effect. In addition, strange females or males introduced into a recently mated female's cage can block implantation during the first 5 days postmating. It has also been documented that altering the cage environment of a pregnant female can cause abortions (Rohrbach, 1982).

Gestation and Birth

Gestation lengths are from 24 to 26 days. Among rodents gerbils have the highest incidence and the greatest extent of implantation delay induced by lactation. There is a well defined linear relationship between the number of young nursing and the length of the gestation. Gestation will be prolonged 1.9 days per pup when 3 or more pups are nursing (Norris and Adams, 1981).

Delivery times are approximately 1 h in length with the female consuming the placenta. Cannibalism of stillbirths does not occur under proper husbandry conditions. Litters range in size from 1–7 with the average being 5. Smaller numbers of young will be born to older or younger gerbils. Prenatal mortality is 32% with the ovulation rate remaining constant throughout the animal's reproductive life. Neonatal mortality has been reported to occur in 35% of litters, with mortality in those litters being 20% (Norris, 1987). Neonates are born hairless and blind, weighing 3–4 g. Ears open from days 3 to 7, hair grows at days 7–10 and eyes open between 14 and 20 days. Sexing the juveniles is done by observing the anogenital distance which is twice as long in males as in females (Fig. 2.1).

Pre-weaning deaths are typically due to a failure in maternal care or lactation ability. Exces-

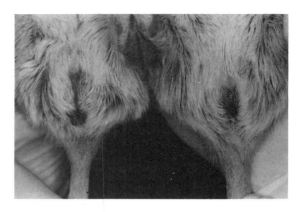

FIG. 2.1 The anogenital distance of the male gerbil (left) is twice that of the female (right).

sive human handling has been suggested as an additional cause for neonatal mortality (Wagner and Farrar, 1987). Offspring will suckle for up to 25 days, but will eat solid food at 14–16 days. Mortality can be significant if the 16–25-day-old gerbils are not offered accessible food and water. Young gerbils can easily eat moistened pelleted rodent food placed in a container on the cage floor.

During the neonatal dependency period, the female marks the nest with the ventral scent gland. Pups are particularly attracted to the odour up to 3 weeks of age and are no longer attracted by 9 weeks (Yahr and Anderson-Mitchell, 1981). The male aids the female in the postpartum care of the offspring, guarding the nest when the female leaves it, as well as helping to retrieve and clean the pups.

Reproductive information is summarised in Fig. 2.12 found at the end of the chapter.

Husbandry

Husbandry and nutrition are major variables that need to be evaluated for any sick gerbil. Many of the clinical symptoms seen may be either directly or indirectly caused by deficiencies in either husbandry or nutrition. Figure 2.2 shows the common clinical symptoms associated with husbandry problems in the gerbil.

The following variables need to be defined for any gerbil presenting with clinical symptoms:

1. What kind of diet does the animal consume? Where does it come from? How is it stored? How often is it fed? What is the milling date? Where is the food and water placed in the cage?
2. What is the temperature/humidity in the room? Where is the cage in the room? What is the temperature/humidity in the cage? How consistent is the temperature/humidity?
3. What type of cage is used? What is the bedding material? How many animals are in the cage? What are the sexes and ages of the cage mates? How often is the cage and water container cleaned? What environmental enrichment devices are contained in the cage?

Answers to these questions will help to determine if husbandry issues are affecting the health status of the animal.

CLINICAL SIGNS ASSOCIATED WITH HUSBANDRY PROBLEMS—GERBILS	
Rough hair coat	Malnutrition Excess humidity Improper cage ventilation Dehydration
Hair loss on tail	Improper handling Barbering
Dehydration	Failure to provide accessible water Failure to provide adequate diet
Neonatal death	Failure to provide accessible food and water to neonates Overcrowding Failure to provide nesting material Excessive handling

Fig. 2.2 Clinical signs associated with husbandry problems—gerbils.

Housing

The ideal housing environment for any animal is one that mimics the animal's natural environment, that accommodates and protects the animal, allows for feeding and watering and provides the opportunity to observe and interact with the animal. The best cage environment for gerbils is one that provides a solid floor and allows enough height for standing, since gerbils spend a good deal of time in an upright posture. The *Universities Federation of Animal Welfare (UFAW) Handbook* recommends a minimum height of 15 cm and 100 cm² floor space per animal for groups. For a breeding pair and their offspring, 700–900 cm² floor space is suggested (Norris, 1987). The 100 cm² floor space per animal corresponds to the mouse floor space recommended in the *Guide for Care and Use of Laboratory Animals*, therefore in a laboratory environment, gerbils are typically housed in rodent shoeboxes with wire top lids. If overcrowding occurs, the animals will stop breeding and aggressive behaviour will increase, indicated by bites to the tail base resulting in focal denudation.

There are numerous commercially available bedding materials; however, hardwood, paper byproducts, or peat are the best choices. Ground corn bedding will be eaten and pine bedding can alter the animal's hepatic physiology and has also been reported to cause matted greasy fur (Norris, 1987). Bedding should be a minimum of 3 cm in depth to allow the gerbil to burrow. Sand should be made available to the gerbil as either a part of the bedding material or in a container placed in the cage. As previously discussed, sand is a critical component of the gerbil's thermoregulatory physiology. The sand will need either to be changed frequently as faeces and food debris accumulate or offered to the animal for short time intervals.

In the wild, gerbils form nests in which to rest and raise young. The nest is not woven, but instead is compacted by the weight of the animal's body. The materials used (bark, twigs and grasses) are chewed into the proper shape and consistency. Choices of nesting material for the caged gerbil include shredded paper, cardboard and rags.

Potential clinical issues related to improper bedding or nesting materials include gastric or anal impaction if the animal eats materials which are not digestible, skin irritation from rubbing against rough bedding or coarse sand, conjunctivitis or rhinitis from dusty bedding, and neonatal mortality if nesting materials are not provided.

Environmental enrichment devices for caged gerbils can include such items as exercise wheels, PVC pipe for animals to run through and twigs they can chew. However, if the goal of the pet owner is to duplicate the animal's natural environment and stimulate typical behaviour patterns, the following housing design may be considered. A mixture of clay, sand and straw resulting in a consistency similar to packed sand is placed in a tall aquarium which has irregularly shaped rocks along the bottom. This housing arrangement mimics the natural environment as it gives the animal the opportunity to spend time making tunnels. New tunnels will continue to be dug as old tunnels are filled. The rocks help maintain the integrity of the tunnels. Nesting material will be carried into the burrows, but will also be used on the surface of the soil. The soil needs to be dampened periodically to maintain its compressibility (Paradise, 1980).

The gerbil's water consumption will vary depending on room humidity and water content in the diet. It is recommended that caged gerbils are provided with 4 ml water per day (Arrington and Ammerman, 1969). In the wild, water *per se* is not consumed, instead fluid requirements are extracted from the food consumed. Because of the gerbil's tremendous ability to concentrate urine and the fact that the water content of the faecal pellets is very low, the need to clean their cages is minimal compared to other rodents. The frequency will depend on the size of the cage used, the absorbency of the bedding material, the ventilation within the cage and the cage population. Once per week is the minimal recommendation for cleaning a typical 20 cm (width) × 40 cm (length) × 15 cm (height) rodent shoebox.

As previously mentioned gerbils live in an environment that has temperature extremes to which they can readily adapt, therefore the traditional room temperature of 20–22.2°C (68–72°F) is acceptable for housing gerbils. As for any animal, dramatic temperature fluctuations should always be avoided. It is important to remember that the temperature and humidity in the room may differ considerably from the interior of the cage. Cage design, bedding material and population density will affect cage temperature and humidity. Humidity is a husbandry variable that can significantly affect the health of the gerbil. It has been documented that humidity levels higher than 50% cause the gerbil's fur to become matted with an increase in grooming behaviour (Schwentker, 1968). As will be discussed under skin problems, this exaggerated grooming behaviour may contribute to nasal dermatitis; therefore, the humidity should be maintained at 40–50%.

Nutrition

The natural diet for the gerbil is seasonally variable and consists of seeds, leaves and roots during the growing seasons and seeds during the winter months. Commercially available pelleted rodent food meets the gerbil's dietary requirement, however it does not provide the dietary moisture the animal is accustomed to. To increase the moisture content and give the animal variety, the diet may be supplemented with seeds, fruits and leafy vegetables. Care must be taken to avoid an excess of seeds in the diet since the animal may preferentially eat these leading to obesity and mineral deficiencies. The most rapid weight gain and greatest food consumption occurs between 4 and 7 weeks of age when animals gain 1.0 g/day. Adult gerbils can consume between 4.0 and 10 g of food per day (Otken and Hall, 1980). Decreased food consumption has been associated with increased longevity in other rodent species, therefore, limiting the gerbil's food availability and avoiding obesity is likely to increase the animal's life expectancy. Food can be placed either in the wire cage lid, making sure that the gerbil can reach it, or placed on the cage floor to enable easier access by juveniles.

Nutritional diseases are relatively rare. Unlike the guinea pig, gerbils are particularly resistant to the effect of vitamin deficiencies, however they are sensitive to valine and choline deficiencies and evidence suggests that they need taurine in their diet (Otken *et al.*, 1985). Arginine is required by growing juveniles, but not adults (Otken and Hall, 1980; Otken *et al.*, 1985). Unlike other rodent species, gerbils are not coprophagous when provided with an adequate diet. If the diet is deficient, however, coprophagy may result (Otken and Scott, 1984).

Problems related to diet are primarily seen in juvenile animals. Weaning begins at around 14 days of age, and food and water should be made available at this time. A gerbil of this age is particularly sensitive to food and water deprivation. Intact rodent pellets are difficult for juveniles to consume, but pellets can be eaten readily if soaked in water. Gerbils, like other rodents, have continuously growing incisors whose length is maintained by gnawing on hard objects like rodent pellets. Although it happens less frequently in gerbils than in rabbits or other rodents, teeth can break and the opposing tooth can overgrow. A thorough oral examination is required for any animal experiencing weight loss. Teeth can be trimmed using a sharp, dedicated 'teeth trimming' pair of nail clippers, rongeurs or a dental drill.

Handling, Injection, Specimen Collection

Handling

Gerbils are quick agile animals capable of making horizontal as well as vertical leaps in any direction. However, they are also curious, tractable animals, generally easy to handle. Unless adverse stimuli are present, they will approach a hand placed into a cage and can then be scooped into the individual's palm. It is always advisable to question the owner as to the frequency of handling, as gerbils not used to human contact will be more difficult to handle.

If they escape from the handler, they are easily re-captured since their instinctive response to freedom is to explore rather than to hide. They can also be picked up with a very gentle touch at the base of the tail taking care not to 'skin' the tail. Animals should not be handled by the tail tip since this can both break the tail and damage the skin (Fig. 2.3).

Injection

Injections can be given intraperitoneally (IP) by holding the gerbil with the head facing toward the ground and injecting into the lower left quadrant of the abdomen with a 25 gauge needle (Fig. 2.4). Positioning the gerbil in this fashion may shift the location of the gastrointestinal tract thereby minimising the risk of perforating the intestine with the needle. IV injections are given either through the lateral tail vein or the saphenous vein. Warming the skin helps to visualise and dilate the vessels. SC injections can be given between the shoulder blades (Fig. 2.5). Intraosseous (IO) administration of fluids via a spinal needle inserted in the trochanteric space is more difficult technically than giving fluids IP, but it may be warranted if long term, slow rate infusion is needed. For a description of the technique, please refer to *Chapter 8*. IM injections can be administered into the quadriceps or the posterior thigh muscles; however, the muscle mass in these animals is very small and can be traumatised easily.

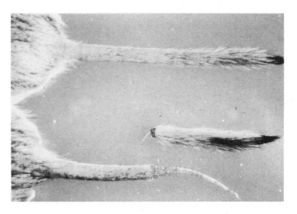

Fig. 2.3 Sloughed tail skin caused by inappropriate handling.

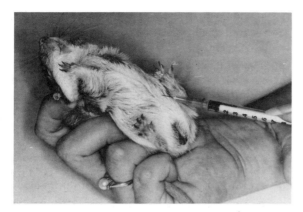

FIG. 2.4 Intraperitoneal injection into the lower left abdominal quadrant of the gerbil.

Specimen Collection

The technique chosen for blood collection will depend on the volume of blood needed. In a 50 g animal, total blood volume will be approximately 3.4 ml. If the animal is to survive, then no more than 10–15% of the circulating volume should be sampled. If 15% of the blood volume is sampled from a compromised animal, fluids need to be administered after the procedure. Larger volumes of blood (greater than 0.5 ml) from larger animals can be obtained by a cardiac tap whereby a 22 gauge needle is inserted into the ventricle of an anaesthetised animal from either a lateral or ventral approach. This procedure should only be used when justified as it may cause iatrogenic cardiac tamponade. Small

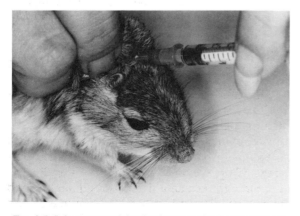

FIG. 2.5 Subcutaneous injection between the shoulder blades.

volumes of blood (0.1–0.3 ml) may be collected from the orbital venous sinus. The animal should be lightly anaesthetised and the head should be stabilised between a thumb and forefinger with pressure being exerted to extrude the eye. The thumb is used to occlude the external jugular vein caudal to the mandible which increases the blood available in the orbital sinus. A microhaematocrit tube can then be placed at the lateral canthus and slid posteriorly and medially and under the eye. Once positioned behind the eye, a sharp thrust should allow blood to flow into the tube. Direct pressure on the eyelid will stop continued bleeding. The haematocrit tube may also be positioned from the medial canthus, however the sinus is most accessible laterally. Another option for small blood volume withdrawal is to place a rubber band tourniquet above the animal's stifle. The hair should be clipped and the limb extended so that the metatarsal vein can be visualised. A 25 gauge needle can be inserted and as the blood flows into the needle hub it can be collected into a microhaematocrit tube.

Handling the animal may stimulate the elimination of urine and faeces, however the amount of urine will be small since gerbils eliminate only 2–3 drops of urine per day.

Radiography Techniques

An X-ray machine that is able to generate 300 mA in 1/120 s with kvp between 40 and 60 is optimal for assessing mammals the size of gerbils (Silverman, 1993). Mammography film can provide exceptional resolution with a Min R (Eastman Kodak) single intensifying screen cassette with Min R single emulsion film giving good results (Hoefer, 1995). To position gerbils for radiographs, they should first be lightly sedated. Diazepam at 5 mg/kg IP works well. The gerbil is positioned directly on the film cassette with tape holding the limbs in place. This allows the animal's entire body to be radiographed and evaluated. Although not yet widely available, magnetic resonance imaging can be very effective in detecting lesions that may be missed using standard radiography techniques (Allen *et al.*, 1993).

When evaluating the radiographs, it is helpful to have a radiograph of a normal gerbil for comparison. On a dorsal–ventral presentation, the thorax is much smaller in width than the abdomen and the stomach usually contains gas and appears rounded. The cardiac silhouette is also rounded and is wider and more cranial relative to what would be seen in a dog. Subtle lung patterns are very difficult to discern but diffuse thoracic opacification resulting from pneumonia can be seen.

Intubation

Commercially manufactured gavage needles (20 gauge) attached to syringes can be used to provide dietary supplementation to sick gerbils. One millilitre can be safely administered per feeding. The substances administered can be a mash of rodent pellets or a mixture of cereal, fruit and vegetable baby food. Caution must always be used to avoid forcing the feeding needle into the animal's oesophagus since tearing or entry into the trachea can occur.

Diseases — An Introduction

Another reason why the gerbil could be considered the ideal pet is that the animal is susceptible to only a few natural infections and unlike the guinea pig and hamster, can be safely treated with a wide spectrum of antibiotics. Viral infections have never been documented in this animal species. The following discussion covers those diseases that are most frequently seen in gerbils. Figure 2.8 found at the end of the chapter summarises the clinical presentations and suggested treatments for the diseases discussed.

One of the challenges of diagnosing diseases in sick rodents is that the animal typically presents with the same signs regardless of the inciting viral, bacterial or husbandry event. A sick gerbil generally has a rough hair coat with ocular porphyrin staining and is hypothermic, lethargic, anorexic and dehydrated.

The clinician must remember the following when treating these animals:

1. The ratio of body surface area to body mass is very large; therefore, dehydration and hypothermia occur quickly and must be treated. Warmed fluids given either IP or SC are necessary to maintain the patient.
2. Rodents have higher metabolic rates and lower energy reserves than larger animals. Gerbils eat up to 8 times per day. Dietary supplementation must be considered in a rodent which has been inappetant for as little as 24 h.

Diseases of the Digestive System

In addition to considering the bacterial agents discussed below, attention to the composition and presentation of the animal's diet should always be included when evaluating animals presented with gastrointestinal clinical symptoms.

Bacterial Diseases

Tyzzer's disease

Agent. The most common infectious disease reported to occur in gerbils is Tyzzer's disease caused by *Clostridium piliforme*. The organism occurs in both vegetative and spore forms. The vegetative form is unstable in the environment, however, spores can survive at room temperature for longer than a year. Infection by the spores can be eliminated with sodium hypochlorite or peracetic acid contact for 5 min. Alcohol or phenolic disinfectants have very little effect on the spores (Ganaway, 1980).

The organism has a worldwide distribution and natural infection probably occurs via ingestion of spore-contaminated food or bedding. An environment that is unsanitary or over-crowded is the ideal setting for a Tyzzer's disease outbreak. To prevent reoccurrences of the disease, a thorough evaluation of the animal's food source, bedding and husbandry conditions should be made.

Hosts. The clinical disease has been reported in mice, rats, gerbils, hamsters, guinea pigs, rabbits, cats, dogs, non-human primates and horses (Committee on Infectious Diseases of Mice and Rats, 1991). Subclinical infections are common in mice and rats.

Clinical signs. The clinical symptoms and pathology associated with infection can easily be related to the spread of the organism. Primary infection occurs in the ileum and caecum followed by spread via the portal vein to the liver. Bacteraemia can then follow resulting in myocardial lesions and suppurative encephalitis. The gerbil is particularly sensitive to the pathology caused by the organism with greatest mortality occurring in 3–7-week-old animals. Signs may vary from acute death with no gross lesions to more chronic disease with the affected animal being lethargic with watery diarrhoea. If the central nervous system is affected, signs may include head tilt, continuous rolling or sudden death (White and Waldron, 1969; Veazey et al., 1992).

Diagnosis. A presumptive diagnosis may be made at necropsy based on finding typical foci of necrosis in the liver and heart together with caecitis. This can be supported by finding the intracytoplasmic bacilli (using a silver stain) located at the border of necrotic foci. An enzyme-linked immunosorbent assay is also available through diagnostic laboratories and allows the veterinarian to make a diagnosis from a serum sample (Motzel et al., 1991).

Treatment. It has been reported that the use of oxytetracycline at 0.1 mg/ml in the water for 30 days has decreased morbidity in colonies (Agren et al., 1989). Animals require supportive care in the way of fluid administration. The best way to treat this disease is to prevent its occurrence by practising good husbandry techniques. If an outbreak has occurred the environment should be decontaminated and an effort made to identify and eliminate the source of infection before introducing other animals. Remember to evaluate food and bedding sources which may be contaminated with spores.

Salmonellosis

Agent. *Salmonella* is a Gram-negative nonspore-forming rod-shaped bacterium. Infection occurs primarily by ingestion of contaminated food, water or bedding. The source of contamination can be other animals including humans.

Hosts. Most animal species including humans can be hosts. Many animals are subclinical carriers of the organism.

Clinical signs. The animal's overall presentation is one of the typical sick rodent, i.e. depression, dehydration, emaciation, rough hair coat. Diarrhoea may or may not be present but gastrointestinal distension is common. Sudden death may occur. Enlargement of the testicles is an indication that *Salmonella* may be the causative organism (Clark et al., 1992).

Diagnosis. The diagnosis can only be made definitively by culturing the organism. The best organs from which to attempt isolation of the organism include liver, spleen and intestines; good isolation is also possible from the faeces and blood. Faeces should be placed in selenite F enrichment broth, followed by a *Salmonella*-specific or brilliant green selective agar. Histological findings include pyogranulomatous meningitis, splenic and hepatic necrosis, ileocaecitis and coagulative necrosis of the testicles.

Control / treatment. It is recommended that animals infected with *Salmonella* should not be treated since the disease is zoonotic and a threat to both human and animal populations. Animals that recover from the disease may become asymptomatic carriers and effectively serve to spread the organism.

Parasitic Diseases

A variety of helminth infections have been reported in the gerbil. However, they occur rarely and the majority are of no consequence as clinical symptoms have not been associated with them.

Pinworms

Agent. The rat and mouse pinworms, *Syphacia muris* and *Syphacia obvelata* can infect the gerbil. These worms have a direct life cycle with ingested ova maturing in the caecum or colon. Female pinworms deposit eggs in the perineal region.

Clinical signs. No clinical symptoms have been documented. However, in other species, heavy infestations of these worms can cause rectal prolapse.

Diagnosis. Detection is best made by placing clear adhesive tape on the perineum, then examining the tape for the presence of ova under a microscope.

Dentostomella translucida

Agent. The oxyurid *D. translucida* may be found in the animal's proximal small intestine.

Clinical signs. No clinical symptoms associated with infestation have been reported.

Diagnosis. The infection may be detected by identifying ova in faecal floats, but the eggs are not shed consistently. The prepatent period is 24 days.

Tapeworms

Agent. The tapeworm *Hymenolepis nana* deserves mention because this parasite has zoonotic potential.

Clinical signs. As with any intestinal parasite, infection can result in an unthrifty animal or intestinal disturbances.

Diagnosis. The eggs of the worm can be transmitted directly through ingestion or indirectly from cockroaches and beetles. Once infected, the animal will start to shed eggs within 24 days. Once an infection is established it can be propagated in closed colonies as autoinfection is common. Diagnosis is made by ova identification. Children handling the animals may become infected via the faecal−oral route.

Treatment for endoparasites

Ivermectin administered orally at 200 μg/kg (Harkness, 1994), or injected SC 11 days apart (Flynn *et al.*, 1989), or mebendazole 2.2 mg/ml for 5 days are effective treatments for most endoparasitic infections in rodent species. The animal may also be treated topically with Ivermectin. One part Ivermectin can be mixed with 10 parts water, then misted over the animal and the cage once weekly for 3 weeks. The animal will groom and ingest the Ivermectin (LeBlanc *et al.*, 1993). A recommended treatment for tapeworm infestation is niclosamide administered at 100 mg/kg for 7 days, then after a treatment-free period of 7 days the gerbil should be fed niclosamide again for 7 days (Hughes *et al.*, 1973).

Diseases of the Nervous System

Non-Infectious Diseases

Seizures

Infectious diseases primarily affecting the gerbil's nervous system have not been reported, however gerbils are prone to epileptiform seizures similar to those described in man. There is a genetic predisposition for the trait and colonies of epileptic gerbils have been bred as models for further studies of the disease. The seizures can be induced by external stimuli such as handling and animals that are seizure-sensitive exhibit more arousal behaviour (rearing and ambulation) whenever they are exposed to a strange environment. It has been theorised that seizures have evolved as a survival mechanism for the gerbil as the seizure activity could confuse potential predators.

Clinical signs. Seizures can start in gerbils by 2–3 months of age with the incidence and severity increasing up to 6 months. Gerbils can experience cataleptic, hypnotic and grand mal seizure types. The components of a major seizure include 16–48 s of clonic tonic activity (i.e. rigid posture with foreleg treading and mouth spasms) followed by extensor immobility, then abnormal behaviour and finally normal behaviour. Seizures can last from 300 to 368 s (Gutler and MacKintosh, 1989).

Diagnosis. The condition is diagnosed by observing the seizure activity. The condition has been related to a deficiency in glutamine synthetase, the enzyme which catabolises glutamate to glutamine. Glutamate serves as one of the nervous system's excitatory amino-acids (Laming *et al.*, 1989).

Control / treatment. It has been documented that even if the animal is genetically predisposed to seizure activity, the frequency and intensity of the episodes can be decreased by frequent handling of the animal early in life. Phenobarbital at 10–20 mg/kg and diphenylhydantoin at 25–50 mg/kg every 12 h are potential drug therapies. Caution should be used when administering either one of these therapies as fatalities can easily occur.

Antibiotic toxicity

The administration of streptomycin is contraindicated in gerbils. The antibiotic interferes with acetylcholine metabolism resulting in neuromuscular blockade and paralysis. Doses of 50 mg per animal have resulted in 80–100% mortality.

Diseases of the Integument and Musculoskeletal System

Infectious Diseases

Ventral scent gland infection / inflammation

Gerbils can present with abdominal skin that appears red and possibly ulcerated. Carcinoma of the ventral scent gland must be considered especially in older animals; however a primary infection of the gland resulting in inflammation should also be considered. Topical antibiotics in combination with steroid cream can be applied, followed by an abdominal bandage wrap to hold the ointment in place. If the lesion is not responsive, removal of the gland is recommended since neoplasia is the probable diagnosis.

Non-Infectious Diseases

Facial dermatitis

Facial dermatitis, commonly referred to as 'sore nose', is one of the more common pathological conditions afflicting gerbils. The problem appears most commonly in postpubertal animals that are housed in a group caged environment and are environmentally stressed by overcrowding and high humidity. The disease initiator is hypersecretion or excess accumulation of Harderian gland secretions. The porphyrin pigment, if allowed to accumulate on the skin, is thought to be an irritant which leads the animal to self-traumatise the area. Disease then follows as the area becomes invaded by *Staphylococcus saphrophyticus* or *Staphylococcus aureus* (Bresnahar *et al.*, 1983; Peckam *et al.*, 1974). *Staphylococcus xylosus* has also been implicated (Solomon *et al.*, 1990).

Clinical signs. The clinical presentations of the disease appear to vary depending on whether or not pathogenic staphylococcal organisms have invaded and propagated. If staphylococcal organisms are involved, the animal presents with a localised moist dermatitis around the external nares which extends to the front paws and legs, then to the ventral thorax and abdomen. As the disease progresses, the animal loses hair. Erythema and scabbing may or may not be present. Sinusitis may also occur. Animals will lose body condition as they may stop eating and drinking and can eventually die. Spontaneous recoveries are also possible. If bacterial organisms are not involved, the facial lesions do not progress and the moist, ulcerative, exudative

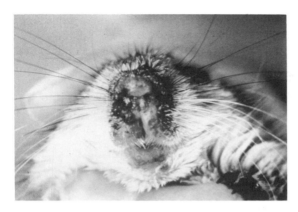

FIG. 2.6 Sore nose in a gerbil.

stage is not present. Figure 2.6 illustrates a gerbil with sore nose.

Diagnosis. The diagnosis is made by observing the typical clinical presentation. Skin cultures will identify if staphylococcal organisms are involved.

Control / treatment. Controlling the disease requires a thorough understanding of the physiology of the gerbil. Harderian gland secretions and the disposition of those secretions are under environmental control. When the gerbil is exposed to cooler temperatures, the animal will groom the secretions over the body with the lipid content insulating the animal and increasing radiant absorption. At higher temperatures, the grooming of Harderian secretions is decreased and the animal will increase the frequency of sandbathing. Sore nose may result if environmental temperatures and or humidity are consistently high and the animal is not provided with the opportunity to sandbathe. Providing optimal husbandry conditions and environmental control should be the first step in preventing the disease. If cultures indicate that a bacterial component is present, a 14-day course of systemic antibiotics such as chloramphenicol, tetracycline or gentamicin is recommended. Topical treatments such as nitrofurazone and povidone−iodine surgical scrub have resulted in lesion regression but recurrence is common (Collins, 1987).

Housing the animals on sand decreases the incidence and severity of the disease and removing the Harderian gland prevents the disease. The long term effect on the gerbil of Harderian gland removal is not known (Thiessen and Pendergrass, 1982; Farrar *et al.*, 1988).

Hair loss

Gerbils may lose tail fur due to improper handling. If this occurs, the tail itself may become necrotic and amputation will be necessary. Barbering can occur if the animal is housed in an overcrowded cage. Hair removal with distinct margins will be observed on the tail base and the head crown. The underlying skin is normal in appearance. If aggression occurs, indicated by bite marks at the tail base and perineal area, secondary bacterial infections can result with irregular hair loss and skin inflammation.

Another condition referred to as 'bald nose' can occur in gerbils fed from wire cage-top feeders. A stripe of hair loss is visible over the muzzle with the underlying skin being normal (Fig. 2.7). This condition has been associated with the feeding behaviour of certain gerbils as they aggressively push their noses through the wires to obtain food. Placing the food within the cage or eliminating the wire bar lid can prevent this hair loss. A similar hair loss may also occur in gerbils with vigorous burrowing habits. Providing the animals with 'cage toys' may diminish this behaviour.

Hair pigmentation

A condition has been reported whereby some gerbils are born having abnormal hair pigmentation with patchy, scanty hair distribution. These animals also have a 'failure to thrive' syndrome. Surviving animals develop a normal hair coat at maturity (Collins, 1987).

Neoplastic Diseases

Neoplasms of the skin occur with high frequency in the aged gerbil. The ventral scent gland is particularly at risk in aged animals for either adenoma or squamous cell carcinoma for-

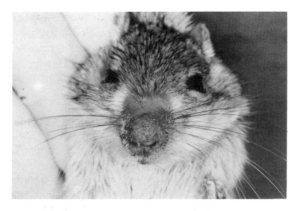

FIG. 2.7 Hair loss on a gerbil's nose associated with feeding from wire top cage lids.

mation. Other neoplastic masses include squamous cell carcinomas and melanomas of the ear and foot.

Ventral scent gland

Clinical signs. Neoplastic processes involving the ventral scent gland initially present as a generalised reddening of the affected gland. Ulceration and secondary bacterial infection is common. Metastases are infrequent (Benit and Kramer, 1965; Vincent *et al.*, 1975; Meckley and Zwicker, 1979).

Treatment. Haemostasis should be ensured during surgical removal of a mass since size and blood supply may be significant compared to the body mass of the animal. The earlier the recognition and removal of the mass, the better the prognosis. The practitioner needs to remember that neoplasms are usually found in aged animals that often have concomitant renal disease.

Parasitic Diseases

Demodectic mange

Agent. Demodectic mange caused by *Demodex merioni* has been reported to occur in the gerbil.

Hosts. The mite is thought to be species-specific and transmitted only between gerbils.

Clinical signs. The animal will present with generalised alopecia, skin ulcerations, scaliness and hyperaemia. Secondary bacterial infection may occur.

Diagnosis. Diagnosis can be made by visualisation of the parasite in skin scrapings with the aid of a microscope.

Control / treatment. If an animal has generalised demodicosis, the overall health of the animal has generally been compromised. Variables to consider are the age of the animal, diet, husbandry and whether or not the animal has concomitant disease. Treatment of the parasite will not be effective unless the other problems have been addressed. Rinsing the animal in an amitraz/water mixture (0.66 ml to 1 pint water) 3–6 times at 2 week intervals is a recommended treatment (Harkness, 1994).

Liponyssoides sanguineous

Agent. *L. sanguineous*, the mouse mite, has also been reported to occur in gerbils, however no clinical signs were observed (Levine and Lage, 1985).

Fungal Diseases

Ringworm

Agent. Ringworm in gerbils occurs most commonly from *Trichophyton mentagrophytes*, however, infections with *Microsporum* sp. can also occur. The fungus can be transmitted from other animals or humans.

Clinical signs. Gerbils typically present with areas of focal hair loss or brittle hair. The underlying skin may appear dry or inflamed and hyperkeratosis may be present.

Diagnosis. A definitive diagnosis is made by taking skin scrapings and culturing the fungus on dermatophyte test media. *Microsporum* sp. will fluoresce when exposed to a Wood's lamp.

Control / treatment. Oral administration of griseofulvin (30 mg/kg PO sid for 3 weeks) is the recommended treatment; however, topical administration of tolnaftate is also an option.

Diseases of Metabolic Origin

Ageing

Gerbils can live in captivity for up to 4 years with the mean survival time being 2–3 years. As the animal ages, certain pathologies occur with increasing frequency. Chronic interstitial nephritis characterised by polyuria, polydypsia and weight loss is the most common and significant disease occurring in aged gerbils. Supportive treatment for this condition includes supplemental fluid administration. After 2 years of age, spontaneously occurring neoplasia is a significant cause of morbidity and mortality with the reproductive tract, the adrenal gland and skin the most commonly affected sites (Ringler *et al.*, 1972). Cystic ovaries occur in approximately 20% of aged female gerbils resulting in infertility and decreased litter sizes. Head tilts caused by aural cholesteatomas occur with high frequency in aged gerbils (Schiffer *et al.*, 1986). The pathology results from the invagination of the tympanic membrane which causes a secondary infection and accumulation of cholesterol crystals. No effective treatment is available for the gerbil. These animals also experience hearing loss that is quantitatively similar to the loss that occurs in humans over the age of 65 (Mills *et al.*, 1990).

Hyperglycaemia

In a certain percentage of the gerbil population, breeding animals can hypersecrete adrenal steroids which can result in hyperlipidaemia, hyperglycaemia and eventually spontaneous diabetes mellitus. Obese gerbils (> 80 g) are predisposed to hyperglycaemia and glucose intolerance with mean fasting blood glucose levels of 101.60 g% (Lucocq and Findlay, 1981).

References

Agren, G., Zhou, O. and Zhong, W. (1989a) Aetiology and social behaviour of Mongolian gerbils, *Meriones unguiculatus* at Xilinhot Inner Mongolia China. *Animal Behaviour* **37**, 11–27.

Agren, G., Zhou, O. and Zhong, W. (1989b) Territoriality, cooperation and resources priority, handling in the Mongolian gerbil. *Animal Behaviour* **37**, 28–32.

Allen, K., Van Bruggen, N. and Cooper, J. (1993) Detection of bacterial sinusitis in the Mongolian gerbil using magnetic resonance imaging. *Veterinary Record* **132**, 633–635.

Arrington, L. R. and Ammerman, C. B. (1969) Water requirements of gerbils. *Laboratory Animal Science* **19**, 503–505.

Benit, K. F. and Kramer, A. W. (1965) Spontaneous tumors in the Mongolian gerbil. *Laboratory Animal Care* **15**, 281.

Bresnahar, J. F., Smith, G. D., Lentsch, R. H. *et al.* (1983) Nasal dermatitis in the Mongolian gerbil. *Laboratory Animal Science* **33**, 258–263.

Brown, R., Hauschild, M., Holmson, S. and Hutchinson, J. (1988) Mate recognition by urine odours in the Mongolian gerbil. *Behavioural and Neural Biology* **47**, 174–183.

Clark, J. D., Shotts, E., Hill, J. and McCall, J. (1992) Salmonellosis in gerbil induced by non-related experimental procedure. *Laboratory Animal Science* **42**, 161–163.

Clark, M., Spencer, C. and Galef, B. (1986) Reproductive life history correlates of early and late survival maturating of female Mongolian gerbil. *Animal Behaviour* **34**, 551–568.

Cocke, R. and Thiessen, D. (1986) Chemocommunication among prey and predator species. *Animal Learning and Behaviour* **14**, 90–92.

Collins, B. R. (1987) Dermatologic disorders of common small non-domestic animals. In: *Contemporary Issues in Small Animal Practice*, Vol. 8, pp. 235–394. Churchill Livingstone.

Committee on Infectious Diseases of Mice and Rats (1991) *Infectious Diseases of Mice and Rats*. National Research Council, National Academy Press, Washington, DC.

Dillon, W. and Glomski, C. (1975) The Mongolian gerbil: qualitative and quantitative aspects of the cellular blood picture. *Laboratory Animals* **9**, 283–287.

Farrar, P., Opsomer, M., Kocen, J. and Wagner, J. (1988) Experimental nasal dermatitis in the Mongolian gerbil: Effect of bilateral Harderian gland adenectomy on the development of facial lesions. *Laboratory Animal Science* **38**, 72–76.

Flynn, B. M., Brown, P. A., Eckstein, J. M. *et al.* (1989) Treatment of *Syphacia obvelata* in mice using ivermectin. *Laboratory Animal Science* **39**, 461–463.

Ganaway, J. R. (1980) Effect of heat and selected chemical disinfectants upon infectivity of spores of *Bacillus piliformis* (Tyzzer's disease). *Laboratory Animal Science* **30**, 192–196.

Guide for the Care and Use of Laboratory Animals (1985) Contract N01-RR-2-2135, ILAR, NIH Bethesda, MD.

Gutler, M. and MacKintosh, J. (1989) Epilepsy and behaviour of Mongolian gerbil: An ethological study. *Physiology and Behaviour* **46**, 561–566.

Harkness, J. (1994) Small rodents in exotic pet medicine. *Veterinary Clinics of North America: Small Animal Practice*, Vol. 24, pp. 84–102.

Holmes, D. (1985) The Mongolian gerbil in biomedical research. *Laboratory Animal Science*, **14**, 923–938.

Hoefer, H. (1995) Small mammal radiography. *The North American Veterinary Conference Proceedings*.

Hughes, H. C., Barthel, C. H. and Lang, C. M. (1973) Niclosamide as a treatment for *Hymenolepis nana* and *Hymenolepis diminuta* in rats. *Laboratory Animal Science* **23**, 72–73.

Laming, P., Cosby, S. and O'Neill, J. (1989) Seizure in Mongolian gerbils are related to differences in glutamine synthetase. *Comparative Biochemistry and Physiology* **94**, 399–404.

LeBlanc, S., Faith, R. and Montgomery, C. (1993) Use of topical ivermectin treatment for *Syphacia obvelata* in mice. *Laboratory Animal Science* **43**, 526–528.

Levine, J. F. and Lage, A. L. (1985) House mouse mites infecting laboratory rodents. *Laboratory Animal Science* **34**, 393–394.

Lucocq, J. M. and Findlay, J. A. (1981) Islet organ blood glucose and glucose tolerance of lean and obese Mongolian gerbils. *Cell Tissue Research* **220**, 623–636.

Meckley, P. and Zwicker, G. (1979) Naturally occuring neoplasms in the Mongolian gerbil. *Laboratory Animal Science* **13**, 203.

Mills, J., Schmidt, R. and Kulish, L. (1990) Age related changes in auditory potentials of the Mongolian gerbil. *Hearing Research* **46**, 201–210.

Motzel, S. L., Meyer, J. K. and Riley, L. (1991) Detection of serum antibodies of *Bacillus piliformis* in mice and rats using enzyme linked immunoabsorbent assay. *Laboratory Animal Science* **41**, 26–30.

Najarian, H. H. (1961) *Haemobartonella* in the Mongolian gerbil. *Texas Reports on Biology and Medicine* **19**, 123–133.

Norris, M. L. (1987) Gerbils. In: *The UFAW Handbook on the Care and Management of Laboratory Animals*, 6th edn, pp. 360–376, Poole, T. (ed.). Agricultural and Food Research Council, Cambridge, England.

Norris, M. L. and Adams, C. E. (1981a) Mating postpartum and length of gestation in Mongolian gerbils. *Laboratory Animal* **15**, 189–191.

Norris, M. L. and Adams, C. E. (1981b) Time of mating and associated changes in the vaginal smear of the post-parturient Mongolian gerbil. *Laboratory Animal* **15**, 193–198.

Otken, C. and Hall, H. (1980) Qualitative amino-acid requirements for Mongolian gerbils, *Nutrition Reports International* **22**, 409–418.

Otken, C. and Scott, C. (1984) Feeding characteristics of Mongolian gerbils. *Laboratory Animal Science* **34**, 181–184.

Otken, C., Dougherty, S. and Servin, M. (1985) A possible need for taurine in the diet of the gerbil. *Nutrition Reports International* **31**, 955–962.

Paradise, P. (1980) *Gerbils*. TFH Publishing Co., Neptune, NJ.

Peckham, J. C., Cole, J. R., Chapman, W. L. *et al.* (1974) Staphylococcal dermatitis in Mongolian gerbils. *Laboratory Animal Science* **24**, 43–47.

Ringler, D. H., Lay, D. M. and Abrams, G. D. (1972) Spontaneous neoplasms in ageing gerbilinae. *Laboratory Animal Science* **22**, 407–414.

Robinson, D. G. (1979) Physiological parameters and selected general data. *The Gerbil Digest* **6**, 1–2.

Robinson, P. F. (1959) Metabolism of the gerbil. *Science* **130**, 502–503.

Rohrbach, C. (1982) Investigation of the Bruce effect in the Mongolian gerbil. *Journal of Reproduction and Fertility* **56**, 411–417.

Ruhren, R. (1965) Normal values for haemoglobin concentration and cellular elements in the blood of Mongolian gerbils. *Laboratory Animal Care* **15**, 313–320.

Schiffer, S. P., Lukas, V. and Crisp, C. (1986) Diagnostic exercise: Head tilt in a gerbil. *Laboratory Animal Science* **36,** 176–177.

Schwentker, P. (1968) *Care and Maintenance of the Mongolian Gerbil.* Tumblebrook Farms, Brant Lake, NY.

Silverman, S. (1993) Diagnostic imaging of exotic pets. *Veterinary Clinics of North America: Small Animal Practice,* Vol. 23, pp. 1287–1299.

Solomon, H., Dixon, D. and Pouch, W. (1990) A survey of *Staphylococci* isolated from the laboratory gerbil. *Laboratory Animal Science* **40,** 316–318.

Thiessen, D. (1988) Body temperature and grooming in the Mongolian gerbil. *Annals of the New York Academy of Sciences* **525,** 27–37.

Thiessen, D. D. and Pendergrass, M. (1982) Harderian gland involvement in facial lesions in the Mongolian gerbil. *Journal of the American Veterinary Medical Association* **181,** 1375–1377.

UFAW (1987) *Handbook on the Care and Management of Laboratory Animals.* Agricultural and Food Research Council, Cambridge, England.

Veazey, R., Paulsen, D. and Schaeffer, D. (1992) Encephalitis in gerbils due to naturally occurring infection with *Bacillus piliformis. Laboratory Animal Science* **42,** 516–518.

Vincent, A. L., Porter, D. D. and Ash, L. R. (1975) Spontaneous lesions and parasites of the Mongolian gerbil. *Laboratory Animal Science* **25,** 711.

Wagner, J. E. and Farrar, P. L. (1987) Husbandry and medicine of small rodents. *The Veterinary Clinics of North America: Small Animal Practice,* Vol. 17, pp. 1061–1087. WB Saunders, Philadelphia, PA.

Wallace, P., Owen, J. and Thiessen, D. D. (1973) The control and function of maternal scent marking in the Mongolian gerbil. *Physiology and Behaviour* **10,** 463–466.

White, D. J. and Waldron, M. M. (1969) Naturally occuring Tyzzer's disease in the gerbil. *Veterinary Record* **85,** 111–129.

Yahr, P. and Anderson-Mitchell, K. (1983) Attraction of gerbil pups to maternal nest odours, duration, specificity and ovarian control. *Physiology and Behaviour* **31,** 241–247.

(Data Tables follow).

Data Tables

COMMON DISEASES—GERBILS						
Disease	Aetiology	Diagnosis	Clinical signs and history	Treatment and control	Zoonotic potential	Comments
Gastrointestinal system						
Tyzzer's disease	*C. piliforme*	ELISA on serum	Weanlings Diarrhoea CNS symptoms Sudden death	0.1–0.8 mg/ml tetracycline Supportive fluids Decontaminate environment	No	This species is very susceptible
Salmonellosis	*Salmonella enteritidis* and *S. typhimurium*	Culture faeces and blood	Gastrointestinal distension Testicular enlargement With or without diarrhoea	None recommended	Yes	
Nervous system						
Seizures	Genetic predisposition	Observation	Seizures	Phenobarbital 10–20 mg/kg Diphenylhydantoin 25–50 mg/kg	No	
Integument and musculoskeletal system						
Sore nose	Excess Harderian gland secretions Staphylococcal organisms	Skin culture	Hair loss on face, front paws Moist appearance to skin, erythema, sinusitis	Chloramphenicol IM or SC 30 mg/kg Tetracycline in water 0.1–0.8 mg/ml Topical iodine scrub Removal of Harderian gland Provide sand Improve husbandry	No	
Aggression	Staphylococcal organisms	Observation	Hair loss, bite marks around tail base	Improve husbandry Decrease number in cage	No	
	Barbering	Observation	Hair loss around tail base and head crown No skin inflammation	Remove dominant animal	No	

Fig. 2.8—continued

COMMON DISEASES—GERBILS						
Disease	Aetiology	Diagnosis	Clinical signs and history	Treatment and control	Zoonotic potential	Comments
Mange	*Demodex merioni*	Skin scraping	Generalised skin ulceration scales, hyperaemia	Amitraz 0.66 ml to 1 pint of water 2 week intervals		
Ventral scent gland inflammation	Cancer Primary infection	Biopsy	Red, ulcerated ventral abdomen	Topical antibiotic, antiinflammatory Gland removal if cancer		
Ringworm	*Trichophyton* sp. *Microsporum* sp.	Skin scraping and culture	Hairloss Skin inflammation	Griseofulvin 1.5 % topically or Griseofulvin 30 mg/kg PO sid, 3 weeks	Potential	
Ageing						
Nephritis	Associated with ageing	Elevated creatinine, BUN Weight loss	Polyuria Polydipsia	Supportive fluids	No	
Aural cholesteatoma	Associated with ageing	Physical examination	Head tilt Hair loss around ears	None	No	

FIG. 2.8 Common diseases—gerbils.

PHYSIOLOGICAL DATA—GERBILS	
Adult weight	50–90 g
Life span	2–4 years
H_2O consumption (adult)	3–4 ml/day (depends on food moisture)
Temperature (rectal)	101–103 °F (38–39 °C)
Food consumption	10–15 g/day
Heart rate	260–600/min
Respiratory rate	70–120/min
Data taken from Canadian Council on Animal Care (1984).	

FIG. 2.9 Physiological data—gerbils.

HAEMATOLOGICAL VALUES—GERBILS		
	Male	Female
RBC $\times$ 10^6/mm^3	8.1	8.6
PCV%	47.5	45.8
Haemoglobin	14.8	14.14
Reticulocytes/1000 RBC	31	33
WBC $\times$ 10^3/mm^3	12	9.7
Neutrophils %	20	26
Eosinophils %	1	1
Basophils %	1	1
Lymphocytes %	78	73
Monocytes %	0.9	1
Platelets $\times$ 10^3/mm^3	400–600	400–600
Blood volume ml/kg	78	78
Data taken from Dillon and Glomski (1975); Canadian Council on Animal Care (1984); BVA/FRAME/RSPCA/UFAW Joint Working Group on Refinement (1993).		

FIG. 2.10 Haematological values—gerbils.

CLINICAL CHEMISTRY VALUES—GERBILS	
	Mean (Range)
Calcium mg/dl	(3.7–6.2)
Phosphorus mg/dl	(3.7–8.2)
Sodium mEq/l	151 (141–171.5)
Chloride mEq/l	(93–118)
Potassium mEq/l	4.54 (3.3–6.3)
Glucose mg/dl	93.78 (40–140.7)
BUN mg/dl	20.88 (16.8–31.3)
Creatinine mg/dl	0.88 (0.5–1.4)
Uric acid mg/dl	1.64 (1.1–2.8)
Total protein g/dl	7.90 (4.8–16.8)
Albumin g/dl	3.08 (1.8–5.8)
Globulin g/ml	4.83 (0.6–14.3)
Cholesterol mg/dl	(90–130)
Alkyl phosphate IU/l	(12–37)
Data taken from Mays (1969).	

FIG. 2.11 Clinical chemistry values—gerbils.

REPRODUCTIVE DATA—GERBILS	
Breeding age	10–12 weeks
Oestrous cycle	Polyoestrous
Duration of oestrous cycle	4–6 days
Gestation	24–26 days
Average litter size	4–5
Birth weight	2.5–4.0 g
Eyes open	14–20 days
Wean	21–24 days
Postpartum oestrus	24 h
Number of mammae	6
Breeding duration	15–18 months
Data taken from Canadian Council on Animal Care (1980–1984) and Wagner and Farrar (1987).	

FIG. 2.12 Reproductive data—gerbils.

3

Hamsters

NEIL S. LIPMAN and CHARMAINE FOLTZ

Introduction

There are 25 species of hamster distributed worldwide, principally in South-East Europe and Asia (Honacki *et al.*, 1982). Only a few species, however, are found as pets or in research colonies. The Syrian or golden hamster *(Mesocricetus auratus)* is by far the most common. Indigenous to a restricted geographical area in North-Western Syria, they live singly in deep, multichambered burrows which provide a cool and humid environment in contrast to the arid desert. All pet and research Syrian hamsters originated from 3 littermates caught in Allepo, Syria which were used to establish a research colony at the Hebrew University, Jerusalem in 1930. Syrian hamsters have undeservedly developed a reputation for being pugnacious and difficult to handle. When handled gently and consistently they can become docile and alluring pets.

Chinese or striped hamsters (*Cricetulus griseus*) which are considerably smaller than the Syrian hamster, are also kept as pets, albeit less frequently. As their name implies they are indigenous to China. Adult males are approximately 10% larger than females and weigh 30–35 g. The females are extremely aggressive and as a result are often difficult to breed. They develop a genetically determined spontaneous diabetes mellitus which has been studied extensively as an animal model for human disease. In addition, they share with several other species of hamsters the distinction of having the fewest number of chromosomes of any mammal ($2N = 22$).

The furry-footed or Djungarian (*Phodopus sungorus*), the Armenian (*Cricetulus migratorius*) and the Turkish (*Mesocricetus brandti*) hamster are found infrequently as pets or in research facilities.

Hamsters have been used extensively in biomedical research because of their susceptibility to a variety of infectious and parasitic diseases, their propensity to develop dental caries when fed a high carbohydrate diet, and their unique anatomical and physiological features. Much of what is known about their biology and diseases has originated from these research efforts.

This chapter will review the biology and medicine of hamsters, including distinctive anatomical and physiological features. This information will be of use both when treating hamsters and when advising clients on their proper care. Additional references, provided at the end of the chapter, may be consulted for a more thorough discussion. **Unless otherwise noted, the review will be limited to the Syrian hamster as it is the species most commonly encountered as a pet.**

Unique Biology

Hamsters are 15–20 cm in length and weigh 85–140 g. Adult females are larger than males. Sex differentiation is easy in adults. The male's large testicles (carried caudally) contribute to a more rounded appearance and smaller appearing tail (Fig. 3.1). It is important to recognise, as with all rodents, that the inguinal canal remains open and the scrotal sack may be empty. Gentle pressure applied to the caudal abdomen will cause the testes to protrude. Sex differentiation in preweanlings can be determined by measuring or comparing the ano-genital distances of littermates. The distance is greater and the genital papilla is larger and pointed in males. The anogenital region of the female is characterised by 3 orifices, the urethral, vaginal and anal (Fig. 3.1).

There is a variety of coat colour phenotypes. The wild type (agouti) is reddish brown, with a pale yellow ventrum. Coat colour varieties include cinnamon, cream, yellow brown, piebald, tortoiseshell and albino (Robinson, 1968). In addition there is a long haired or 'teddy bear' variety. Coat phenotypes are inherited as autosomal or sex-linked traits. The cream variety is considered the most gentle, whereas mottled or spotted varieties are the most aggressive.

The dental formula of the hamster is $2(I \frac{1}{1} C \frac{0}{0}$

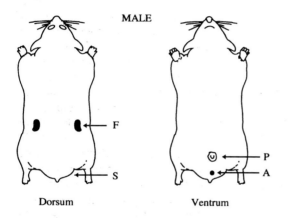

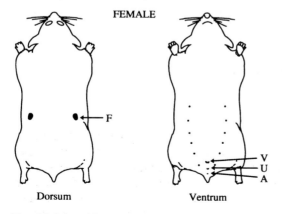

FIG. 3.1 Schematic representation of the dorsum and ventrum of a male and female hamster. (F) flank gland; (S) scrotum; (P) prepuce; (A) anus; (V) vulva; (U) urethra.

$P \frac{0}{0} M \frac{3}{3}$). Incisors are open rooted and continue to grow, although irregularly, throughout life. The occlusal surfaces are sharpened by the opposing incisor pair. Malocclusion, with incisor overgrowth and penetration of oral structures, may be associated with ptyalism and weight loss.

Cheek pouches, which are highly distensible evaginations of the lateral buccal wall, are well developed in hamsters. They are devoid of glands and are 'immunologically privileged' sites because transplantation of foreign tissue does not engender immunological rejection. They are used to transport and store food or conceal a newborn litter when danger is present. Owners may report that the dam has eaten her litter. If the owner is advised to leave her alone, the pups may reappear.

Hip glands, also referred to as costovertebral, flank, or scent glands, are sebaceous and are more prominent in males (Fig. 3.1). In young animals the area is small and unpigmented. With age, especially in males, the area becomes darkly pigmented and becomes covered with coarse fur. The glands are easily visible following clipping. When the male becomes sexually excited, the fur over the gland becomes wet. The secretions appear to be irritating, as the hamster scratches and rubs the area. There is evidence that the glands are secretory in the oestrus female as males are frequently observed investigating the area.

The hamster's stomach is unusual. A distinct constriction divides the stomach into two portions: the cardiac or non-glandular region, lined by squamous epithelium, and the glandular region. There is a narrow passageway between the two sections. The oesophagus enters the cardia just cranial to the constriction and so near the pylorus that the lesser curvature of the stomach is almost non-existent. Vomition is not possible because of these anatomical features.

The hamster's gastrointestinal and renal systems are adapted to an arid environment. The duodenum, jejunum and colon are long. The kidney has an extremely long papilla which extends into the ureter. Hamster urine is cream coloured and thick, presumably as a result of adaptation for water conservation; however, its consistency does not change substantially when water is provided *ad libitum*.

As in other rodents, the male reproductive system is complex, with numerous accessory sex glands, including the coagulating, prostate, ampullary, bulbourethral and large vesicular glands. Large fat bodies overlie the testes. Females have a duplex uterus.

Physiological data are presented at the end of the chapter (Fig. 3.7). Haematology and clinical chemistry reference values (Figs 3.8 and 3.9) at the end of the chapter should be scrutinised carefully. Differences in genotype, age, diet, investigation method, sampling technique and circadian rhythm may lead to varying results. Preferably, normal values should be established for individual laboratories. Serum cholesterol levels are of interest as they are the highest among common laboratory animals (Lee *et al.*, 1959); the changes that occur in the haemogram during hibernation are also worthy of note.

Behaviour

Little is known about the behaviour of hamsters in the natural environment (Siegel, 1985). They live singly in chambered burrows in close proximity to other hamsters, communicating with ultrasonic auditory signals. The burrows are generally less than 0.5 m deep, have 1 or 2 chambers and include an entrance and an escape route. Hamsters are nocturnal, however the light cycle is frequently interrupted with short periods of activity. They are extremely territorial, and should not be picked up directly from their nests. Hamsters have the tendency to seek dark, protected areas (Walker *et al.*, 1964). Females are dominant to males and can be very aggressive. Ideally, hamsters should be housed singly because of potential aggression towards cagemates. Group housing is most successful when same-sex littermates are housed together from weaning; mixed sex housing may lead to aggression once the animals reach reproductive age. Breeders may group-house hamsters in polygamous breeding systems but aggression and injury may be observed. Anaesthetising prospective cagemates and allowing them to recover in a neutral cage has been recommended when establishing new groups (Harkness and Wagner, 1983). Hamsters frequently exercise at night, therefore an exercise wheel should be provided. Female hamsters will run up to 8 km a day when provided with the opportunity (Richards, 1966). Hamsters are skilled at escape and should be housed in cages with tight-fitting lids.

Hamsters are 'permissive hibernators', they have the option of hibernating in response to decreased environmental temperatures ($< 4.5\,°C$, $< 40\,°F$), availability of food, the duration of light provided and other variables (Gumma *et al.*, 1967). In a large group, exposed to the same environmental conditions, some animals will hibernate while others will not. Hibernation is not a continuously maintained state; hamsters alternate between 2–3 days of hibernation and periods of arousal and normal homeothermic existence. During hibernation, they have lowered body temperature, heart and respiratory rates but remain sensitive to tactile stimuli and can be aroused. Distinct clinical pathological changes occur during hibernation, including increases in RBC count, Hb concentration and PCV. Haemogram changes are a result of retardation of RBC senescence and the absence of RBC destruction. White cells are also decreased. The provision of constant temperature throughout the year ($21–22\,°C$, $70–74\,°F$) and lighting (12–14 h of light) are recommended.

Reproduction

Mating

Hamsters reach sexual maturity at approximately 6 weeks of age. However, it is not uncommon to find them reproducing as young as 1 month. Maximum reproductive efficiency is achieved if breeding is delayed until female hamsters are 8–10 weeks and males are 10–12 weeks of age (Balk and Slater, 1987). Hamsters are seasonally polyoestrous. The female has a

96 h oestrous cycle which takes place over 5 days. Which stage in the oestrous cycle the hamster is at can be ascertained, as in other species, by examining the cytological features of the vaginal smear. The end of the cycle is marked by the appearance of a copious viscous white postovulatory discharge that fills, and may exude from the vagina and has a distinct odour. Females can be bred during the evening of the third day following the discharge; ovulation occurs between midnight and 1 a.m. Females are most receptive just before and after ovulation. Receptivity is demonstrated by lordosis in the presence of a male. Repeated copulation occurs for 20–60 min. A copulation plug, composed of secretions from the vagina and the male's accessory sex organs, may be observed in the vaginal vault or in the cage the morning following breeding. Pregnancy is confirmed by the absence of the postovulatory discharge at days 5 and 9 postmating and the observation of a distended abdomen and marked weight gain at 10 days of pregnancy. Pseudopregnancy may occur with an infertile mating. It lasts for 8–12 days and resembles a normal pregnancy except there is a decrease in body weight during the last 2 days.

A variety of mating systems have been utilised for breeding. The preferred technique is **hand-mating**. Two hours after initiation of the dark cycle a female in oestrus is placed in the male's cage for 15–60 min. The female is removed if copulation is not observed within 5 min or if the female is aggressive. If mating occurs, they are left together until the next light cycle. **Monogamous** mating involves placing a prepubertal pair together permanently. Fighting and pup loss may occur. **Harem** or group mating schemes can be employed in which multiple females are housed with one or several males. There can be as few as 1 male and 2 females, to groups of 3–5 males and 10–12 females. They are housed together for 7–14 days. Females are individually caged for gestation and lactation. Fighting frequently occurs with this system. It is not advisable to keep potential breeding females in all-female groups because they fail to exhibit normal mating behaviour despite having normal oestrous cycles (Brown and Lisk, 1978). Reproductive

data can be found in Fig. 3.10 at the end of the chapter.

Gestation and Birth

The normal gestation period is 15.5 days but it may range from 15 to 18 days. Pregnant females should be placed individually in a clean cage on the 13th day of pregnancy and provided with nesting material. Just prior to parturition the female becomes restless and alternates between nest-building, grooming and eating. A bloody vaginal discharge may be evident before delivery of the first foetus. The young are altricious: they are hairless, blind and have undeveloped limbs and closed ears. However, they do have sharp teeth. The average litter size is between 5 and 9.

Cannibalism is common during the first week of life, with a higher incidence among primiparous females. Cage changing or animal handling should not be performed between the last 2 days of pregnancy and approximately 10 days following birth. If the dam must be disturbed or young handled during the first week of life, provide fresh palatable food and attempt to mask human scent by applying a non-toxic fragrance to the dam's nose. Cross-fostering is rarely successful if young are abandoned.

Pups weigh 2–3 g at birth. Their ears and eyes open at 5 and 15 days, respectively; hair growth begins at 10 days. They begin to eat and should be provided with solid food as early as 7–10 days. Pups require fluid intake in excess of that provided by the dam. Sipper tubes should be 1–2 cm above the level of bedding in cages with litters 10–20 days of age (Slater, 1972). Pups are weaned at 21–28 days when they weigh 35–40 g. Two to 18 days post weaning a fertile oestrus occurs (Harkness and Wagner, 1983). Reproductive senescence develops after 14 months of age.

Husbandry

Housing

A variety of caging systems which are available to house rodents can be utilised successfully for maintaining hamsters. Cages should be smooth, indestructible and have tight-fitting lids with a positive latching mechanism. Hamsters burrow and gnaw, frequently escaping from inadequate caging. Caging should be made of rigid plastic or stainless or galvanised steel, with rounded corners that cannot be chewed. Wood and aluminium should not be used. While open wire-mesh-bottomed caging has been used, solid bottom caging provided with suitable contact bedding is preferred, especially for breeding. A variety of commercially available hamster caging systems employ plastic tubes for environmental enrichment and a dark hiding place or nest box into which the animal can retreat. A running wheel should be provided for exercise. Caging should be non-porous so it can be adequately sanitised. Figure 3.2 shows specific space requirements for laboratory hamsters which can be used as a guide for housing pets.

A variety of contact bedding materials is available. Wood shavings or chips, beet pulp, ground corncob, or cellulose products can be used. Cedar bedding has been associated with the induction of hepatic microsomal enzymes which may increase drug metabolism rates. Tissue paper or cotton wadding should be provided for nesting material.

Hamsters produce minimal excrement or odour. Urine output is limited and they urinate in the same area, generally a corner, in the cage. Cages should be sanitised weekly and fresh bedding provided. However, the cage can be left unchanged for 2 weeks as recommended for breeding.

Feeding and watering implements used for other rodents are suitable for hamsters. Water bottles with metal sipper tubes are recommended; glass tubes should not be used as they are frequently broken by chewing. A variety of feeders may be used. If feed is provided from slotted sheet metal or wire bar hoppers, the slots should be at least 11 mm wide to enable the hamster's blunt nose to reach the feed with minimal trauma.

Nutrition

Hamsters are omnivorous and hoard feed by nature. Adult hamsters of both sexes consume between 5.5 and 7 g of feed per day. They frequently remove feed from feeders and relocate it to the corner of the cage opposite the one used for defaecation and urination. If hamsters are fed fresh feed, hoarded food should be removed several times a week to prevent spoilage. They are coprophagic; ingestion of faecal material containing nutrients produced by intestinal microflora reduces the demands for particular essential nutrients. Consequently, the potential for toxicity from the ingestion of pharmaceuticals or metabolites which are excreted in the faeces should be recognised.

There is less known about nutritional requirements for hamsters than for rats and mice. The

SPACE RECOMMENDATIONS—HAMSTERS		
	Minimum floor area/animal (cm)	Height (cm)
< 60 g b.w.	64.52	15.24
60–80 g b.w.	83.88	15.24
80–100 g b.w.	103.23	15.24
> 100 g b.w.	122.59	15.24
Nursing female with litter		
Syrian	780.45	15.24
Chinese	161.25	15.24
Data taken from US Department of Health and Human Services (1985) and CFR (1993).		

FIG. 3.2 Space recommendations—hamsters.

hamster forestomach is ultrastructurally and physiologically similar to a ruminant's, providing the hamster with fermentative capabilities which affect nutrient utilisation. The pelleted diet used for rats and mice is satisfactory for hamsters and is preferred over mixed seed diets available through pet stores in which the animal may select favourite components and not receive a balanced diet. However, the protein content of rodent diets is generally greater than 20% which exceeds the 13.7–16.7% dietary protein shown to be most beneficial for hamsters (Arrington *et al.*, 1979). Supplementation of pelleted rodent diet with 25% pelleted rabbit chow will provide more fibre and reduce the proportion of dietary protein consumed. Fresh feed should be supplied weekly. Pelleted commercial diet should be stored in a cool and dry place and should be consumed within 6 months of production. The provision of commercially available treats, fresh fruits and vegetables should be done sparingly as it may preclude the animal from receiving a balanced diet. If provided, fruits and vegetables should be thoroughly washed to remove potential microbiological and chemical contaminants. Water should be provided *ad libitum*. A hamster's daily water consumption is 10 ml/100 g body weight. Although the hamster has been used experimentally to induce a variety of nutritional diseases caused by both deficiency and excess, spontaneous nutritional diseases are not well characterised. Nutritional diseases would be expected to resemble those observed in other species. Specific nutritional diseases are described later in the chapter.

Handling, Injection, Specimen Collection

Handling

As discussed previously, hamsters are considered by some to be difficult to handle. Males are generally more docile than females. If simple precautions are taken however, hamsters can be routinely handled with minimal stress to the animal and handler. Awakening the animal from sleep will frequently be met with an aggressive response. They can be removed from their cage or transferred between sites with the use of a small can or cup which they will usually enter; they can be scooped out with cupped hands; or they can be lifted by gently grasping the loose skin over the dorsal cervical region (Fig. 3.3). There are several handling techniques that can be utilised for restraining the hamster. It can be grasped around the head and abdomen with the thumb directed toward the hind quarters or, once placed on a flat surface, the palm of the hand may be placed down over the hamster with the thumb near the head and the excess skin grasped and bunched into the hand until the body wall is reached. The animal will be immobile and will not be able to turn its head to bite.

Injection

Subcutaneous (SC) injections are administered as in other species. Injections can be given in the

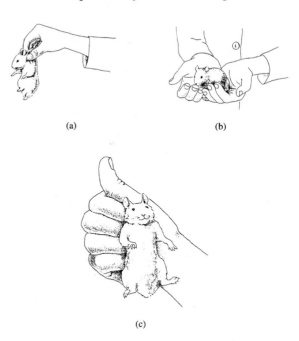

(a)   (b)

(c)

FIG. 3.3 Techniques for moving or restraining hamsters. Hamsters may be moved by gripping the excess skin in the interscapular region (a) or may be cupped in the palm of the hand (b). Hamsters can be restrained by gripping the excess skin over the dorsum into the hand until the body wall is reached (c). Reprinted with permission from the *Training Manual Series Volume 1*, American Association for Laboratory Animal Science.

interscapular and inguinal regions. The SC space in the hamster is copious because of the excess amount of loose skin.

Intramuscular (IM) injections can be administered into the quadriceps or the hamstring muscles caudal to the femur. If the hamstrings are used, the needle should be directed caudally away from the sciatic nerve. Careful consideration should be given to the volume, concentration and material administered as the muscle mass is small and necrosis may result. We recommend that no more than 0.25 ml be given IM.

Intraperitoneal (IP) injections are frequently administered in hamsters. The animal should be firmly restrained with its head tilted downward to the floor. Injection should be made to either side of the midline in the inguinal region, caudal to the umbilicus, to avoid the large caecum. The needle should be inserted approximately 5 mm toward the head at an angle of 45° with respect to the body wall. The plunger should be withdrawn to determine if an abdominal viscus has been penetrated. Warmed replacement fluids are frequently administered IP or SC.

Intravenous (IV) injections are extremely difficult in the hamster because of the lack of easily accessible veins. The lateral vein of the tarsus, the anterior cephalic vein and the lingual vein have been utilised. The fur overlying the areas, if present, should be clipped and a tourniquet applied above the stifle or elbow to dilate the veins. Needles recommended for use are 27–30 gauge. Fluid volumes up to 2.0 ml have been administered over a 1 min interval; extreme caution should be taken when administering large volumes. When IV administration is necessary but not possible in critical patients, fluids and parenteral therapeutics can be administered by intraosseous injection. A 22 gauge spinal needle with a quincke type point is inserted into the tibial crest. General or local anaesthesia may be required for placement.

Drugs can be administered directly into the stomach using an 18 gauge, 4.0 to 4.5 cm ball-tipped feeding needle. With the animal firmly restrained, the needle is advanced into the mouth over the tongue until it is swallowed. Passage should meet little resistance. The needle should be advanced to the last rib. Oral administration of liquids can also be performed with an eye dropper. Extreme care should be taken because hamsters can bite through glass or plastic.

Specimen Collection

Urine and faeces can frequently be collected from the perineal region following restraint. Metabolic cages designed specifically for excrement collection are commercially available.

Blood collection is relatively difficult in the hamster. Small volumes of blood can be collected from the veins described above. One method is to use a needle without an attached syringe, followed by collection of blood from the needle's hub with a microhaematocrit tube. Toe nail clip or puncture of a foot pad or pinna can be used to collect very small quantities. Larger volumes can be collected from the orbital venous sinus in anaesthetised animals. A schematic representation of the sinus is presented in Fig. 3.4. The sinus is located within the orbit and surrounds the globe. The hamster is anaesthetised and the tip of a microhaematocrit tube is inserted through the conjunctiva at the lateral canthus and directed medially into the sinus (Timm, 1989; Silverman, 1987). Pressure is needed to penetrate the tissues surrounding the sinus. Gentle pressure applied over the ipsilateral jugular vein inhibits blood flow from the

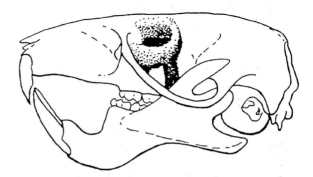

FIG. 3.4 Schematic representation of the orbital venous sinus from the hamster. The sinus depicted by the shaded area is located within the orbit and surrounds the globe. Reprinted with permission from *Laboratory Animal Science* (1989) **39**, 262–264.

sinus and causes its engorgement. Blood can be collected by holding the animal over a collection vessel as the blood flows from the tube. Following collection, the haematocrit tube is removed and pressure is applied over the eye with gauze to ensure adequate haemostasis. Retrobulbar haemorrhage and exophthalmus are potential complications. The circulating blood volume of the hamster is 78 ml/kg; up to 10% of this volume can be withdrawn at a single time from a healthy adult hamster with minimal adverse effect (Morton *et al.*, 1993).

Techniques and agents used for anaesthesia are described in *Chapter 7*. Methods for euthanasing hamsters are similar to those used with other small laboratory rodents. Commonly used techniques include carbon dioxide asphyxiation or overdose with a volatile or injectable anaesthetic. Volatile anaesthetics can be used by placing the anaesthetic liquid on a pledget of cotton or gauze pad and placing the anaesthetic with the animal in a closed jar. Care should be taken to avoid having direct contact between the anaesthetic and the animal. An overdose of pentobarbital sodium (120 mg/kg) can be administered IP.

Diseases

An overview of the diseases discussed below can be found in Fig. 3.6 at the end of the chapter.

Diseases of the Respiratory System

The hamster is not unique with respect to the clinical conditions and diseases that affect the respiratory system. However, they appear to be more resistant to infectious respiratory disease than other rodents. Treatment for infections, notably bacterial pneumonias, must be considered carefully as *Clostridium difficile* enterotoxaemia is a relatively common and almost always fatal complication of antibiotic administration.

Bacterial Diseases

Bacterial respiratory infections, including pneumonia and otitis, are reported to be the second most common disease after gastrointestinal disorders in hamsters, however they are still uncommon.

Agents. Both Gram-negative and Gram-positive organisms, including *Pasteurella pneumotropica*, other *Pasteurella* sp., *Streptococcus pneumoniae*, *Streptococcus agalactiae*, *Staphylococcus aureus*, *Klebsiella pneumoniae*, *Bordetella* sp. and *Salmonella* sp., have been isolated from affected animals.

Hosts. Most of these organisms reside as normal flora in the respiratory and gastrointestinal tracts of a variety of rodent and non-rodent species and can cause opportunistic infections.

Clinical signs. A variety of stresses, such as poor nutrition, inadequate environmental control and husbandry failures leads to a weakening of host defences and disease. Clinical signs are similar to those observed in other small laboratory animals and may include rough hair coat, head tilt, nasal discharge, chattering, huddling, inactivity, tachypnoea and dyspnoea.

Control / treatment. Antimicrobial treatment should be selected based upon the sensitivity of the organism and should be balanced against the potential pitfalls. Chloramphenicol, trimethoprim−sulphamethoxazole or enrofloxacin may be beneficial in bacterial pneumonias of undetermined aetiology.

Viral Diseases

Hamsters are susceptible to infection by a number of viruses which have a predilection for respiratory epithelium. Although serological evidence of exposure has been detected, spontaneous clinical disease of viral aetiology is extremely rare. Hamsters have been found with circulating antibodies to Sendai virus, Pneumonia Virus of Mice (PVM) and Simian Virus 5

(SV5). Of these, Sendai virus is the only agent of potential concern.

Sendai virus

Agents. Sendai virus, a paramyxovirus, is extremely contagious and is transmitted by the aerosol route.

Hosts. Sendai virus infects a number of rodent species, notably mice and rats, which may develop clinical or inapparent disease and are likely sources of infection for hamsters. Serological evidence of infection has been demonstrated in guinea pigs, but its significance remains unknown.

Clinical signs. Although Sendai virus infects respiratory epithelium, tissue destruction is mediated by the host's immune response and clinical disease is likely due to secondary bacterial infection. Nasal exudate, roughened hair coat, dyspnoea and tachypnoea may occur.

Diagnosis. Exposure to Sendai virus can be demonstrated by serological monitoring. The ELISA and IFA tests are commercially available. However, titres will not reflect active infection.

Control / treatments. Control can be achieved by restricting contact with infected rodents. Treatment is limited to supportive care e.g. subcutaneous fluids, nutritional support and antimicrobial therapy for secondary bacterial infections.

Neoplastic Diseases

Neoplasia of the respiratory tract is uncommon in the hamster. When it occurs, benign tumours (nasal polyps) of the nasal cavity and proximal trachea are more common. There are no reports of polyp removal or the likelihood of their reoccurrence.

Diseases of the Cardiovascular System

Non-Infectious Diseases

Atrial thrombosis

Atrial thrombosis is common in Syrian hamsters with incidence increasing with age. Females tend to develop the condition earlier than males. Early myxomatous and fibrotic valvular changes and myocardial degeneration are associated with the development of thrombosis, frequently in the left atrium. Clinical signs include hyperpnoea, tachycardia and cyanosis. No specific treatments have been described.

Calcifying vasculopathy

Mineralisation of the elastic layers of the aorta, coronary, renal and gastric arteries is a common and progressive condition of hamsters. In severe cases, calcification may also involve the basal laminae of respiratory epithelium and the connective tissues of various organs. In late stages, the disease may be associated with hyperplasia or adenomas of the parathyroid gland. The exact aetiology of the disease has not been determined but there is evidence to support hereditary and dietary causes (Pour and Birt, 1979).

Cardiomyopathy

An inbred strain of albino hamsters (BIO 14.6) develops a spontaneous cardiomyopathy, however, the incidence in the pet population has not been well established.

Diseases of the Gastrointestinal System

Gastrointestinal (GI) disease is clearly the most significant contributor to morbidity and mortality in hamsters, especially in weanlings. 'Wet tail' is the term that has been applied to hamsters with enteric disease, as the perineum is frequently contaminated with diarrhoea. 'Wet tail' is not a single entity or disease, rather, it is a clinical feature associated with a variety of syndromes, only a few of which have been defined aetiopathologically. Most of the diseases below have similar clinical presentations, making diagnosis difficult, especially in clinical practice. As in other species, provision of an adequate diet is essential in preventing GI disease.

Bacterial Diseases

Proliferative ileitis

Proliferative ileitis (PI) is the most commonly recognised and significant disease of hamsters. The syndrome has also been referred to as regional enteritis, terminal ileitis, enzootic intestinal adenocarcinoma, atypical ileal hyperplasia and hamster enteritis.

Agent. The definitive aetiologic agent has not been identified, although a bacterium is likely. The role of other agents or cofactors has also been postulated. A considerable number of bacterial species including *Campylobacter jejuni*, *Escherichia coli* and *Chlamydia trachomatis* strain SFPD have been implicated in the syndrome (Fox *et al.*, 1993). A *Desulfovibrio* sp. may finally prove to be the definitive aetiology as the organism has been identified using 16S rRNA sequence analysis (Fox *et al.*, 1994).

Hosts. The syndrome generally affects weanling hamsters 3–8 weeks of age, although PI has been observed infrequently in adults. Although the affected anatomical sites differ, the proliferative bowel diseases of swine, rabbits and ferrets are similar to PI in the hamster and are likely to be also caused by the *Desulfovibrio* sp.

Clinical signs. Early disease is characterised by lethargy, anorexia, irritability, ruffled hair coat and weight loss. Later, a foetid watery diarrhoea occurs, causing matted fur, dehydration, inactivity and abdominal pain (hunched posture). Rectal prolapse and intussusceptions are relatively common and are often accompanied by haematochezia. Thickened bowel segments may be palpated. Mortality is high and may occur within 24–48 h after the appearance of clinical signs.

Diagnosis. Diagnosis is based upon patient profile, the ability to palpate thickened bowel and clinical signs. The disease is characterised by segmental proliferative ileitis. The distal 4–8 cm of ileum and occasionally the caecum and proximal colon are affected (Fig. 3.5). Involved areas are turgid, thickened, oedematous and may be friable; peritoneal adhesions are frequently present. Subserosal nodules may be observed on the ileum. Peyer's patches and mesenteric lymph nodes are enlarged, oedematous and hyperaemic. Chronic lesions are characterised by a circumferential fibrotic scar which may cause partial or complete obstruction.

Microscopic findings depend on the stage of disease. Proliferative lesions are characterised by marked mucosal hyperplasia. Villus necrosis and leucocytic infiltration of the lamina propria are common. There is a distinct demarcation between affected and normal ileum. In chronic cases, marked hypertrophy of muscle layers develop and diverticula of mucosa can be found in the submucosa and subserosa. A slightly curved bacillus, referred to as an intracellular campylobacter-like organism (ICLO) because of its physical resemblance to bacteria of the genus *Campylobacter*, can be demonstrated in Warthin–Starry stains of affected mucosa. The organism is probably the *Desulfovibrio* sp.

Control / treatment. The prognosis is guarded at best. Several antibiotic regimens have been

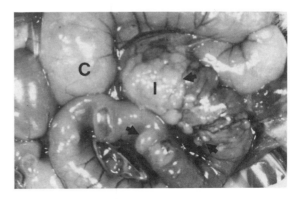

FIG. 3.5 Distal ileum (I) and caecum (C) from a hamster with proliferative ileitis. The ileum is turgid and thickened with numerous subserosal nodules (arrowed).

reported which reduce mortality in affected colonies. Antibiotic administration should be accompanied by supportive therapy. Based upon success in the ferret with proliferative colitis, chloramphenicol palmitate (PO) would be the treatment of choice (Krueger *et al.*, 1989). Tetracycline and neomycin, both of which can be administered in the drinking water, have been reported to be successful in hamsters.

Antibiotic-associated colitis

Antibiotic-associated colitis (AAC) or clostridial enterotoxaemia is a major cause of morbidity and mortality in hamsters; it presents a significant challenge to the clinician whose armentarium to fight bacterial disease is markedly reduced.

Agent. The aetiology and pathogenesis of the disease has been clearly elucidated. Following treatment with antibiotics, *Clostridium difficile*, an anaerobic, Gram-positive, spore-forming bacterium, colonises the intestinal tract and produces a cytotoxin and enterotoxin. Colonisation occurs as a result of antibiotic-induced suppression of competitive micro-organisms.

Hosts. Although a small percentage of hamsters carry *C. difficile* as part of the normal GI flora, most hamsters are infected from environmental sources including feed and water. As has been observed with resistance to *Clostridium botulinum* toxin in young children, young hamsters appear to be resistant to the effects of the toxins. A long list of antibiotics has been implicated in the disease, including ampicillin, carbenicillin, a variety of first and second generation cephalosporins, chlortetracycline, clindamycin, gentamicin, lincomycin, penicillin and tetracycline (Small, 1987). Even antibiotics routinely recommended for use in hamsters can potentially induce the syndrome. Other stressors such as surgery and dietary or housing change have been implicated in initiating disease.

Clinical signs. Clinical signs include anorexia, ruffled fur, dehydration, depression, diarrhoea and death. The prognosis is grave and death may occur suddenly. Disease generally develops 4–10 days following administration of the offending pharmaceutical agent.

Diagnosis. Definitive diagnosis of AAC is based upon detection of the cytotoxin in caecal contents or faeces. However, a history of antibiotic administration and subsequent development of clinical signs and characteristic pathological changes are strongly suggestive of AAC. The syndrome is characterised pathologically by a haemorrhagic ileocaecal colitis. The caecum and often the distal ileum and proximal colon are dilated with fluid and gas and the serosa is congested or haemorrhagic. Microscopically, severe congestion of the villous and submucosal capillaries and venules are observed. An inflammatory infiltrate is often present in the lamina propria and while the mucosal surface frequently remains intact, the cells on the tips of the villi may be necrotic and the villi are often distended with an exudate. *C. difficile* cytotoxin can be detected by placing sterilised caecal contents or faeces onto a variety of cell lines and observing for cytopathic effect (CPE). Neutralisation of CPE by a specific antitoxin is confirmatory. Caecal or faecal samples can be sent to many commercial laboratories who routinely perform the assay from material of human origin.

Control / treatment. Treatment should include aggressive fluid administration and supportive care. Humans develop a similar syndrome associated with *C. difficile* and can be treated with vancomycin (to which the bacterium is sensitive), however, hamsters will generally die unless the antibiotics are administered indefinitely since the normal microflora which suppresses *C. difficile* growth is not re-established during vancomycin administration (Boss *et al.*, 1994). Transfaunation (PO) with a faecal slurry from healthy hamsters may be helpful. Cholestyramine resin which has been used successfully to treat AAC in the rabbit is not effective in the hamster (Lipman *et al.*, 1992).

Tyzzer's disease

Agent. Tyzzer's disease, caused by *Clostridium piliforme*, has been infrequently reported in hamsters. The aetiological agent is a Gram-negative, sporeforming bacterium which cannot be grown on artificial media, making routine isolation extremely difficult. The organism forms spores which are transmitted by the faecal–oral route. Spores are resistant to adverse environmental conditions making environmental control difficult.

Hosts. Disease has been observed in a variety of species in addition to hamsters, including mice, rats, gerbils, guinea pigs, cats and dogs.

Clinical signs. The disease in hamsters is characterised by high morbidity and mortality. Pale yellow diarrhoea, ruffled hair coat, lethargy, anorexia and dehydration are observed. Animals may die within 24–48 h after onset, or suddenly without premonitory signs.

Diagnosis. Diagnosis is usually made at necropsy. The caecum and colon are filled with yellow foamy fluid and the serosa is hyperaemic. Hepatomegaly with multifocal small (1–2 mm) yellow white foci are observed. Multiple, small (2–5 mm) white nodules may be observed bulging from the epicardial surface of the heart. Microscopically, catarrhal inflammation with focal mucosal erosions are observed in the affected areas of the gastrointestinal tract; multifocal hepatic and myocardial necrosis may also be observed. Organisms are demonstrated using Warthin–Starry stain in cells adjacent to erosions and necrotic foci.

Control / treatment. Successful treatment has not been reported; tetracycline could be used in the face of a colony outbreak. Fresh fruits and vegetables should be avoided as they may be contaminated with spores from wild rodents. If

these items are provided they should be thoroughly washed. Leafy vegetables should be avoided as their veins may contain contaminated fluid.

Salmonellosis

Agent. Salmonellosis is only rarely observed in hamsters, due to improved husbandry and sanitation practices. Both *S. enteritidis* and *S. typhimurium* have been isolated from hamsters.

Host. *Salmonella* is transmitted by the faecal–oral route primarily via contaminated feed and bedding, although numerous species, including humans, are potential reservoirs.

Clinical signs. Clinical signs resemble those seen with other enteric diseases and include lethargy, anorexia, rough hair coat, dyspnoea, conjunctivitis and weight loss. Faeces may be normal or soft. Pathological findings include catarrhal enteritis, septic pulmonary thrombophlebitis and hepatosplenomegaly. Numerous small white foci may be observed in the liver and spleen. Bacterial septicaemia or toxaemia is thought to damage the venous intima, inciting thrombus formation.

Diagnosis. Diagnosis is based on isolation and identification of the organism from the faeces or blood.

Control / treatment. Treatment has not been reported, but if attempted should be based on microbial sensitivity. Fresh fruits and vegetables, if provided, should be thoroughly washed in order to minimise the risk of infection. Salmonellosis is zoonotic and an asymptomatic carrier state may result following treatment.

Other Bacterial Gastrointestinal Diseases

A variety of other bacteria has been implicated in hamster gastrointestinal disease. However, the frequency of their isolation and their role in disease may be disparate. The intestinal flora of healthy hamsters consists principally of Gram-positive organisms. The isolation of *Escherichia coli* from diarrhoea should raise suspicions. Enteroinvasive *E. coli* was isolated from a hamster with PI-induced acute enteritis in experimentally inoculated weanlings (Frisk *et al.*, 1981). Treatment should consist of supportive and antimicrobial therapy.

Campylobacter jejuni has been isolated from hamsters with PI, however experimental infection rarely causes disease. The hamster must be considered a potential reservoir of campylobacteriosis for humans and other species for which *C. jejuni* is an enteric pathogen. Erythromycin is the drug of choice in humans; its therapeutic effectiveness has not been evaluated in hamsters.

Although clinical disease has not been observed, hamsters have been shown to be a natural reservoir of *Campylobacter cinaedi*, which has been associated with disease in immunosuppressed persons (Gebhart *et al.*, 1989).

There have been several reports of caecal hyperplasia associated with clinical disease in hamsters. Caecal hyperplasia has been observed in adult hamsters which died of clostridial enterotoxaemia that was not associated with antibiotic administration. The authors were not able to determine the cause of the caecal pathology but postulated that *Clostridium difficile* colonisation occurred as a result of the alteration of the caecal microflora which resulted from cytoarchitectural changes (Ryden *et al.*, 1991). Caecal hyperplasia has also been associated with high mortality in sucklings and weanlings (Barthold *et al.*, 1978). The aetiology was not determined.

Viral Diseases

Surprisingly, no viral aetiology has yet been incriminated in hamster diarrhoeic disease. As rotaviruses and coronaviruses have been identified in most mammalian species it is probably only a matter of time until a virus is associated with GI disease in the hamster. Toolan H-1, a parvovirus of rats, has been associated with an epizootic of high mortality with malformed and missing incisors in weanling and suckling hamster pups (Gibson *et al.*, 1983).

Parasitic Diseases

There are a variety of protozoal and helminth parasites of clinical importance in hamster enteric disease. Protozoans are abundant in the hamster. Most protozoans are commensals or at best opportunists. As protozoans prefer a liquid environment, it is not surprising to find an increase in their numbers in cases of diarrhoea.

Giardiasis

Agent. *Giardia muris*, whose life cycle is similar to other *Giardia* spp., resides in the anterior small intestine of the hamster.

Host. There are a number of *Giardia* spp. which infect a variety of mammals including man. It remains unclear whether animal-to-animal or animal-to-human transmission occurs with all *Giardia* spp., but evidence suggests these possibilities exist.

Clinical signs. Although infections usually do not cause clinically significant enteritis, they have been observed to cause a catarrhal enteritis in weanlings.

Diagnosis. Diagnosis is made by detection of cysts or trophozoites in the faeces.

Control / treatment. Treatment can be attempted with the administration of metronidazole.

Other Protozoa

The role of *Spironucleus muris* and *Balantidium coli* in 'wet tail' are not clear. Treatment with metronidazole may be considered in cases where a definitive aetiology is lacking.

Pinworms

Agent. Pinworms are the major nematode of significance in hamsters. While a variety of species have been identified including *Syphacia muris*, *S. mesocriceti* and *Aspicularis tetraptera*, *S.*

obvelata is most commonly found. The life cycle is direct. Following ingestion of ova, the larvae hatch and migrate to the caecum or colon where they reach sexual maturity. Fertilised females migrate to the anus and oviposit adhesive-coated eggs on the perineum (*Syphacia* spp.) or reside in the large bowel and release ova into the faeces (*Aspicularis* sp.). Prepatent periods have not been determined for the hamster but in other rodents range from 11 to 23 days, depending on the particular pinworm species.

Hosts. As pinworms frequently infect mice and rats, they are a likely source of infection for hamsters.

Clinical signs. Clinical signs have not been reported in the hamster but would be expected to resemble those observed with pinworm parasitism in other rodents. Infection is usually of no clinical significance unless accompanied by a heavy parasite burden.

Diagnosis. Ova are detected by sticking a piece of clear cellophane tape to the perineum, removing it and adhering it to a microscope slide to observe banana-shaped ova (*Syphacia* sp.) or by performing a faecal flotation and detecting strongyle-like eggs (*Aspicularis* sp.).

Control / treatment. Piperazine citrate (10 mg/ml in the drinking water) administered for two 7-day courses separated by a 5 day interim has been shown to be effective in eradicating *S. obvelata* in hamsters (Unay and Davies, 1980). Although not reported for the hamster, a regime of 2 doses of ivermectin (200 μg/kg SC) administered 11 days apart has been used to treat pinworms in mice (Flynn *et al.*, 1989).

Hymenolepis nana

Agent. Infections with the cestode *H. nana*, the dwarf tapeworm, can be a significant clinical and public health problem in hamsters. *H. nana* can have both a direct and indirect life cycle. Autoinfection can result in large worm burdens.

The worms, which are 25–40 mm long, reside in the small intestine.

Hosts. The host range is broad and includes a variety of rodent species and man.

Clinical signs. Infection may be inapparent or can lead to unthriftiness, intestinal occlusion, or impaction. Catarrhal enteritis and abscessation of mesenteric lymph nodes have been observed.

Diagnosis. Diagnosis is made by identification of ova in faeces. The oval egg (37–47 × 50–55 μm) contains an oncosphere enclosed in an inner envelope which has two polar thickenings with 4–8 filaments attached to each. The oncosphere contains three pairs of hooklets (Wagner, 1987). *H. nana* must be differentiated from *H. diminuta*, which may also be detected in hamsters but is not of public health significance because it has an indirect life cycle. The spherical ova of *H. diminuta* are twice as large as those of *H. nana* and they do not have filaments. The adults of *H. diminuta* (60 × 2–3 cm) are also considerably larger than *H. nana* and the scolex is unarmed.

Control / treatment. One method of treatment is the use of niclosamide fed at 1 mg/g of feed (100 mg/kg body weight) for two 7-day periods with a 1-week interim (Hughes *et al.*, 1973). The use of praziquantel has also been suggested (no dose provided) (Wagner, 1987). Infected hamsters should be handled with extreme care to prevent potential zoonotic transmission.

Neoplastic Diseases

Neoplasia of the gastrointestinal system is relatively uncommon in the hamster. Tumours do not differ from those observed in other species.

Non-Infectious Diseases

Constipation in preweanling hamsters is frequently observed when fluids are not provided in addition to the dam's milk. If water bottles are not available to young hamsters, thoroughly washed succulent fruits and vegetables should be supplied.

Cheek pouch impactions have been described following overstuffing and desiccation of material placed into the pouch (Holmes, 1984). Large persistent swellings are noted on one or both sides of the face. The pouches should be carefully emptied with forceps and flushed with a syringe and water. The cheek pouches can be everted for examination under anaesthesia. Abrasions can be treated with topical antibiotic ointment.

Anorexia, weight loss and ptyalism may result from an overgrowth of incisor teeth resulting from malocclusion. Overgrown teeth can be trimmed with guillotine-type nail clippers, bone cutters, or a rotary cutting tool. If malocclusion is present, teeth will require regular trimming for the animal's lifespan.

Diseases of the Genitourinary System

Neoplastic Disease

The incidence of neoplasia of the female hamster's reproductive tract varies from colony to colony. Granulosa cell tumours and thecomas have been reported to occur frequently. These tumours generally occur unilaterally. Endometrial adenocarcinomas are reported commonly in Chinese hamsters (Strandberg, 1987). They typically occur in animals older than 100 weeks of age. Uterine polyps, leiomyomas, leiomyosarcomas, cervical carcinomas and squamous papillomas of the vagina have all been reported to occur in the hamster. Tumours of the reproductive tract of males have been infrequently reported. Renal and bladder tumours are rare.

Non-Infectious Diseases

Arteriolar nephrosclerosis

Arteriolar nephrosclerosis or hamster nephrosis is an important ageing lesion which can cause significant morbidity and mortality. The syndrome resembles nephrosis in the aged rat. The aetiopathogenesis has not been clearly elucidated but appears to be related to the level of dietary protein. Affected animals develop uraemia, proteinuria and polyuria. The disease frequently progresses to endstage renal failure. Treatment has not been reported in the hamster, but would be similar to treatment of chronic renal disease in other species. At post-mortem examination, the kidneys are pale tan with an irregular surface. Histologically, there is extensive interstitial inflammation and fibrosis and glomerulosclerosis. Proteinaceous casts are found in dilated tubules. Amyloid deposition frequently occurs concurrently.

Squamous metaplasia of the vagina and periarteritis of ovarian, uterine and broad ligaments is commonly reported in females. The clinical relevance of these lesions is minimal.

Diseases of the Nervous System

Non-Infectious Diseases

Vitamin E deficiency

Vitamin E deficiency in pregnant dams has been associated with haemorrhagic necrosis of the central nervous system of foetal hamsters and should be a consideration in evaluating foetal losses in hamsters (Keeler and Young, 1979).

Diseases of Sensory Organs

Non-Infectious Diseases

Ophthalmic disorders

Spontaneously occurring ocular disorders are rare in the hamster. Keratoconjunctivitis may occur with trauma or unsanitary bedding conditions. Tooth root abscesses may result in facial swelling or exophthalmus. The prognosis is poor due to the need for antibiotic therapy and the consequent risk of antibiotic-associated enteritis (Kern, 1989). Chinese hamsters may develop diabetes-related ophthalmic disorders such as cataracts and glaucoma.

Diseases of the Integument and Musculoskeletal System

Bacterial Diseases

Bacterial organisms associated with disease of the hamster's skin are the same as those isolated from other domestic species e.g. *S. aureus* and *Streptococcus* sp.

Actinomycosis

Agent. *Actinomyces bovis* is a Gram-positive, filamentous agent that causes 'lumpy jaw' in cattle. Although rarely reported, salivary gland abscesses in the hamster may be caused by this organism.

Hosts. Besides cattle and hamsters, this agent can cause disease in dogs, elks, horses and humans.

Clinical signs. Actinomycosis in the hamster typically causes enlarged salivary glands containing purulent fluid. Histologically there is liquefactive necrosis, often with sulphur granules (clumps of bacteria) similar to that seen in 'lumpy jaw' in cattle.

Diagnosis. Diagnosis is based on demonstration of the organism in anaerobic culture. The presence of sulphur granules is strongly suggestive of actinomycosis, but they are not always seen.

Control / treatment. Treatment consists of lancing and draining the abscess and debriding all affected tissue. Long-term antibiotic therapy, based on antimicrobial sensitivity, is necessary for effective treatment of this anaerobic organism and may lead to the development of AAC in the hamster. Penicillin, erythromycin and cephaloridine, which are frequently effective in other species for the treatment of actinomycosis, have all been associated with AAC in the hamster.

Cutaneous bacterial abscesses

Agents. Cutaneous bacterial abscesses may be caused by a number of organisms, including *S. aureus, Streptococcus* sp., *A. bovis* and *P. pneumotropica*. *S. aureus* is the most frequently isolated and has also been associated with ulcerative dermatitis.

Hosts. These bacteria are frequently part of the hamster's enteric flora and are ubiquitous environmental agents.

Clinical signs. The most common location for cutaneous abscesses in the hamster is the head, sometimes involving the cheek pouches. The development of cervical lymphadenitis may be associated with chronic cutaneous lesions; these animals are usually severely debilitated.

Diagnosis. Aerobic and anaerobic bacterial cultures provide the definitive aetiological diagnosis.

Control / treatment. Abscesses should be lanced and debrided and appropriate antibiotic therapy should be instituted. Treatments with enrofloxacin or ciprofloxacin have been reported to be effective for staphylococcal pyodermas (Harkness, 1994). These lesions are frequently associated with fighting or substandard caging. Caging should be examined for sharp edges or protruding wires. If wounds are due to fighting, hamsters should be separated.

The flank glands, especially in males, may become inflamed. Inflammation is best treated by clipping and cleaning the area and applying topical antibiotic with corticosteroid. Male hamsters with inflamed flank glands may be candidates for castration (Burke, 1992). Castration may reduce the secretory activity of the flank glands and may be considered as a potential treatment for affected males.

Streptococcal mastitis

Agent. Beta-haemolytic *Streptococcus* spp. have been associated with acute bacterial mastitis in hamsters.

Hosts. Beta-haemolytic *Streptococcus* spp. reside as normal flora in the gastrointestinal tract and are ubiquitous in the environment.

Clinical signs. The onset of mastitis occurs approximately 7–10 days following parturition. The involved glands are firm with a haemorrhagic exudate. Affected females may cannibalise their litters. The incidence of reoccurrence is not established.

Diagnosis. Culture of the agent from affected glands.

Control / treatment. Antimicrobial therapy is based on culture and sensitivity.

Fungal Diseases

Dermatophytosis / ringworm

Agents. Ringworm in hamsters occurs as in other domestic species and is frequently caused by *Trichophyton mentagrophytes* or *Microsporum* sp.

Hosts. Both agents have a wide host range that includes, man, cats, dogs, chinchillas, guinea pigs, rabbits, mice and rats.

Clinical signs. Infection may be asymptomatic. Dry scaly circular lesions or encrustations with broken hair may be observed.

Diagnosis. Diagnosis is made by culture and examination of hair shafts cleared with 10% potassium hydroxide. Examination of affected areas with a Wood's (ultraviolet) lamp may reveal the presence of *Microsporum canis*.

Control / treatment. Treatments include topical fungicides, clipping hair from affected areas and treating with povidone–iodine scrubs, or systemic griseofulvin at dosages indicated for the cat (Burke, 1992).

Viral Diseases

Epithelioma

Agent. Hamster papovavirus (HapV) is related to other papovaviruses (Shope papilloma, polyoma and SV40).

Hosts. The hamster is the only known host for this virus.

Clinical signs. The virus causes epitheliomas in hamsters 3 months to 1 year of age. The incidence of epitheliomas has been reported to be 5% in a research colony of hamsters, however the incidence in the pet population is unknown.

Diagnosis. Keratinised neoplasms arising from hair follicles in hamsters 3 months to 1 year of age are suggestive of this viral agent.

Control / treatment. There is no information to support the progression of epitheliomas to squamous cell carcinoma or spontaneous resolution as has been demonstrated in papovaviral-induced neoplasms in other species.

Parasitic Diseases

Demodicosis

Agents. *Demodex criceti* may be distinguished from *D. aurati* by its shorter rounder appearance (87–103 μm in length) compared to the thinner and longer *D. aurati* (183–192 μm in length). *D. criceti* feeds on surface epithelium while *D. aurati* is present in hair follicles (Wagner, 1987). Both agents are common inhabitants of hamster skin.

Hosts. *D. criceti* and *D. aurati* have been reported in hamsters only.

Clinical signs. Clinical signs of demodicosis, as in other species, are associated with ageing, intercurrent infection, stress, or immune suppression. The *D. aurati* burden is thought to be heavier in males than in females. Skin lesions associated with demodicosis include alopecia over the dorsum, predominantly the rump, with dry scaly skin. These lesions are generally not pruritic.

Diagnosis. For demodicosis, diagnosis is readily made with skin scrapings or plucking hair from alopecic areas and examining for mites. For light infestations, diagnosis by digestion of hair in 10% KOH or NaOH may be necessary; males are preferred for sample collection. The maximum numbers of mites are usually present over the dorsum. It is important to rule out bacterial infections, other parasites, trauma and dermatophytes in establishing a primary diagnosis of demodicosis, as the parasites are frequently found in hamsters without clinical signs of disease.

Control / treatment. Control of demodicosis is achieved by minimising stress, maintaining high levels of sanitation, avoiding exposure of overtly infected animals to asymptomatic animals and treating those affected. Presumably treatments used for demodicosis in other animals, such as amitraz, would be appropriate for the hamster (Burke, 1992). Toxicity in hamsters has not been determined and caution should be exercised when administering this agent to hamsters.

Other Mites

Agent. *Notoedres notoedres* (hamster ear mite), *N. cati* (cat mange mite) and *Ornithonyssus bacoti* (the tropical rat mite) occur in the hamster.

Host. *N. notoedres*, the hamster ear mite, is not known to affect other species (Flynn, 1973). *N. cati* demonstrates less host specificity than some mites and will affect cats, rabbits and hamsters. *O. bacoti* has a wide host range which includes wild rodents and small mammals. The tropical rat mite will bite humans.

Clinical signs. Exudative crusting lesions associated with *N. notoedres* and *N. cati* are found on the ears, snout, extremities, anus and genitalia. *O. bacoti* mites do not reside on the host for extended periods and bites may be the only skin lesion observed. However, if infection is heavy, anaemia may occur.

Control / treatment. *Notoedres* sp. infestations are treated with ivermectin at doses of 300–400 μg/kg SC, repeated every 2 to 3 weeks until the mites are eliminated (Burke, 1992). As *O. bacoti* spends a great deal of time off the host, infestation can be controlled by frequent cage and bedding changes. Spraying bedding with 5 ml of a 1% suspension of malathion at 2–4 week intervals has been reported to be effective (Wagner, 1990).

Neoplastic Diseases

Tumours of the integument and musculoskeletal systems are uncommon. Melanomas appear to be the most frequently reported skin tumour but benign tumours of the hair follicles and sebaceous glands, keratoacanthomas, squamous papillomas and carcinomas and basal cell tumourshave also been reported. Adenomas of the Harderian glands occur. Lymphosarcomas of the skin may appear as ill-defined draining lesions in older hamsters (Burke, 1992).

Non-Infectious Diseases

Osteoarthritis

Osteoarthritis of the femoro-tibial articulation is frequently observed in older hamsters, usually animals greater than 2 years of age.

Cage paralysis

Cage paralysis is a nutritional myopathy that may develop with diets deficient in Vitamin E or D. Hamsters fed primarily table scraps are more likely to develop this disorder. It is uncommon in hamsters fed nutritionally balanced commercial diets (Holmes, 1984).

Trauma

Fighting among adults and cannibalism of litters are common among hamsters. Prevention of fighting and mating strategies have been discussed previously. Traumatic injuries are treated as in other species, with careful attention to the selection and administration of antibiotics.

Bedding-associated dermatitis

Degenerative lesions of the feet have been observed in both Syrian and Chinese hamsters housed on wood shavings. The lesions, primarily of the footpad, are characterised by degeneration and atrophy of the digits, with a granulomatous inflammatory response. Wood shavings are observed in the dermis and subcutis on histological examination. The footpad is suspect as the portal of entry with subcutaneous migration to proximal sites (Meshorer, 1976).

Diseases of Multiple Systems

Included among the agents causing multi-system disease are several important zoonotic agents. Zoonotic conditions include pseudotuberculosis, tularaemia and lymphocytic choriomeningitis. Special consideration should be made with respect to the risk to the pet owner when evaluating hamsters that are suspected to be infected with zoonotic pathogens.

Bacterial Diseases

Pseudotuberculosis

Agent. A member of the family Enterobacteriaceae, *Yersinia pseudotuberculosis* is a Gram-negative enteric pathogen transmitted directly in the faeces of wild rodents and birds.

Hosts. Pseudotuberculosis is a zoonotic disease infecting many other species including man, rabbits, mice, deer, cats, swine, monkeys, sheep, goats, chinchillas, mink, horses and many exotic mammals.

Clinical signs. Pseudotuberculosis may manifest as acute septicaemia or chronic disease characterised in its latter stages by diarrhoea and cachexia. The chronic form is more common in the hamster. Multifocal greyish-white discrete nodules can be observed grossly in several organs. Areas of necrosis are observed histologically in the intestine, mesenteric lymph nodes, liver, spleen and lungs.

Diagnosis. The disease can be definitively diagnosed by culture. Serological detection of antibody to the organism is suggestive of infection in the absence of positive culture results.

Control / treatment. A colony that is infected with the organism should be depopulated and the facilities disinfected. Treatment is not recommended as the organism is a zoonotic pathogen. Wild rodents and birds should not have access to hamster housing.

Tularaemia

Agent. There is a single report of a fatal epizootic disease in hamsters due to *Francisella tularensis* (Frisk, 1987). The Gram-negative bacterium may be transmitted directly or indirectly by arthropod vectors.

Hosts. *F. tularensis* has a wide host spectrum that includes humans, wild rodents and lagomorphs.

Clinical signs. In a single reported outbreak 4–6-week-old hamsters in a closed breeding colony were affected. Clinical onset of disease was rapid with most animals found moribund or dead. Premonitory signs were limited to 'huddled' behaviour and roughened hair coat. Pathology was observed in the lungs, which were mottled with subpleural petechial and ecchymotic haemorrhages; the liver, which was enlarged and pale with miliary white foci; the intestines, which had prominent Peyer's patches; and lymph nodes, which were enlarged. Microscopically, lymphoreticular necrosis associated with Gram-negative bacteria was observed.

Diagnosis. Bacterial culture, Gram-stained impression smears and histopathology are suitable for diagnosis. Ancillary diagnostics include inoculation of bacterial isolates into laboratory animals (i.e. mice).

Control / treatment. The disease is prevented by eliminating contamination by wild rodents. Possible exposure through supplemental foods such as lettuce, carrots and apples was suggested in the outbreak. Mortality was 100% in the reported outbreak and no effective treatment was described.

Viral Diseases

Lymphocytic Choriomeningitis

Agent. Lymphocytic Choriomeningitis Virus (LCMV) is an enveloped RNA Arenavirus.

Hosts. LCM is an important zoonotic disease which can produce 'flu-like symptoms, which may progress to choriomeningitis in man. Historically, the natural host of LCMV, the wild house mouse (*Mus musculus*), was considered to be the primary reservoir. However, most human exposures have been associated with exposure to pet and laboratory hamsters (Biggar *et al.*, 1975). The virus infects a wide host range including humans, monkeys, mice, rats, rabbits and chickens.

Clinical signs. As in the mouse, the disease may manifest in several forms depending upon the age of the hamster when infected, the strain of virus, the immunological status of the host and the infectious dose. LCMV may produce a tolerant persistent infection in which the animal sheds virus in the urine and saliva for extended periods of time (6 months to one year) but has no clinical signs of disease.

Natural infection may result in viraemia/viruria with clearance of the virus and only a transient lymphocytic infiltration of visceral organs; more commonly, the virus produces chronic, subclinical disease with prolonged viraemia. Adult hamsters exposed to the virus will usually clear the infection within 4 weeks of exposure (Biggar *et al.*, 1975). Hamsters exposed as neonates may develop acute illness with symptoms of rough hair coat, blepharitis and facial oedema accompanied by chronic convulsive seizures. Animals may recover or may die. Young hamsters that do not clear the virus will begin to show clinical signs of disease beginning in the seventh week of life; this progresses over months to a wasting disease caused by immune complex glomerulonephritis. Lymphocytic infiltration occurs in many organs including meninges, brain, kidney, liver, spleen and pancreas.

The mechanism of transmission is not known but evidence suggests that injuries associated with bites or scratches are a more likely route of infection than aerosol or oral spread (Harkness, 1994).

Diagnosis. Care should be exercised in collection of blood or handling of tissues from an animal suspected of having LCMV due to its zoonotic potential. Diagnosis of LCMV is most practically done serologically by ELISA or IFA. However, persistently viraemic animals may bind circulating antibody resulting in undetectable levels. A newer sensitive ELISA method decreases this possibility, but negative serology does not definitively rule out infection and shedding. Direct inoculation of tissues or blood from suspect cases into virus-free animals is required to detect persistent tolerant infections. Diagnosis can be made using tissue culture in combination with direct or indirect immunofluorescent antibody tests. An indirect immunofluorescence assay on infected tissue can also be used.

Control / treatment. Control of LCMV is best achieved by purchasing hamsters from colonies known to be free of the agent and by preventing exposure of hamsters to wild mice. There is no treatment for LCMV and, given its zoonotic potential, any animal diagnosed with this disease should be humanely euthanased followed by decontamination of the environment. As an enveloped virus the agent is sensitive to lipid solvents as well as detergents, acid treatment (pH 5.5), heat and radiation (UV or gamma).

Non-Infectious Diseases

Amyloidosis

Amyloidosis is a common ageing lesion in hamsters. It is associated with an immune system defect that results in deposition of immunoglobulin fragments in subendothelial locations in various organs, primarily the liver, kidney, spleen and adrenal glands. Clinical signs are associated with organ failure. Nephrotic syndrome (proteinuria/hypoproteinaemia, anasarca/oedema, hypercholesterolaemia, hypergammaglobulinaemia) is a common presenting sign (Murphy *et al.*, 1984). Female hamsters have a higher incidence of disease and may have significant organ compromise by 1 year of age. Most hamsters will have some evidence of amyloidosis by 18 months of age. Affected organs are pale, enlarged and irregular in appearance. Amyloid can be detected histologically in tissue sections stained with Congo red, and show a characteristic green birefringence under polarised light. No treatment for amyloidosis has been described.

Polycystic disease

Polycystic disease is a benign congenital condition in which cysts are frequently observed incidentally in old hamsters; they are generally hepatic but they may also be observed in the ovary, epididymis and adrenal glands. The cysts vary in size from 0.5 to 3 cm, are filled with amber fluid and are not generally associated with clinical signs.

Diseases of the Haematopoietic System

Few diseases of the haematopoietic system are unique to the hamster. Malignant lymphomas are a common and important disease of this species.

Neoplastic Diseases

The haematopoietic system is the most frequent site of neoplasia in the hamster. Malignant lymphomas can occur in different forms (Toft, 1992). Intestinal lymphoma is the most common, but animals may present with peripheral lymphadenopathy. Other organs such as liver, spleen and kidneys may also be involved. The frequency of occurrence and epizootic presentation are suggestive of a viral aetiology. Horizontal transmission has been documented and hamster papovavirus has been implicated as the causative agent (Percy and Barthold, 1993).

Diseases of Metabolic Origin

Adrenal cortical tumours are among the more common and significant metabolic diseases of the hamster. Diabetes mellitus is a spontaneous disease observed in specific genetic lines of Chinese hamsters and should be included as a differential diagnosis in that species.

Neoplastic Diseases

Endocrine tumours of the adrenal cortex are a common spontaneous neoplasm of the hamster. These tumours are more common in males and generally occur in aged animals (2–3 years of age) (Strandberg, 1987; Wagner and Farrar, 1987). Tumours of the thyroid, parathyroid, pituitary and pancreatic islets have also been reported, but are uncommon. The endocrine imbalance caused by these tumours may cause alopecia, altered behaviour, Cushing's syndrome and hypothyroidism (Wagner and Farrar, 1987). The incidence of endometrial adenocarcinoma also increases in animals greater than 100 weeks of age. Islet cell hyperplasia is a change found in aged hamsters that has not been identified with any clinical symptoms.

Non-Infectious Diseases

Diseases of Ageing

As previously mentioned, ageing hamsters may present with symptoms related to atrial thrombosis, arteriolar nephrosclerosis, osteoarthritis of the femoro-tibial articulation and amyloidosis resulting in multiple organ failure.

Diabetes mellitus

Diabetes mellitus is an inherited trait in Chinese hamsters. It is believed to be inherited as an autosomal recessive trait in some lines of animals and polygenic in others. Animals are generally not obese and have glucose intolerance, mild to severe hypoglycaemia, polyuria, glycosuria, occasional ketonuria and are hypoinsulinaemic. Chinese hamsters have been used as a model for Type I diabetes mellitus in man. Clinical evidence of diabetes is observed in affected animals by 90 days of age. Treatment includes insulin administration as well as dietary restriction. In prediabetic animals, dietary restriction can delay the onset of glucosuria, while in the overtly diabetic animal, it can reduce the severity of hyperglycaemia.

Pregnancy toxaemia

There is a single report describing pregnancy toxaemia due to shipping stress in the hamster (Richter et al., 1984). The syndrome resembles pregnancy toxaemia in man and guinea pigs as it was associated with disseminated thrombi in organs and placenta without evidence of an infectious aetiology. Pregnancy toxaemia in the hamster differs from that observed in other species in which diet, obesity and anorexia contribute to the development of ketoacidosis. In the guinea pig uteroplacental ischaemia is thought to initiate disseminated intravascular coagulation (DIC). A similar pathogenesis is suggested in the hamster. In the animals dying in this report there were no clinical signs except lethargy, with affected animals dying suddenly within 24 h of arrival. A caesarian-section may prevent death if this condition is diagnosed promptly.

References

Arrington, L. R., Ammerman, C. B. and Franke, D. E. (1979) Protein requirement of hamsters fed a natural diet. *Laboratory Animal Science* **29**, 469–71.

Balk, M. W. and Slater, G. M. (1987) Care and management. In: *Laboratory Hamsters*, pp. 61–67, Van Hoosier, G. L. Jr and McPherson, C. W. (eds). Academic Press Inc, Orlando.

Barthold, S. W., Jacoby, R. O. and Pucak, G. J. (1978) An outbreak of caecal mucosal hyperplasia in hamsters. *Laboratory Animal Science* **28**, 723–727.

Biggar, R. J., Woodall, J. P., Walter, P. D. *et al.* (1975) Lymphocytic choriomeningitis outbreak associated with pet hamsters. *Journal of the American Medical Association* **232**, 494–500.

Bivin, W. S., Olsen, G. H. and Murray, K. A. (1987) Morphophysiology. In: *Laboratory Hamsters*, pp. 9–14, Van Hoosier Jr, G. L. and McPherson, C. W., (eds). Academic Press, Orlando.

Boss, S. M., Gries, C. L., Kirchner, B. K. *et al.* (1994) Use of vancomycin hydrochloride for treatment of *Clostridium difficile* enteritis in Syrian hamsters. *Laboratory Animal Science* **44**(1), 31–37.

Brown, S. M. and Lisk, R. D. (1978) Blocked sexual receptivity in grouped female golden hamsters, the result of contact induced inhibition. *Biology of Reproduction* **18**, 829–833.

Burke, T. J. (1992) Skin disorders of rodents, rabbits and ferrets. In: *Kirk's Current Veterinary Therapy*, Vol XI, pp. 1170–1175, Kirk, R. W. (ed.). WB Saunders Co., Philadelphia.

Burns, K. F. and de Lannoy, C. W. (1966) Compendium of normal blood values of laboratory animals with indication of variations. I. Random-sexed populations of small animals. *Toxicology and Applied Pharmacology* **8**, 429–437.

Code of Federal Regulations (CFR) (1993) *Animal Welfare*. Office of the Federal Register, Washington.

Desai, R. G. (1968) Hematology and microcirculation. In: *The Golden Hamster: Its Biology and Use in Medical Research*, pp. 185–194, Hoffman, R. A., Robinson, P. F. and Magalhaes, H. (eds). Iowa State University Press, Ames.

Flynn, B. M., Brown, P. A., Eckstein, J. M. *et al.* (1989) Treatment of *Syphacia obvelata* in mice using ivermectin. *Laboratory Animal Science* **39**, 461–463.

Flynn, R. J. (1973) *Parasites of Laboratory Animals*. Iowa State University Press, Ames.

Fox, J. G., Dewhirst, F. E., Fraser, G. J. *et al.* (1994) The intracellular Campylobacter-like organism from ferrets and hamsters with proliferative bowel disease is a *Desulfovibrio* sp. *Journal of Clinical Microbiology* **32**, 1229–1237.

Fox, J. G., Stills, H. F., Paster B. J. *et al.* (1993) Antigenic specificity and morphologic characteristics of *Chlamydia trachomatis*, strain SFPD, isolated from hamsters wth proliferative ileitis. *Laboratory Animal Science* **43**, 405–410.

Frisk, C. (1987) Bacterial and mycotic diseases. In: *Laboratory Hamsters*, pp. 111–133, Van Hoosier, G. L. Jr and McPherson, C. W. (eds). Academic Press, Orlando.

Frisk, C. S., Wagner, J. E. and Owens, D. R. (1981) Hamster (*Mesocricetus auratus*) enteritis caused by epithelial cell-invasive *Escherichia coli*. *Infection and Immunity* **31**, 1232–1238.

Gebhart, C. J., Fennell, C. L., Murtaugh, M. P. *et al.* (1989) *Campylobacter cinaedi* is normal intestinal flora in hamsters. *Journal of Clinical Microbiology* **27**, 1692–1694.

Gibson, S. *et al.* (1983) Mortality in weanling hamsters associated with tooth loss. *Laboratory Animal Science* **33**, 497.

Gumma, M. R., South, F. E. and Allen, J. N. (1967) Temperature preference in golden hamsters. *Animal Behaviour* **15**, 534–577.

Harkness, J. E. (1994) Small rodents. *Veterinary Clinics of North America: Small Animal Practice* **24**, 89–102.

Harkness, J. E. and Wagner, J. E. (1983) *The Biology and Medicine of Rabbits and Rodents*, 2nd edn. Lea & Febiger, Philadelphia.

Hoffman, R. A., Robinson, P. F. and Magalhaes, H. (1968) *The Golden Hamster: Its Biology and Use in Medical Research*. Iowa State University Press, Ames.

Holmes, D. D. (1984) *Clinical Laboratory Animal Medicine*. Iowa State University Press, Ames.

Honacki, J., Kinman, K. and Koeppl, J. (1982) *Mammal Species of the World*. Allen Press Inc. and the Association of Systematics Collections, Lawrence.

Hughes, H. C., Barthel, C. H. and Lang, C. M. (1973) Niclosamide as a treatment for *Hymenolepis nana* and *Hymenolepis diminuta* in rats. *Laboratory Animal Science* **23**, 72–73.

Keeler, R. F. and Young, S. (1979) Role of vitamin E in the aetiology of spontaneous haemorrhagic necrosis of the central nervous system of fetal hamsters. *Teratology* **20**, 127–132.

Kern, T. J. (1989) Ocular disorders of rabbits, rodents and ferrets. In: *Current Veterinary Therapy*, pp. 681–685, Kirk, R. W. (ed.). WB Saunders Co., Philadelphia.

Krueger, K. L., Murphy, J. C. and Fox, J. G. (1989) Treatment of proliferative colitis in ferrets. *Journal of the American Veterinary Medical Association* **194**, 1435–1436.

Lee, C. C., Herrman, R. G. and Froman, R. C. (1959) Serum, bile and liver total cholesterol of laboratory animals, toads and frogs. *Proceedings of the Society of Experimental Biology and Medicine* **102**, 542–544.

Lipman, N. S., Weischedel, A. K., Connors, M. J. *et al.* (1992) Utilisation of cholestyramine resin as a preventive treatment for antibiotic (clindamycin) induced enterotoxaemia in the rabbit. *Laboratory Animal* **26**, 1–8.

Maxwell, K. O., Wish, J. C., Murphy, J. C. *et al.* (1985) Serum chemistry reference values in two strains of Syrian hamsters. *Laboratory Animal Science* **35**, 67–70.

Meshorer, A. (1976) Leg lesions in hamsters caused by wood shavings [brief report]. *Laboratory Animal Science* **26**, 827–829.

Mitruka, B. M. and Rawnsley, H. M. (1977) *Clinical Biochemical and Hematological Reference Values in Normal Experimental Animals*. Masson, New York.

Moore, W. (1968) Hemogram of the Chinese hamster. *American Journal of Veterinary Research* **27**, 608–610.

Morton, D. B., Abbot, D., Barclay, R. *et al.* (1993) Removal of blood from laboratory mammals and birds. *Laboratory Animal* **27**, 1–22.

Murphy, J. C., Fox, J. G. and Niemi, S. M. (1984) Nephrotic syndrome associated with renal amyloidosis in a colony of Syrian hamsters. *Journal of the American Veterinary Medical Association* **185**, 1359–1362.

Percy, D. H. and Barthold, S. W. (1993) *Pathology of Laboratory Rodents and Rabbits*. Iowa University Press, Ames.

Poole, T. (ed.) (1987) *The UFAW Handbook on the Care and Management of Laboratory Animals*, 6th edn. Longman, Essex.

Pour, P. and Birt, D. (1979) Spontaneous diseases of Syrian hamsters—their implications in toxicological research: Facts, thoughts and suggestions. *Progress in Experimental Tumour Research* **24**, 145–156.

Richards, M. P. M. (1966) Activity measured by running wheels and observation during the oestrous cycle, pregnancy and pseudopregnancy in the golden hamster. *Animal Behaviour* **14**, 450–458.

Richter, A., Lausen, N. and Lage, A. (1984) Pregnancy toxemia (eclampsia) in Syrian golden hamsters. *Journal of the American Veterinary Medical Association* **185,** 1357–1358.

Robinson, R. (1968) Genetics and karyology. In: The *Golden Hamster: Its Biology and Use in Medical Research*, pp. 41–72, Hoffman, R. A., Robinson, P. F. and Magalhaes, H. (eds). Iowa State University Press, Ames.

Ryden, E. B., Lipman, N. S., Taylor, N. S. *et al.* (1991) *Clostridium difficile* typhlitis associated with caecal mucosal hyperplasia in Syrian hamsters. *Laboratory Animal Science* **41,** 553–558.

Schuchman, S. M. (1989) Individual care and treatment of rabbits, mice, rats, guinea pigs, hamsters and gerbils. In: *Current Veterinary Therapy*, Vol X, pp. 738–765, Kirk, R. W. (ed.) WB Saunders, Co., Philadelphia PA.

Siegel, H. I. (1985) *The Hamster — Reproduction and Behaviour*. Plenum Press, New York.

Silverman, J. (1987) Biomethodology. In: *Laboratory Hamsters*, pp. 69–93, Van Hoosier, G. L. Jr and McPherson, C. W. (eds). Academic Press, Orlando.

Slater, G. M. (1972) The care and feeding of the Syrian hamster. *Progress in Experimental Tumour Research* **16,** 42–49.

Small, J. D. (1987) Drugs used in hamsters with a review of antibiotic-associated colitis. In: *Laboratory Hamsters*, pp. 179–168, Van Hoosier, G. L. Jr and McPherson, C. W. (eds). Academic Press, Orlando.

Strandberg J. D. (1987) Neoplastic diseases. In: *Laboratory Hamsters*, pp. 157–168, Van Hoosier, G. L. Jr and McPherson, C. W. (eds). Academic Press, Orlando.

Timm, K. I. (1989) Orbital venous anatomy of the Mongolian gerbil with comparison to the mouse, hamster and rat. *Laboratory Animal Science* **39,** 262–265.

Toft, J. D. (1992) Commonly observed spontaneous neoplasms in rabbits, rats, guinea pigs, hamsters and gerbils. *Seminars in Avian Exotic Pet Medicine* **1**(2), 80–92.

Unay, E. S. and Davis, B. J. (1980) Treatment of *Syphacia obvelata* in the Syrian hamster (*Mesocricetus auratus*) with piperazine citrate. *American Journal of Veterinary Research* **41,** 1899–1900.

U.S. Department of Health and Human Services (1985) *Guide for the Care and Use of Laboratory Animals.* Institute of Laboratory Animal Resources (ILAR), Washington.

Van Hoosier, G. L. and McPherson, C. W. (1987) *Laboratory Hamsters*. Academic Press, Orlando.

Wagner, J. E. (1987) Parasitic diseases. In: *Laboratory Hamsters*, pp. 135–156, Van Hoosier, G. L. Jr and McPherson, C. W. (eds). Academic Press, Orlando.

Wagner, J. E. and Farrar, P. L. (1987) Husbandry and medicine of small rodents. *Veterinary Clinics of North America: Small Animal Practice* **17,** 1061–1087.

Walker, E. P., Warnick, F., Lange K. I. *et al.* (1964) *Mammals of the World*, Vol. 2. Johns Hopkins Press, Baltimore.

(Data Tables follow).

Data Tables

COMMON DISEASES—HAMSTERS						
Disease	Aetiology	Diagnosis	Clinical signs and history	Treatment and control	Zoonotic potential	Comments
Respiratory system						
Sendai virus pneumonia	Sendai virus— paramyxovirus	Serology	Respiratory disease Any previously unexposed hamster	None	No	Secondary bacterial pneumonia may occur
Bacterial respiratory infections	P. pneumotropica Pasteurella sp. Streptococcus pneumoniae S. agalactiae Staphylococcus aureus; K. pneumoniae Bordetella sp. others	Bacterial culture	Respiratory disease Any animal; however, predisposing stresses play an important role	Appropriate antibiotic therapy	No	Chloramphenicol and enrofloxacin are good first choice antibiotics
Cardiovascular system						
Atrial thrombosis	Aetiology not defined	Suggested by clinical signs	Tachycardia; hyperpnoea; cyanosis Incidence higher in females and increases with age	Common ageing lesion	No	
Calcifying vasculo- pathy	Aetiology not defined	Pathology	Incidence increases with age	Dietary modification may be useful (?)	No	
Cardio- myopathy	Inherited in some inbred strains	As in other species	Heart failure	None reported; treat as in other species	No	
Gastrointestinal system						
Proliferative ileitis	Multifactorial— various infectious aetiologies implicated (Desulfovibrio sp. is the likely aetiology)	Palpation Pathology	Wet tail Generally weanling hamsters 3–8 wks of age	Supportive; chloramphenicol palmitate; tetracycline; neomycin	No	Poor prognosis

Fig 3.6—continued

COMMON DISEASES—HAMSTERS						
Disease	Aetiology	Diagnosis	Clinical signs and history	Treatment and control	Zoonotic potential	Comments
Gastrointestinal disease						
Antibiotic-associated colitis (AAC)	Clostridial enterotoxaemia (*C. difficile*)	Cytotoxin assay	Wet tail High mortality Antibiotic therapy Environmental stresses	Supportive Transfaunation Vancomycin (indefinitely)	No	Poor prognosis
Tyzzer's disease	*Clostridium piliforme*	Pathology	Diarrhoeic disease High mortality Colony outbreaks associated with exposure to contaminated feeds or wild rodents	Tetracycline	No	Poor prognosis
Salmonellosis	*Salmonella enteritidis*, *Salmonella typhimurium*	Bacterial culture	Diarrhoea Dyspnoea Exposure to contaminated feed or animals (including man)	Not recommended as asymptomatic carrier state can result	Yes	
Giardiasis	*Giardia muris*	Faecal flotation	May cause catarrhal enteritis in weanlings	Metronidazole	?	*Giardia* spp. are host-adapted but may infect other species
Pinworms	*Syphacia muris*, *Syphacia mesocriceti*, *Syphacia obvelata*, *Aspicularis tetraptera*	Anal tape Faecal flotation	May result with exposure to mice or rats	Piperazine Ivermectin	No	
Hymenolepiasis	*Hymenolepis nana* (dwarf tape-worm)	Faecal flotation	Unthriftiness Impaction	Niclosamide Praziquantel	Yes	
Genitourinary system						
Arteriolar nephro-sclerosis	Aetiology not defined Associated with high protein diet	Clinical signs suggestive of chronic renal disease	Polyuria; polydipsia Incidence increases with age	None specific to hamster; treat as in other species with renal disease	No	

Fig. 3.6—continued

COMMON DISEASES—HAMSTERS						
Disease	Aetiology	Diagnosis	Clinical signs and history	Treatment and control	Zoonotic potential	Comments
Nervous system						
CNS haemorrhage in foetal hamsters	Vitamin E deficiency	Pathology Response to vitamin E	Foetal losses Reproductive failure	Supplement dams with vitamin E	No	
Integument and musculoskeletal system						
Actinomycosis	*Actinomyces bovis*	Anaerobic bacterial culture	Cervical swelling	Lance/drain Antibiotic therapy	No	Long term antibiotic therapy has high risk of of AAC development
Cutaneous bacterial abscesses	*S. aureus* is organism most frequently reported Also *Streptococcus* sp., *Actinomyces bovis*, *P. pneumo-tropica*	Bacterial culture	Usually present with swelling in the cervical area Often associated with fighting or substandard caging	Enrofloxacin or ciprofloxacin for staphylococcal pyoderma	No	
Streptococcal mastitis	*β*-Haemolytic *Streptococcus*	Bacterial culture	Usually observed 7–10 days following parturition	Antibiotic therapy	No	
Dermato-phytosis	*Trichophyton menta-grophytes Microsporum* sp.	Fungal culture	Typical skin lesions	Topical fungicides Povidone–iodine Griseofulvin	?	Zoonotic in other species, although not reported from hamster
Epithelioma	Hamster papovavirus	Pathology	Epitheliomas Hamsters 3 months to 1 year of age		No	

Fig. 3.6—continued

COMMON DISEASES—HAMSTERS						
Disease	Aetiology	Diagnosis	Clinical signs and history	Treatment and control	Zoonotic potential	Comments
Demodicosis	*Demodex criceti* *Demodex aurati*	Skin scraping	Alopecia; dry scaly skin Aged, stressed, or immunosuppressed animals for clinical symptoms	Amitraz	No	Also found in healthy hamsters
Other mites	*Notoedres notoedres* (hamster ear mite)	Skin scraping	Colony problem may affect all age groups	Ivermectin	No	
	Notoedres cati (cat mange mite)				Yes	Infests cats and rabbits
	Ornithonyssus bacoti (tropical rat mite)		Environmental problem; owner may experience bites	Frequent cage changes; spray with malathion	Yes	
Osteoarthritis	Degenerative disease	Palpation Radiograph	Animals > 2 years of age	Soft bedding	No	
Cage paralysis	Nutritional myopathy associated with vitamin E or D deficiency	History Clinical signs	Dietary insufficiency	Supplement as necessary; feed fresh commercially formulated diets	No	
Systemic diseases						
Pseudo-tuberculosis	*Yersinia pseudo-tuberculosis*	Bacterial culture Serology	Epizootic with high morbidity and mortality	Depopulate colony and sanitise environment	Yes	Infects other species
Tularaemia	*Francisella tularensis*	Bacterial culture	Epizootic affecting 4–6-week-old hamsters	Prevent by eliminating sources of contamination (wild rodents or feed)	Yes	
Lymphocytic chorio-meningitis	Lymphocytic chorio-meningitis virus (LCMV)	Serology IFA on infected tissue	Sudden deaths in young hamsters or chronic wasting disease	Prevent by buying from LCMV-free suppliers Euthanasia of animals is recommended	Yes	

Fig. 3.6—continued

COMMON DISEASES—HAMSTERS						
Disease	Aetiology	Diagnosis	Clinical signs and history	Treatment and control	Zoonotic potential	Comments
Amyloidosis	Immune dysfunction resulting in immuno-globulin fragment deposition in various organs	Suggested by clinical signs, pathology	Nephrotic syndrome Higher incidence in females, but affects most hamsters > 18 months of age	None described	No	Poor prognosis
Polycystic disease	Inherited		Incidental necropsy finding	None	No	
Haematopoietic system						
Lymphoma	Viral aetiology Hamster papovavirus	As in other species	May be epizootic	None described	No	
Other systems						
Adrenal cortical tumours			Alopecia Altered behaviour, usually older males	None described in hamsters	No	
Diabetes mellitus	Inherited in lines of Chinese hamsters	As in other species	Clinical signs usually evident by 90 days of age	Insulin-responsive Dietary restriction	No	
Pregnancy toxaemia	Uteroplacental ischaemia		Stress induced in last trimester of pregnancy	None described, avoid stress in near term females	No	One reported case

FIG. 3.6 Common diseases—hamsters.

PHYSIOLOGICAL DATA—HAMSTERS		
	Syrian	Chinese
Adult weight: Males	85–130 g	30–35 g
Females	95–150 g	27–32 g
Life span: Average	18–24 months	30–36 months
Maximum	36 months	—
H_2O consumption	100 ml/kg	4 ml/day
Temperature (rectal)	37–38 °C	—
Food consumption	5.5–7 g/day	2.5–3.5 g/day
Heart rate	280–412/min	—
Respiratory rate	33–127/min	—
Blood volume	78 ml/kg	—
Blood pressure (mean)	97.8 mm/Hg	—
Urine volume	5.1–8.4 ml/24 h	—
Urine pH	basic	—
Data taken from Bivin et al. (1987), Poole (1987) and Harkness and Wagner (1983).		

FIG. 3.7 Physiological data—hamsters.

HAEMATOLOGICAL VALUES—HAMSTERS		
	Syrian	Chinese
$RBC \times 10^6/mm^3$	5.5–8.9	7.12
PCV %	44.1–53.9	—
Haemoglobin g/dl	14.5–18	12.4
Reticulocytes %	1.3–3.7	—
$WBC \times 10^3/mm^3$	6.3–10.1	5.5
Neutrophils %	18.6–32.1	17–21
Eosinophils %	0.46–1.22	1.0–2.4
Basophils %	0–3	0.11–0.19
Lymphocytes %	59.4–81.9	75
Monocytes %	1.4–2.4	1.8–2.4
Platelets $\times 10^3/mm^3$	339–485	—
Data taken from Mitruka and Rawnsley (1977), Moore (1966) and Desai (1968).		

FIG. 3.8 Haematological values—hamsters.

CLINICAL CHEMISTRY VALUES—HAMSTERS (Syrian)		
	Mean	Range
Calcium mg/dl	11	9.8–13.2
Phosphorus mg/dl	7.1	3.0–9.9
Sodium mEq/l	129	—
Chloride mEq/l	95	—
Potassium mEq/l	4.6	2.3–9.8
Glucose mg/dl	127	37–198
BUN mg/dl	18.9	12–26
Creatinine mg/dl	0.58	0.4–1.0
Total bilirubin mg/dl	0.35	0.1–0.9
Uric acid mg/dl	3.8	1.4–6.3
Total protein g/dl	6.1	5.2–7.0
Albumin g/dl	4.2	3.5–4.9
Globulin g/dl	3.4	2.7–4.2
Cholesterol mg/dl	115	55–181
Triglycerides mg/dl	128	72–227
Alkyl phosphate IU/l	131	86–187
SGOT IU/l	57	28–122
SGPT IU/l	48	22–128
LDH IU/l	224	140–412
CPK IU/l	476	263–1031
Data taken from Burns and de Lannoy (1960); Maxwell *et al.* (1985) and Mitruka and Rawnsley (1977).		

FIG. 3.9 Clinical chemistry values—hamsters (Syrian).

REPRODUCTIVE DATA—HAMSTERS		
	Syrian	Chinese
Breeding age	6–8 weeks	7–14 weeks
Oestrous cycle	polyoestrus	polyoestrus
Duration of oestrous cycle	4 days	4 days
Gestation	15.5 days	20.5 days
Average litter size	5–9	4–5
Birth weight	2 g	1.5–2.5 g
Eyes open	15 days	—
Wean	21–28 days	21 days
Postpartum oestrus	2–18 days post weaning	4 days post weaning
Number of mammae	14–22	8
Breeding duration	10–12 months	—
Data taken from Poole (1987), Hoffman *et al.* (1968), Harkness and Wagner (1983) and Van Hoosier and McPherson (1987).		

FIG. 3.10 Reproductive data—hamsters.

4

Guinea Pigs

MICHAEL J. HUERKAMP, KATHLEEN A. MURRAY and SUSAN E. OROSZ

Introduction

Cavia porcellus, the domestic guinea pig or cavy, is a compact, tailless, short-legged hystrico-morph rodent originally indigenous to South America and closely related to the chinchilla, nutria, capybara and porcupine. The modern breeds of guinea pig originated from wild ancestors native to the mountains and grasslands of Peru, Argentina, Brazil and Uruguay that were semi-domesticated by the Incas for use as a food animal. Permanent importation of guinea pigs to Europe was done by Dutch sailors over 400 years ago and they became immediately popular with collectors and fanciers. After their introduction to Europe, *C. porcellus* became extinct in the wild, but, following domestication, were disseminated internationally.

Since the mid-19th century, guinea pigs have been bred widely as pets and research animals. Over the course of domestication, numerous varieties of guinea pig have been developed. The three most common breeds include the English or American (short, smooth, caudally directed hair), Peruvian (long, silky hair) and Abyssinian (rosette or whorled hair pattern). Because the varieties are often interbred, an abundance of colours and hair lengths exists. In addition to albinism and solid coloration, guinea pigs may be bicoloured or tricoloured. Through selective breeding for showing, many additional colour patterns have been developed including agouti, brindle, Himalayan, Dalmatian and tortoiseshell. Guinea pig coat colour genetics are complicated and governed by at least six main coat colour loci.

The origin of the name 'guinea pig' is obscure and remains the subject of much speculation. 'Guinea' may be derived from the fact that, early in the pet trade, they were sold in the UK for the price of a guinea coin and 'pig' may have been inspired by their resemblance to a suckling pig when prepared for the table and their squealing, messy deportment.

In veterinary practice, guinea pigs may be encountered as pets, show animals, in small production colonies for the pet trade or show ring, or in large production colonies for research. As pets, guinea pigs present few problems as they are easily handled, have little odour and are disinclined to escape. They tend not to climb and their jumping ability is poor. Guinea pigs rarely bite, but may struggle against handling. Because they are inexpensive to acquire, easy to maintain, docile, quiet and relatively free of odours, guinea pigs are popular first pets and are often kept in primary schools. However, because of the risk of injury to the animal, children under 4 years of age should only handle guinea pigs under direct adult supervision.

Unique Biology

Hystricomorph rodents differ from myomorph rodents, such as rats and mice, by having a long gestation period, precocious offspring and a cellular membrane that closes over the vaginal orifice, except in oestrus and parturition. The family Caviidae, to which guinea pigs belong, is characterised by one pair of mammary glands, 3 clawed digits on the hind feet and 4 on the front feet. Although age and genetics may cause some variability, at maturity, non-obese, adult male guinea pigs range from 900 to 1200 g and females from 600 to 800 g. The guinea pig lifespan is typically 3–5 years reaching a maximum, in rare cases, of 8 years.

Guinea pigs are morphophysiologically unique in that the functional thymus is found both in the mediastinum and subcutaneously in the neck, the adrenals and spleen are disproportionately large and the bronchioles are exquisitely sensitive to histamine-induced constriction. The inguinal canals are open. Both sexes have two inguinal nipples, although only females have mammary glandular tissue. Despite this, litters of four or more can be raised without difficulty. Males have an os penis and extremely large seminiferous vesicles that extend 10 cm into the abdomen from the pubis, and for the inexperienced, can be confused with uterine horns on laparotomy. The exposed penis has two prongs of equal length at the tip. Guinea pig urine is alkaline, opaque, creamy yellow and contains calcium carbonate and ammonium phosphate crystals which will accumulate as scale on cage surfaces. The ears have large tympanic bullae and four cochlear coils, giving the guinea pig exquisitely sensitive hearing. Colour discrimination and olfaction are also well developed. There are supracaudal sebaceous glands and anal marking glands.

The haematology profile of the guinea pig is unique because of the presence of Foa–Kurloff cells. These mononuclear cells, presumably of thymic origin, contain intracytoplasmic mucopolysaccharide inclusions and proliferate during oestrogenic stimulation (Fig. 4.1); they are found in highest numbers in the trophoblastic region of the placenta. It has been theorised that they protect the foetus from maternal rejection, but may also be found in the lungs, spleen and peripheral circulation, particularly during pregnancy, where they may function as natural killer cells. The lymphocyte is resistant to steroids and, as with other rodents such as rats, mice, hamsters and gerbils, is the predominant peripheral blood cell.

Guinea pigs are monogastric herbivores with an intestinal tract typical of other rodents including a large caecum and colon. The stomach is undivided and lined with glandular epithelium. The gastric emptying time is approximately 2 h and the gastrointestinal transit time, apart from the effects of coprophagy, spans 8–30 h. The caecum is 15–20 cm long, thin-walled and divided into pouches by the action of smooth muscle. It contains up to 65% of the total gastrointestinal capacity and lies in the central and left portions of the abdominal cavity where it may be an accidental target of misdirected intraperitoneal injections. Caecal fermentation is a source of high energy, volatile fatty acids. The small intestine lies coiled on the right side. The colon may comprise 40% of the total length of the intestinal tract. Gram-positive anaerobes and lactobacilli are the predominant intestinal species, but coliforms, streptococci, yeast, *Sarcina* and soil bacteria, including clostridia, may be present in small numbers. A large variety of protozoans, particularly trichomonads, *Giardia* and *Entamoeba*, normally inhabit the lower intestinal tract, but rarely cause disease unless guinea pigs are debilitated or stressed from improper care.

The teeth are open-rooted, erupt continuously (hypsodontic) and are present in the following formula: $2(I_1^1 C_0^0 P_1^1 M_3^3)$. The incisors are chisel-like, while the molars and premolars are flattened for grinding. The roots of the maxillary molars and premolars incline buccally, while those of the mandibular teeth are angled lingually. Malocclusion of the cheek teeth is common in aged animals.

Figures at the end of the chapter detail the physiological, haematological and clinical chemistry profiles of the guinea pig.

Behaviour

Guinea pigs are cursorial, timid and gregarious. In the wild, related species live in male-dominated, polygamous social hierarchies in groups of 5–10 animals and seek shelter in burrows abandoned by other animals. Guinea pigs move, eat and rest in groups, with the young following adults and the males following oestrous females, and then lie in contact under, over, or alongside cagemates. Although they are most active at twilight, guinea pigs in captivity show little diurnal rhythm and are generally active through the day and night. Sleep periods occur throughout the day and night and are

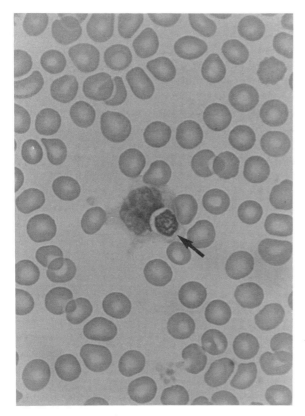

FIG. 4.1 Peripheral blood smear of the guinea pig showing a Foa–Kurloff cell (arrowed).

will not fight with females. Females are less antagonistic and, if maintained in groups without males, will develop either a weak and flexible social hierarchy or none at all. Fighting is most likely to occur in unstable groups of recently mixed adult animals or in established hierarchies in competition for food, water, females or territory. For rodents, guinea pigs are quite vocal and have a repertoire of vocalisations that correlate with different social behaviour. They may be especially vocal, emitting a low or tweeting whistling sound, at the sight of an owner or caretaker when hungry or when separated from conspecifics. There are vocalisations for defence (chutter, whine), exploration (chutt), seeking contact (purr), distress (scream, squeal) and fear (drr) (Harper, 1976).

As a consequence of fear or startling, guinea pigs manifest scatter and immobility responses that can lead to injury. Scattering generally occurs in response to sudden movement and is characterised by stampeding in all directions, jumping and rapid circling. To prevent this behaviour, guinea pigs should be kept in enclosures that permit viewing of the external environment and should be forewarned of approaches. Freezing or immobility lasting several seconds to 20 min can be engendered by either sudden noises or environmental changes.

Reproduction

Mating

Differentiation of the sexes can be difficult for the uninitiated, because variability in body weight makes it a poor determinant and the appearance of the external genitalia is similar for both sexes. The guinea pig sow has a vaginal closure membrane that can be exposed by gentle digital stretching of the genital ridge that extends from the anus to the vulva. The relaxed membrane will be seen as a shallow, U-shaped crease between the anal and urethral openings. It is imperforate except for 3–4 days during prooestrus and oestrus and at parturition. The male guinea pig has no break in the ridge between the

short, usually lasting less than 5 min at a time. If left undisturbed in a cage, guinea pigs will huddle alert, but quiet, in groups next to a wall, except when feeding, during intermittent sleep periods or when agitated by elevated ambient temperatures. Guinea pigs themselves do not dig and do not hibernate, but do seek cover and will spend most of the time in a shelter, if it is provided. They venture infrequently to the centre of their enclosure.

Hierarchies are maintained within territorial limits delineated by anal and supracaudal gland secretions and by urine, vocalisation, agonistic displays and occasional physical combat. Most confrontations between males are resolved without fighting, but males will fight each other over females, often with fatal consequences; males urethral orifice and the anus. The penis can be palpated in the midline and digital pressure applied to this region will extrude the ensheathed penis. Photographs of the external genitalia are shown in Fig. 4.2.

Boars reach sexual maturity at 8–9 weeks of age, but will begin mounting and thrusting at 30 days of age. Most sows reach puberty at 10 weeks of age, although they may begin the oestrous cycle by 4–5 weeks of age. Sows are best bred at 6–12 weeks of age when they reach a body weight of 400–600 g (Harkness and Wagner, 1989; Ediger, 1976). For maximum production, boars should not be bred until they weigh 650 g at approximately 10–16 weeks of age. Virgin females should be mated before 6–8 months of age or the symphysis pubis will fuse in

a narrow configuration that will effectively occlude the passage of a foetus through the pelvic canal. This situation invariably causes a fatal dystocia. Consequently, nulliparous females older than 8 months of age should never be housed with an intact boar. For high production, selecting breeders from parents with high success in rearing total young to weaning, rather than litter size, is the best parameter (Sutherland and Festing, 1987).

Guinea pigs can be bred in monogamous or harem arrangements. The most productive system is to mate animals in polygamous groups of 1 boar and 4–8 sows per breeding pen (Sutherland and Festing, 1987; Manning *et al.*, 1984). Polygamous mating maximises production per boar and takes advantage of communal rearing,

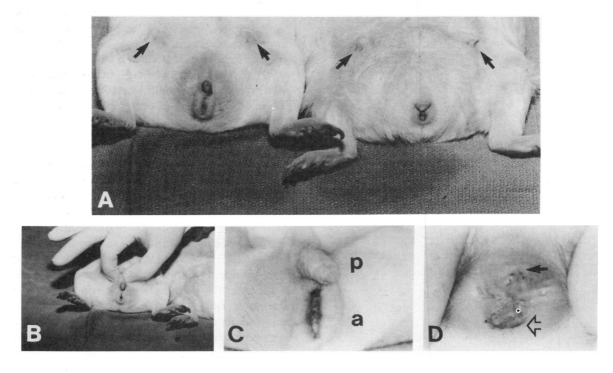

FIG. 4.2 Sexual differentiation of guinea pigs in dorsal recumbency showing (A) side-by-side male (left) and female (right) external genitalia. The teats are indicated by arrows. (B) Palpation of the midline of the boar to detect the sheathed penis. (C) Manual extrusion of the penis (p) of the dorsally recumbent boar. The anus (a) is also shown. (D) Lateral manual retraction of the vulvar lips of the dorsally recumbent female showing the vaginal closure membrane. The closed arrow indicates the ventral commissure and the open arrow designates the dorsal commissure.

while monogamous mating generally results in higher weaning rates. In order to take advantage of breeding at the postpartum oestrus and maximise production, a breeding group should remain intact, except for weaning pups and culling infertile sows, for 18 months (Harkness and Wagner, 1989). If continuously exposed to a fertile boar, sows will have 3–5 litters per year and will wean pups at a mean rate of 12 per year (Ediger, 1976; Townsend, 1975). However, in this system the young are at risk of trampling if the adults are crowded or become excited and older animals may also chew the ears of pups. Consequently, to protect the pups from bullying and competition for milk and to permit easier identification of breeding lines, sows should be removed to a nursery before parturition (Manning *et al.*, 1984). For more intensive production, the postparturient sow can be transiently reintroduced to the harem for several hours to permit postpartum breeding followed by return to the nursery pen. Otherwise, the sow can be reintroduced to the group for breeding after the pups are weaned.

Guinea pigs are polyoestrous and breed all year round. The duration of the oestrous cycle may range from 13 to 20 days, but most commonly is 15–17 days. The cycle is divisible into the standard stages of pro-oestrus, oestrus, metoestrus and dioestrus. The oestrous period itself lasts 24–48 h, but females are receptive to coitus during the night for a period of only 6–15 h (Harper, 1976; Harkness and Wagner, 1989; Manning *et al.*, 1984; Flecknell, 1991). Ovulation is spontaneous and occurs approximately 10 h after the onset of oestrus. Most sows have a 3–4 h oestrous period 2–15 h postpartum, of which approximately 70% of matings are fertile (Harkness and Wagner, 1989; Ediger, 1976; Manning *et al.*, 1984). Because breeding animals are typically housed together continuously, detection of oestrus is not necessary unless timed matings are desired. If timed pregnancies are desired, mating can be confirmed by the observation of the perforated vaginal membrane, the postcoital vaginal plug, or, for several hours only after mating, sperm in a vaginal smear.

Males will purr, sway and run around the sow, often brushing against her. This is followed by anogenital sniffing or licking, pursuit, mounting and intromission. Sows in oestrus will mount others and, when exposed to a boar, will arch their back and elevate the hindquarters. Following dismounting by the male, the female briefly cleans the genitalia in a doubled-over posture. Females ward off unwanted advances with avoidance, a warning spray of urine, rearing on the hindquarters and baring teeth, or lunging and swatting the male on the nose. While guinea pigs may remain fertile for up to 4 years, the optimal breeding life ends at 2 years of age. Generally, litter sizes decrease and reproductive complications begin to increase after 18–28 months of age. Additionally, infertility can be induced by obesity, metritis, wire flooring, environmental temperatures in excess of 29°C, inadequate light intensity, short day length (less than 10–12 h per day), chronic disease, crowding, penile malformations, oestrogen-contaminated feeds, cystic ovaries and vitamin E and other nutritional deficiencies. Bachelor males aged 1 year or more show decreased libido and, where small particle contact beddings are used, they may adhere to the genitalia and prevent copulation by mechanical impedance and irritation.

Gestation and Birth

The gestation period typically lasts 63–69 days with a range of 59–72 days. The length of gestation is inversely related to the number of foetuses. Implantation occurs on days 6–7 and placentation is haemomonochorial, lacunal and discoidal. The endocrine control of gestation is similar to that of primates in that the 9–10 week gestation period may be divided into three equal trimesters. The placenta begins secreting progesterone on day 15 and assumes the maintenance role for the latter half of pregnancy. The guinea pig receives all maternal antibody from the placenta and none from the colostrum. Pseudopregnancy is rare in guinea pigs, but, when it does occur, it lasts approximately 17 days. Superfoetation has been reported (Richardson, 1992). Exercise is particularly important for pregnant sows to prevent pregnancy toxaemia and maintaining body condition conducive to uneventful parturition. Exercise can be promoted by keeping the sow in a spacious pen with the food kept at a distance from drinking water and from the nesting area. However, towards the end of pregnancy the foetal mass may be so large as to impede ambulation. In this case, food and water should be kept in proximity to the sow. In order to prevent eclampsia and ketosis, calcium supplementation (4 mg/kg/day PO) may be given in late gestation (Richardson, 1992).

During pregnancy, the sow may double her body weight, and food consumption will triple over baseline maintenance levels. The foetuses may be palpated during the interval 2–6 weeks post-mating by controlling the sow in a prone position with the nondominant hand holding the thorax. With the guinea pig facing away, the thumb of the dominant hand should be placed on the contralateral iliac crest and the first two fingers on the ventral midline. Simultaneously, the thumb should be slipped lateral to the iliac crest and the two fingers pressed gently upward and laterally. Foetuses will be firm, rounded and essentially immobile, but will slip between the digits. Kidneys and faecal pellets are readily mobile and faecal pellets are elongated rather than rounded. From 6 weeks post-mating until 7 days before term, the foetuses can be felt by gently cupping the abdomen of the sow in the palm of the hand. The ossified foetal skeletons are visible radiographically at 6 weeks.

During the latter half of gestation, the pubic symphysis, under the influence of relaxin, gradually separates until a palpable gap of 1.5 cm is present 48 h prepartum. At parturition, the opening may expand to 2–3 cm in diameter. If an animal has been regularly palpated, parturition typically occurs 18–20 days after foetal movements are first detected. Parturition can be induced by administering oxytocin if the sow is at day 66 or more of gestation and is adequately dilated. The onset of labour is abrupt and can be at any time of the day, but usually occurs at night. It lasts for 10–30 min with a span of 5–10 min between pups. The sow squats while delivering and cleans the pups. Normally, the placenta and membranes are eaten by the sow or other animals in the group, including boars. Guinea

pigs deliver between 1 and 6 young with 3–4 being an average litter. Healthy newborns weigh 60–100 g, while pups weighing less than 50–60 g usually die (Ediger, 1976). The young are born with eyes open, teeth erupted and the body covered with hair. The periparturient sow does not build a nest and, other than anogenital grooming, the newborns receive only cursory maternal attention.

In breeding colonies, foetal wastage and maternal mortality are the greatest barriers to high production and are caused by many conditions including embryonic resorption, uterine haemorrhage, dystocias and, rarely, exhaustion from prolonged labour. Subclinical ketosis contributes insidiously to this problem. While the incidence of stillbirths is 9–11% in outbred animals in peak production, the rate of neonatal deaths should be less than 1% in a well managed colony. Stillbirths and abortions are highest in primiparous females, immature sows, where gestation is less than 66 or more than 72 days, in conjunction with large litters, and where sows are stressed by loud noises, ambient temperatures in excess of 26–28°C, exposure to potential predators or destabilisation of a social group. The presence of other nursing sows may stimulate premature labour. Numerous infectious and metabolic diseases, as well as food restriction during late pregnancy, may also cause prenatal deaths. Blood on the vagina or on the nose, secondary to grooming, may be a presenting complaint for abortion. Sows that abort should be given 2 months sexual rest before breeding is attempted (Elward, 1980).

Dystocia is relatively uncommon in sows in good health and condition, but common and often fatal in obese sows, those bred for the first time after 6–8 months of age, and sows with large foetuses. Feeding diets containing 22% or more protein is correlated with excessively large foetuses, prolonged gestation and dystocia. The risk of dystocia is compounded by the fact that parturition is difficult to predict because of the variability in gestation length, the lack of nest-building and the abrupt onset of delivery. Consequently, pregnant sows should be closely monitored by the owner for decreases in appetite or activity, the onset of labour and the presence of bloody or green–brown vaginal discharges suggestive of dystocia. Oxytocin administration and attempts to lubricate and deliver pups are rarely successful due to the fact that the condition is invariably caused by physical factors, such as intrapelvic fat or a fused pelvic symphysis, that prevent the neonate from passing through the pelvis.

A caesarean section is indicated if the pubic symphysis is not adequately dilated and where a sow strains unsuccessfully for more than 20 min, strains intermittently over the course of 2 h, or if a pup is not delivered within 10–15 min of oxytocin administration. Pup and maternal survival is dependent upon immediate surgical intervention, because the well developed pups have a high immediate demand for oxygen and are sensitive to carbon dioxide. Consequently, pups detached from the maternal blood supply will die in the uterus within several minutes and the sows will die subsequently of related complications. Pups that are delivered alive from a dystocia often have irreversible anoxic brain damage and will be uncoordinated and unable to suckle.

Milk production peaks 5–8 days postpartum at 65 ml/day and ceases by day 18–23. Sows nurse in a sitting posture and typically lose 50–150 g body weight during lactation. Mammary involution will occur in sows that have not been nursed for 24 h. Transient agalactia, lasting less than 24 h, may occur in sows that have had an exhaustive parturition. Nursing does not begin until 12–24 h after birth and continues for 2–3 weeks. Pups will start to drink water and eat solid food within a few days of birth, but, for normal growth and health, they should nurse for a minimum of 15 days (Manning *et al.*, 1985; Sisk, 1976). Pups should be weaned at 150–240 g body weight or 15–28 days of age. It is especially important that female offspring be weaned by 21 days of age and isolated from boars, because they may come into oestrus by 4–5 weeks of age and may be bred. Pregnancy in immature sows is rarely carried to term and invariably leads to stillbirths, abortion or dystocia, often with uterine prolapse. As a consequence, the young sow often dies as well.

In harem mating systems, large pups will suckle newly freshened sows and deprive neonates of milk. Consequently, weanlings should be promptly removed from intact breeding groups or sows with nursing pups should be isolated in a nursery cage. Such isolation also serves to reduce the risk of traumatic injuries. Following weaning, development is rapid and weanlings grow at a rate of 25–50 g/week to 2 months of age. Weight gain continues at a lesser rate until the adult body weight is attained.

Orphans

Because pups begin eating solid food during the first few days postpartum, hand-rearing is not as difficult as with altricial species such as rats, mice and rabbits. However, mortality is significantly higher in pups under 4–7 days of age as compared to older counterparts (Manning *et al.*, 1984). In general, orphan-rearing is approximately 50% successful. Because they will not accept their first meal until 12–24 h following birth, orphans will lose weight initially due to dehydration, but rapidly make compensatory gains. Parenteral fluid therapy or benign neglect, in lieu of force-feeding, is indicated at this time. From birth until 4 days of age, orphans should be permitted to lap a creamy mixture of 10 g ground guinea pig pelleted diet, 10 g rolled oats, 1 g dextrose, 0.5 g salt, 1.5 g whole dry active yeast, 10 mg ascorbic acid, 0.5 mg thiamine and 100 ml water from a spoon. Pups should consume 1–2 ml of mixture per feeding. Feeding should be done during daylight hours every 2–3 h. Chopped vegetables or cow's milk are inappropriate substitute diets for newborn and growing pups. Evaporated milk, diluted 1:2 with tap water, is too low in protein and too rich in complex carbohydrates that predispose to indigestion and cataracts, but can be used in an emergency as a temporary diet. Protein-deficient pups will develop facial and forelimb oedema and alopecia (Bell *et al.*, 1978). During the first 7 days postnatally, stimulation for urination and defaecation with a warm, moistened cotton cloth should be done several times daily and the pups kept in a container that is partially warmed with a heating pad placed under the floor. Woollen fabric makes a good nesting material. Pups attempting to nurse each other may induce rectal prolapse. After 4 days, the pups can be weaned by offering both dry chow pellets and ground guinea pig chow softened with water.

Cross-Fostering

When given the opportunity, the young will also nurse other lactating sows. Most sows, especially if kept in a social group, will nurse pups that are not theirs. Consequently, orphans often can be cross-fostered onto another sow. If a sow is reluctant to permit cross-nursing, move it to a bedded box with one of its pups, keep the other pups in the original cage, rub the orphaned pups with the bedding and pups of the foster dam and move them into the box containing the foster dam. If the sow nudges the pups away, she is rejecting them. In such cases, gradually move the pups to her until acceptance occurs or rub the pups and the chin of the sow with mentholated vapour rub to mask the odour of the new pups. In some cases, primiparous sows or those that have had a difficult parturition will develop a hysterical fear of their newborns. The gradual approximation technique and administration of anxiolytic drugs to the sow should be used to reintroduce the pups.

The reproductive data for guinea pigs are listed in Fig. 4.13 at the end of the chapter.

Husbandry

Housing

Guinea pigs are adaptable to many housing systems and may be kept in pens, cages, aquaria, or in large bins on the floor or in racks or tiers. As a rule of thumb, adult guinea pigs should be provided with a minimum of 700 cm^2 floor space per animal and a sow with a litter should be given 1500 cm^2 (Harkness and Wagner, 1989; Manning *et al.*, 1984). These recommendations are somewhat arbitrary, but are helpful in preventing the adverse behavioural and environmental effects of overcrowding. In general, the larger the floor space per animal, the less cleaning will be required. Housing enclosures should be constructed of plastic, stainless steel, or wire and should have smooth, sanitisable surfaces

that are impervious to moisture. Permanent structures made of brick or concrete are wasteful of space, difficult to clean and poorly insulated and are not recommended. Unsealed wood will become soaked with urine and is difficult to clean. The surface integrity of sealed wooden structures, although impervious to moisture, is susceptible to gnawing.

Because they are easy to clean and generally safe, solid-bottomed cages or pens used with contact bedding are preferred for housing guinea pigs. Glass aquaria or plastic bins are particularly convenient housing enclosures for pets and facilitate efficient cleaning and sanitation. However, opaque plastic bins afford poor visibility for the guinea pig and both types of enclosure will be poorly ventilated requiring more frequent sanitation. Because sudden noises or movements are frightening to guinea pigs and may lead to stampeding or jumping, cages should be rectangular in configuration and open pens should have sides that are at least 40 cm high. Cages or pens constructed with a solid 10–15 cm lower wall with a wire upper wall offer the advantage of greater visibility with less likelihood of startling, are reasonably ventilated and will retain contact bedding. To permit normal postural movements, cages with lids should have sides at least 18 cm high.

Contact bedding should be provided to a depth of 2–5 cm and must be clean, nonabrasive, nonaromatic and nontoxic. Substrates such as hardwood chips, shredded paper, peat moss, dried corn cobs, rice hulls, or other materials of plant origin are recommended. Sawdust and other small particle beddings should not be used because the fine particles can adhere to the vulva, scrotum and prepuce and cause irritation and occlusion. Coarse straw or hay carries the risk of causing trauma, especially to the eyes. Aromatic beddings, such as cedar or pine, are not appropriate, because they are known to activate hepatic microsomal enzyme systems.

Wire flooring, although labour-saving from a sanitation perspective, presents numerous problems. It is discouraged as a flooring surface because it can cause limb fractures, acute lacerations and chronic ulceration of the skin and feet and has been associated with alopecia, infertility, chilling (especially of pups) and wastage of spilled feed. Pregnant females and obese animals are particularly prone to pododermatitis when kept on wire flooring. Where wire flooring is used, it should be smooth, free of sharp projections, rectangular (0.5 cm × 1.0–1.6 cm) and 9–10 gauge. Stainless steel is preferred over galvanised metals, because it is more durable and rust-resistant. To introduce naive animals to wire, a piece of cardboard placed on the floor will ease the transition to the surface. By the time the guinea pigs have chewed the cardboard, they will have adapted to the wire. Where animals are kept permanently on wire, a large, solid-bottomed tray or pan containing contact bedding and placed in a section of the pen will permit some relief from constant exposure to the mesh.

Guinea pigs should be kept out of direct sunlight (Richardson, 1992; Sirois, 1989) ideally at temperatures of 21 ± 1°C although they will tolerate a temperature range of 16–24°C (Harkness and Wagner, 1989; Manning *et al.*, 1984; Percy, 1984; Anderson, 1984). Relative humidity should be kept at 40–70% (Harkness and Wagner, 1989; Manning *et al.*, 1984; Percy, 1984; Anderson, 1984). Guinea pigs can withstand cold temperatures provided they are gradually acclimatised, are housed in groups and are provided with shelter and plenty of bedding. However, they should not be kept outdoors all year round in temperate climates but, if not kept indoors, should be kept in an enclosed area such as a garage or shed. Pups are at risk of fatal chilling at temperatures less than 17°C. Low temperature extremes, as well as high humidity, will also promote respiratory disease. Guinea pigs are less resistant to overheating, and temperatures in excess of 27°C may cause sterility and heat prostration. Guinea pigs housed indoors should be provided with a minimum of 10–12 h of light per day.

Although guinea pigs are fairly hardy and can tolerate a diversity of living conditions, housing enclosures must be kept dry, free of dramatic fluctuations in temperature and relative humidity and be adequately ventilated, but protected from drafts. Environmental stressors can be profoundly immunosuppressive and poor sanitation, overcrowding, improper temperature and humidity control and even a simple change in the location of a cage can cause stress that can contribute to disease susceptibility. Where bedding is used, it should be changed at least twice weekly to prevent detectable ammonia production. Ammonia formed through the interaction of excreted urea with bacteria in the bedding is immunosuppressive and irritating to the upper respiratory tract. Cages, including food and water, must be protected from wild rodents and insects. Scale can be removed by scrubbing with acetic acid (i.e. vinegar) or a weak solution of muriatic acid (i.e. swimming pool cleanser) prior to washing, but acids will corrode poor quality metals.

A pen of approximate size 1 × 1 × 0.35 m is adequate for several animals. The pen should be kept out of direct sunlight, away from potential predators and moved to fresh patches as needed. Fresh water should always be available. Precautions must be taken to ensure that the animals are not grazed on areas exposed to automobile exhaust, herbicides, lawn chemicals, or animal droppings which carries the risk of paratenic or aberrant parasitism.

Enrichment

Guinea pigs are social, cautiously exploratory, gnawing animals that live furtively in burrows and in deep grass. Consequently, attempts at environmental enrichment should be directed at satisfying behaviour that would be expressed under these conditions. Guinea pigs are generally sedentary and are unlikely to use devices intended for exercise such as running wheels. With the exception of immature animals, voluntary explorative behaviours are rare because guinea pigs are suspicious of novel objects. Pups will explore and play and enjoy running around and climbing low barriers placed in the cage, but these behaviours are outgrown by adulthood.

Guinea pigs of all ages enjoy burrowing in large quantities of loose hay which offers protective insulation for animals kept outdoors and may provide a distraction that reduces barbering. The feeding of hay is controversial from a nutritional standpoint and hay is messy indoors. The need for seclusion can also be met by using a 20–25 cm high nest box with a 10 × 15 cm entry or large bore PVC pipe tunnels. Gnawing behaviours can be satisfied by providing clean poplar, willow or fruitwood twigs. During periods of temperate weather, guinea pigs can be grazed outdoors on green grass and clover in a covered mesh pen. Dandelion consumption should be minimised as it will cause diuresis and diarrhoea.

The most enriching provision for guinea pigs is that of companionship (Anderson, 1987). Clients owning pet guinea pigs should be encouraged to keep single-sex groups in order to avoid production of large numbers of offspring. To prevent fighting, males kept in groups should have been raised together since weaning or, less ideally because of the anaesthetic risk, be castrated. To introduce new animals into an existing social group with minimal trauma, move the group to neutral and novel surroundings and dab mentholated vapour rub on the chin of each animal. Solitary guinea pigs will bond closely with a human and close interaction with a human caretaker is an adequate substitute for a conspecific. Guinea pigs should not be exposed to other rodents, rabbits, dogs or cats because they are stressed by the novelty, are likely to panic and are subject to attack, even by rabbits. Additionally, guinea pigs are highly susceptible to pneumonia caused by *Bordetella bronchiseptica* which can be carried subclinically by dogs, cats and rabbits.

Nutrition

Guinea pigs are naturally herbivorous and related wild species live on a range of grasses, seeds, fruits and roots. The domesticated guinea pig will thrive on a freshly milled, properly stored, pelleted, complete commercial diet that has been formulated specifically for guinea pigs. Pelleted diets adequate for other rodents, such as rats and mice, are generally too large and firm for guinea pigs and do not contain vitamin C. Rabbit chow, while devoid of vitamin C, also contains excessive levels of vitamin D. With the exception

of scurvy, nutritional diseases are rare in guinea pigs fed complete commercial diets.

As a rule, guinea pig rations should contain 18–20% protein, 12–16% fibre, 3–4% fat and 0.8–3.0 g/kg vitamin C. Vitamin C deficiency is the most common but also the most easily preventable disease of the domestic guinea pig. Guinea pigs, like primates, lack L-gluconolactone oxidase in the glucose–vitamin C pathway, cannot store vitamin C (ascorbic acid) for appreciable periods and must have a dietary source of ascorbic acid. Vitamin C is essential in hydroxylase reactions forming hydroxyproline and hydroxylysine which are necessary in maintaining collagen molecules and for the catabolism of cholesterol to bile acids. On a body weight basis, the daily dietary requirement for vitamin C is 10 mg/kg for maintenance and 30 mg/kg for pregnancy.

The importance of vitamin C in maintaining normal health cannot be over-emphasised and should be reviewed with every client. The disease is entirely preventable by feeding fresh, commercially milled guinea pig diet. To prevent premature vitamin C degradation, fortified diets must be stored in a cool, dry, well-ventilated area and be fed within 90 days of milling. Because 50% of the activity of vitamin C is lost in the feed in 6 weeks, owners purchasing food from pet or feed shops should regularly buy small quantities that have been on the shelf for no longer than 4–6 weeks from the milling date rather than buying large quantities that are subsequently stored for extended periods in the home. Diets purchased from pet shops are often stored for prolonged periods under dubious conditions and may not have verifiable milling dates. In cases where quality pelleted diet cannot be obtained reliably, daily fortification of the drinking water with 0.2–1.0 g/l vitamin C is a valuable preventive practice that should be recommended to clients. The highest concentrations should be given when the water source may be hard or alkaline. Vitamin C given to excess is not toxic and is harmlessly excreted in the urine. Fresh solutions of vitamin C must be prepared daily using deionised or distilled water because vitamin C is oxidised by copper leached from plumbing and the aqueous solution is highly unstable and loses its potency within 24 h. The activity of vitamin C decreases as much as 50% in a 24-h period in water in an open container and even faster if metal or organic material is present or the room temperature is elevated.

Because many metals will accelerate the decomposition of the vitamin, water bottles should be used with sippers made of stainless steel or pyrex, but not glass, which will shatter when gnawed. Soft metals, such as brass, are also destroyed by gnawing. Guinea pigs suffering from deficiency will respond dramatically to daily tissue saturation doses (50–100 mg/kg) of vitamin C given by injection in the hospital or orally at home. Oral multivitamin drops carry the risk of overdosage of other vitamins and should only be used for periods of a few days. Complete clinical resolution of signs takes approximately 7 days. Because vitamin C is retained in the tissues for a maximum of 4 days, anorexia from any cause carries the risk of contributory scurvy and the stress of illness will also increase the metabolic demand for vitamin C. Consequently, all ill animals should receive vitamin C supplementation.

Guinea pigs will eat a wide variety of foodstuffs, but in general reject sweet, salty or bitter foods. They are particularly fond of alfalfa, good quality hay or green grass. Additionally, fresh kale, cabbage, chicory, peppers and spinach are rich in vitamin C and are often recommended as dietary supplements. However, it is not necessary to supplement a good quality, complete commercial pelleted diet with hay, vegetables or minerals. Roughage supplementation will increase the importance of feeding a high quality pelleted diet because the intake of vitamin C may be reduced. Hay is also messy in the home and often difficult to acquire in urban areas. Coarse hay may be abrasive to the oral mucosa and facilitate bacterial infections. Alfalfa and many other forages are high in calcium which will increase hypercalciuria and compound problems of cage scale while predisposing to urolithiasis.

Soiled, damp or mouldy hay may be a source of maldigestion, aflatoxicosis, mucormycosis and oestrogens. Mucormycosis, caused by *Absidia ramosa* and *Absidia corymbifera*, causes mesenteric or cervical lymphadenopathy, while *Aspergillus flavus* and *Aspergillus fumigatus* can cause aflatoxicosis, allergy, pneumonia, cancer, or asymptomatic infection. In weanling guinea pigs, in particular, aflatoxins may cause high mortality in association with abdominal pain, listlessness, ruffled fur, intussusception and hepatic lipidosis. Breeding sows will show stillbirths and deliver weakened newborns. Consequently, roughage supplementation with loose or cubed hay is indicated only for animals fed diets containing less than 16% fibre or for animals kept out of doors. Guinea pigs should never be fed grass clippings as they cause bloat and indigestion.

Preparing and feeding fresh produce is a time-consuming and expensive source of vitamin C that also carries the risk of bacterial (i.e. *Salmonella, Yersinia*), parasitic (i.e. trematodes) and chemical contamination. Although guinea pigs will consume a variety of vegetables and fruits, if fed in large amounts, these foodstuffs may overwhelm the digestive system and cause diarrhoea. Some foodstuffs may be directly deleterious. For instance, peanuts may be contaminated with aflatoxins, lettuce contains laudanum which may be toxic, cabbage may contain goitrogens and certain greens (i.e. spinach, beet tops) and vegetables are high in calcium and oxalates that may promote urolithiasis. Supplementation of the diet with fresh vegetables rich in vitamin C is recommended only in cases where a quality commercial diet cannot be obtained regularly, ascorbic acid supplementation in the drinking water is impractical, or where establishing a diversified diet is important from a medical perspective such as the use of bananas as a vehicle for oral medication. If this is the case, 20–30 g of fresh produce should be given daily and care must be taken to ensure that the source, selection and storage of greens or fruit is of a means that will not introduce pathogens or intoxicants. An acceptable criterion for selection is to feed only those materials considered fit for human consumption; discarded greens from groceries or institutional kitchens should be avoided. Perishable foodstuffs, as well as twigs provided for gnawing, can be cleaned by soaking for 10 min in a freshly prepared solution of 4 ml household bleach per litre of tap water (200 ppm free chlorine) and then rinsed.

Guinea pigs will eat their faeces, although the quantity of faeces ingested and the contribution to total dietary needs are unknown. Coprophagy is a source of B vitamins, vitamin K and probably serves to conserve minerals. Faecal pellets are usually eaten directly from the anus, but obese or pregnant animals may eat the pellet from the floor. Young animals eat the faeces of adults, usually the dam, and thereby inoculate their intestinal tract with autochthonous flora. If coprophagy is prevented, guinea pigs may lose weight, digest less fibre and develop marginal mineral deficiencies (Hintz, 1969).

Intake of food and water will vary with the ambient temperature, breeding status, food and water wastage and relative humidity. As a general rule, mature guinea pigs will eat 60–70 g/kg/day, but growing and pregnant animals will consume double or triple those levels, respectively. Guinea pigs consume feed in several small meals during the day and night interspersed with rest periods and generally must be fed *ad libitum*, because they do not adjust readily to restricted meal feeding. Scattering feed and defaecating in the feeder are common guinea pig vices. These problems can be reduced by using a J-type feed hopper with inward lips. Animals that habitually waste food can be fed meals two or three times daily, but body weight and food consumption should be monitored closely. Food hoppers must be cleaned frequently to prevent the accumulation of stale or contaminated food, and soiled hay and perishable foods should be removed daily. To reduce aggression, two or more feeders should be provided to animals housed in groups.

A supply of fresh drinking water should be available at all times. As a rule of thumb, water consumption will range from 100–200 ml/kg/day. However, guinea pigs are notoriously playful with their drinking water and wastage may increase the demand up to 400 ml/kg/day. This activity may cause excessive wetting of bedding or even floods. Bowls, pans and crocks should not be used for guinea pig waterers if solid-bottomed cages with bedding are used because the waterers readily become contaminated with faeces and bedding. Because guinea pigs readily learn to drink from sippers, water should be

provided in a suspended inverted glass or plastic bottle with a stainless steel sipper tube. Guinea pigs gnaw on the end of the sipper to drink and will mix food and water in their mouths and expectorate the slurry back into the sipper tube. This will discolour the drinking water, block the tube or cause it to drip. Sipper tubes with ball bearings in the tip help reduce this problem, but water bottles may need to be rinsed and refilled one or more times daily and should be cleaned at least 2–3 times weekly. Although automatic watering can be used advantageously, guinea pigs may need to be shown how to drink from the valves. With guinea pigs it is important to use valves located outside the cage or other devices to divert spilled or leaked water to the outside of the cage. A further advantage of automatic waterers is that they ensure that guinea pigs are not without water for long periods, as may occur after they characteristically drain their water bottle. Automatic waterers must be checked frequently, cleaned and flushed periodically.

Water deprivation in the face of seemingly adequate water supply can occur when animals are presented novel drinking devices, the device is out of reach, the device is unworkable due to air or foreign material in the sipper tube, or the water tastes or smells different. Territorialism on the part of dominant animals may prevent more timid animals from drinking.

Consistent feeding practices are as important as the diet. Guinea pigs are fastidious eaters that establish food preferences early in life. Sudden changes in the diet or the way in which it is presented, such as using a new feeder or changing from a water pan to a bottle, may cause the animal to stop eating or drinking, with serious medical implications. Consequently, any changes that are done such as replacing a waterer, converting from vitamin C supplementation in the diet to the drinking water, or eliminating forages or vegetables should be done gradually. Changing the dietary habits of a guinea pig requires patience and acceptance may require several weeks. If a diverse diet is to be fed, it should be done so early in life and consistently thereafter. When a foodstuff is removed from the diet, guinea pigs will develop a rigid aversion to it over time (Harper, 1976).

Handling, Injections, Specimen Collection

Handling

Guinea pigs should always be restrained using both hands (Fig. 4.3). One hand should gently, but securely, grasp the dorsothorax with the fingers on one side and the thumb on the contralateral side at the level of the pectoral limbs. The second hand should support the hindquarters. This is particularly important with large or pregnant animals as, if suspended from one hand they may suffer internal injuries. The same grip may be used to immobilise the animal, but the hind legs should be grasped and extended while the animal is placed in dorsal recumbency on a flat surface. If animals become fractious, subdued lighting and covering the eyes often have a calming effect.

Among small rodents, guinea pigs are easy to examine clinically. They should be brought to the clinic in a small, covered box with a minimum of bedding. This provides security to the guinea pig in the intimidating environment of the waiting room and will protect it from direct contact with potential pathogens. A cardboard shoe box is ideal for these purposes.

Injection

Subcutaneous injection is the most frequently used and easiest injection route for guinea pigs. The method for a subcutaneous injection is the same as that for other species. A 25 gauge needle should be inserted under the lifted loose skin over the scapulae and parallel with the underlying muscle. As the skin of the guinea pig is very loose, subcutaneous injections of up to 35 ml can be made in a wide range of sites. Subcutaneous administration of fluids will be facilitated by the use of hyaluronidase (0.2–1.0 U/ml fluids) permitting larger volumes to be given painlessly in a solitary site.

No method of intravenous injection is entirely satisfactory in the guinea pig. In general, vascu-

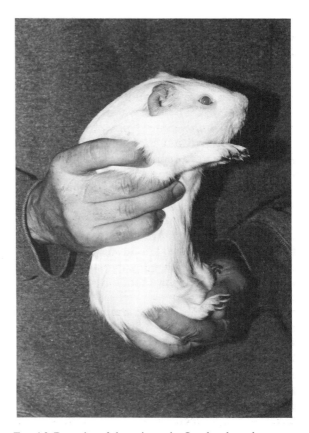

FIG. 4.3 Restraint of the guinea pig. One hand gently grasps the dorsothorax and the second hand supports the hindquarters.

lar access is poor due to the friability, mobility, short length and small size of vessels, and injections or catheterisation are technically challenging. Except for injection of the vessels of the pelvic limbs, sedation or anaesthesia will be required in almost all other cases of intravenous injection. For pelvic limb injection, the guinea pig can be comfortably immobilised by wrapping it in a towel with only the hind legs exposed. Injection volumes of up to 1 ml may be given to sedated adult animals via the marginal ear veins using a 26–30 gauge needle. The injection should be done in a warm room. Local heat and topical application of alcohol will help to distend the vein, which can be further enlarged by slight pressure at the base of the ear. Veins can be discerned from arteries by blanching the ear with general digital pressure and then monitoring the refilling pattern. The caudal branch of the medial saphenous vein of mature animals is visible without occlusion following clipping of the hair on the medial pelvic limb and can be entered with a 23–25 gauge needle (Carraway and Gray, 1989). The lateral saphenous vein can be injected at the point 1 cm proximal to the hock (Sutherland and Festing, 1987). However, the vessel is friable and mobile and access usually requires anaesthesia and a surgical cutdown. In extreme circumstances, attempts can be made to inject the dorsolateral penile vein of an anaesthetised boar. In most cases, either SC or IP administration will be adequate substitutes for IV injection. However, if chronic venous access is absolutely essential, a jugular catheter should be placed following aseptic cutdown under anaesthesia. Alternatively, fluids can be given intraosseously by inserting a spinal needle into the femur through the trochanteric fossa.

For IP injection, the restrained guinea pig should be held on its back with the head slightly lower than the hindquarters to allow the stomach and intestines to fall cranially. A second individual should insert a 21–23 gauge needle at a 45° angle through the skin and abdominal wall slightly to the right of the midline approximately 2.5 cm in front of the pubis. For animals in poor health, a less stressful technique is to maintain them in a quadruped stance and gently insert a 22 gauge catheter into the lateral aspect of the right mid-abdomen. After removal of the stylet, appropriate positioning should be confirmed by aspiration and then warmed fluids can be administered. Volumes of up to 20 ml can be given by this route.

IM injections are frequently associated with self-mutilation and are discouraged. Where intramuscular injection is essential, injections of a volume not to exceed 0.3 ml should be given into the quadriceps muscle approximately 1 cm proximal to the knee with a 22–27 gauge needle.

Oral administration

Small volumes of fluid, not to exceed 5 ml, can be given gently by pipette or dropper to awake animals. Larger volumes of liquid can be given by stomach tube or small bore endoscope. Various designs of tube can be used. Soft pliable rubber or plastic tubes 1.5–6 mm in diameter can be used to dose lightly anaesthetised cavies. The tube should be passed from the mouth down the oesophagus into the stomach. In cases where gastric intubation is not obvious, proper placement can be confirmed by injecting air through the tube while auscultating the stomach. Where sedation is undesirable, a two-person technique can be used where one individual restrains the animal and a second passes the oral catheter through parallel holes in the side of a syringe barrel that has been inserted in the space between the incisors and premolars. Alternatively, one person can gavage a conscious animal using a stainless steel, ball-tipped gavage cannula. A 8–10 cm curved 12 gauge catheter with a blunted, 6 mm ball tip can be introduced through the interdental space and advanced gently by rotating it over the tongue and into the oesophagus. Drugs can be given using drinking water or feed as vehicles; however, this is imprecise. Depending on their level of consumption, guinea pigs may be over- or under-dosed. Medicated food or water should only be used where animals are consuming normally and should not be used where healthy animals may consume it. To achieve an effective dose, the animal must be consuming food and water, and drug concentrations should be at maximal safe levels (based on estimated consumption), freshly prepared and renewed on a daily basis, with all residual feed or water being discarded.

Topical treatment

The application of topical drugs is of little value, unless grooming is prevented by an Elizabethan collar, because they will be inadvertantly consumed. Guinea pigs adapt readily to bathing such as that required to treat ectoparasitism. The guinea pig should be placed in a tub or sink containing warm water to a depth of 5 cm with towelling on the bottom to give traction. Prior to bathing, protective ointment should be placed in the eyes to prevent chemical keratitis. After bathing, the animal should be rinsed and dried gently with a towel or warm air blower.

Specimen Collection

Small quantities of blood (0.5 ml or less) may be collected by nicking an ear vein using a mechanically activated lancet centered over a vessel. Cutting a nail will give up to 0.25 ml blood, however, nail bed laceration may be restricted in some localities, may cause chronic discomfort and should only be used in cases where vascular access by other routes have been unsuccessful. Samples of up to 3 ml may be collected by venepuncture of the saphenous veins with a 25 gauge needle as described above, but these procedures are complicated by the same problems that are encountered in IV injection. Jugular venepuncture can be attempted using techniques similar to those employed for cats. The sedated guinea pig should be placed in ventral recumbency with the forelimbs extended below the edge of a table and the head and neck extended directly upward. A 22–23 gauge needle can then be inserted in the jugular furrow. Cardiac puncture and venepuncture of the cranial vena cava are not recommended due to the attendant risk of subsequent internal bleeding. The volume of blood collected should never exceed the equivalent of 1% of the body weight.

Faecal samples can be collected from the cage or directly from the anus. Urine collection can be done by manual expression of the bladder, cystocentesis or a specialised metabolism cage.

Radiographic Techniques

Radiographic techniques should approximate those used for cats. Stockinettes or radiolucent plastic cylinders are useful for restraint of unanaesthetised guinea pigs.

Diseases—An Introduction

The limited number of pets per family serves to reduce the incidence of infectious diseases in guinea pigs. Consequently, ageing diseases, traumatic injuries or conditions related to inadequate care are likely to be seen in pets, while infectious diseases are more common in colonies and in show animals. The guinea pig is subject to relatively few viral or helminthic diseases. The frequency of neoplasia in the general population of guinea pigs ranges from 0.06 to 0.30% (Manning *et al.*, 1984; Debout *et al.*, 1987; Manning, 1976). With the exception of skin tumours and malignancies of the haematopoietic system, neoplasia is virtually nonexistent in animals less than 4–5 years of age, but, in aged animals, the incidence of cancer approaches 15–30%. Inbred animals account for 75% of all reported cases and most cases of lymphoreticular neoplasia. In non-inbred guinea pigs under 3 years of age, the skin and heart account for almost all cases of neoplasia. One third of all neoplasms are malignant, but metastatic disease is almost unheard of and most neoplasms are solitary. The reason for the low incidence of cancer and metastases in guinea pigs remains unresolved, but Foa–Kurloff cells and serum asparaginase, uniquely found in guinea pigs, may be protective (Manning *et al.*, 1984; Wriston and Yellin, 1973).

Many diseases are the consequence of improper care and a thorough review of the animal's normal habitat and diet, as well as the owner's husbandry practices, must be done. The type of cageing, particularly with regard to wire flooring and its location (i.e. indoors versus outdoors, in direct sunlight, near an air vent or door, temperature ranges) will aid in identifying potential stressors. Thorough questioning regarding the type and source of feed including storage practices, frequency of purchase, vitamin C supplementation and the feeding of hay, vegetables or table scraps is paramount to the complete history. Dermatological disease and malocclusion, two of the most common afflictions of guinea pigs, are often a consequence of marginal diets. A history of handling by small children will aid a diagnosis of trauma and contact with other pets may be suggestive of interspecies disease transmission. If multiple guinea pigs are owned, questioning the owner regarding the health status of other conspecifics and the addition of new animals will be useful in ruling-out infectious diseases. Although breed disease predilections have not been established, questioning regarding the known genetics, particularly with regard to inbreeding is important. Cross-breeding with Abyssinians may give the artificial appearance of unthriftiness, for example.

Initially, guinea pigs should simply be examined for general appearance and behaviour in a quiet room in a walled container such as their transport box or a deep, dry sink. Normal guinea pigs will show prominent, bright eyes, a nose free of exudates and a smooth, regular coat of low lustre hair. An animal in ill health will be inactive and appear hunch-backed with piloerection and dull eyes. The body temperature can be assessed with a rectal thermometer and all external body orifices, except the mouth and auditory canals, are easy to examine. With respect to disease incidence, the respiratory and digestive systems are the most commonly affected.

Body weight monitoring is valuable for non-invasive detection of early abnormalities and it should be done in the home and clinic. Weight loss may go undetected for an extended period of time in long-haired animals that are not handled, because the hair coat obscures the loss of condition. Malocclusion and hypovitaminosis C are the most common causes of weight loss. However, neophobia of feed or feeding devices, infectious diseases, neoplasia and end stage organ failure may also cause loss of weight. For optimal health and production, nonpregnant sows should be maintained at a weight of at least 500 g, but no more than 900 g. Although body condition is relative and is influenced by numerous factors including age and inheritance, obesity should be suspected in any unbred sow weighing over 900 g.

Although many diseases are preventable through good husbandry, guinea pig fanciers will often only bring an animal to a veterinarian after unsuccessful treatment attempts on their part and pet owners often wait until late in the course of disease, when the prognosis for response to therapy is poor, before seeking veterinary attention. Consequently, the emphasis to clients concerning disease control must be on prevention rather than treatment. Where treatment is attempted, the clinician should be forewarned of several caveats. Foremost, doses of pharmaceuticals for guinea pigs are largely empirical and usually a product of shared anecdotal experiences. In many cases, published dosages are based on limited, uncontrolled clinical trials.

Rarely have such dosages been determined using valid pharmacologic studies. In general, smaller animals require more drug given more frequently to mimic the regimen of larger species and drug dosages for small rodents that are extrapolated linearly from dog and cat doses will usually be underestimated. Drug dosage extrapolation between species is complicated and, if generalised, may be imprecise and risk unforeseen toxicities. However, in cases of emergency, it may be the only option. In such instances, pharmacokinetic equivalency may be approximated by extrapolating on a body surface area to body weight ratio basis. By this method, doses given to guinea pigs should be approximately 5 times that of humans and 3 times that of dogs per unit body weight.

From a clinical standpoint **the guinea pig's marked, often lethal sensitivity to antibiotic therapy, cannot be overemphasised.** The anaerobic flora is exquisitely sensitive to antibiotics with a Gram-positive spectrum, particularly those with biliary excretion (George, 1984; Percy *et al.*, 1993). Disturbances of the flora caused by antibiotics may cause an overcolonisation of clostridia, especially *Clostridium difficile*. At the time of weaning, the lack of development of appropriate digestive enzymes coupled with dietary transition may cause maldigestion and changes in the intestinal milieu that promote clostridial overgrowth. The sequence of events is alteration of the normal flora, colonisation of the bowel by pathogenic clostridia and elaboration of toxin leading to clinical disease and death. There is considerable variation and inconsistency in antibiotics associated with this syndrome and the spore-contaminated environment plays a substantive role in the disease.

Antibiotics alone will not cause disease in pathogen-free guinea pigs (Percy, 1984). In the practical setting of the clinic, however, the use of penicillins, ampicillin, bacitracin, erythromycin, spiramycin, lincomycin, gentamicin, clindamycin and vancomycin at therapeutic doses carries the risk of causing the syndrome. Cephalosporins probably carry the same level of risk as penicillins, but have not been incriminated and tetracyclines have been variably implicated. Even the use of topical antibiotics should be considered carefully, because these agents can be consumed in the course of grooming. Antibiotics that appear to have a low risk of inducing the syndrome include chloramphenicol, aminoglycosides, sulphonamides and the quinolones. However, the use of antibiotics should never be cavalier and this is especially so with guinea pigs. Treatment on a colony-wide basis or prescription of antibiotics without a definite clinical indication is a recipe for disaster. Where antibiotics are used therapeutically, concomitant dietary supplementation with lactobacilli (i.e. live yogurt), B vitamins and vitamin K should be done and continued for 5 days after antibiotics are halted.

Guinea pigs do not adapt easily to changes in their routine or environment and should be hospitalised only if critically necessary. The usual diet and water bottle should accompany all admitted patients. Supportive care, including forced-feeding, must be given in all cases of decreased food and water consumption. Oxygen therapy and quiet rest, while minimising the stress of handling, are important (Collins, 1994).

Unfortunately, due to small size, difficulties in gaining access to blood vessels, the fulminant nature of many diseases and challenges in treatment, many definitive diagnoses are made at necropsy.

Figure 4.8 at the end of the chapter summarises the clinical signs, diagnoses and treatments for the diseases discussed below. An additional figure provides an alphabetical listing of clinical signs with differential diagnoses clinicians should consider.

Diseases of the Respiratory System

Healthy guinea pigs breathe through the nose, while laboured or mouth breathing indicates respiratory distress consistent with pneumonia, overheating, vitamin C deficiency, gastric torsion, or injuries sustained from improper handling such as pneumothorax and diaphragmatic hernia. Pneumonia, primarily that caused by bacteria, is the most frequent cause of death in guinea pigs. Guinea pigs are easily palpated and auscultated, although the heart rate is very rapid. The most accurate method of diagnosis of respiratory conditions is through radiography and cytology and bacterial culture of exudates. Radiography is helpful in characterising pulmonary lesions and ruling-out pneumothorax, diaphragmatic hernia and gastric torsion/volvulus as differential diagnoses. Transtracheal washes are difficult and may be highly stressful for all involved. Consequently, antemortem diagnosis of bacterial pneumonia may have to be based on clinical signs and less ideal nasal or conjunctival discharges.

The principles of pneumonia treatment are the same as for other species, but, unfortunately, the response to treatment is uniformly poor. Fluid therapy, quiet rest in a well ventilated, but draught-free cage, oxygen therapy, appropriate antibiotics and topical mentholated vapour rub should be used. Consideration should be given to nebulisation of antibiotics.

Bacterial Diseases

Bordetellosis

Agent. The causative agent is *Bordetella bronchiseptica*, a Gram-negative aerobic bacterium and the most common cause of pneumonia in guinea pigs. It is distributed worldwide and transmitted by direct contact with diseased animals, aerosol, carrier hosts and contaminated fomites. The incubation period is 3–7 days. *Bordetella* preferentially colonise ciliated regions of the respiratory tract and cause disease opportunistically in animals receiving suboptimal care. Haematogenous dissemination to distant organs can occur. Clinical disease tends to occur most commonly in the winter and most frequently in younger animals. Infection in a colony is maintained by carriers.

Hosts. Dogs, cats, rabbits, pigs, nonhuman primates, rats, birds and humans are natural hosts for the bacterium.

Clinical signs. Guinea pigs frequently die of sepsis without prodrome or may have vague and nonspecific signs such as fever, anorexia and weight loss. Infrequently, dyspnoea, sneezing, conjunctivitis, mucopurulent to blood-tinged rhinorrhoea, deafness and vaginal discharge secondary to metritis may be seen. Pregnant sows will either die, abort or deliver stillborn pups. Clinically silent, but palpable, pyosalpinx has been documented.

Diagnosis. The diagnosis of respiratory diseases should be based on bacterial culture and sensitivity obtained from transtracheal washes, nasal or conjunctival discharges, or necropsy specimens. Radiography will demonstrate bronchopneumonia and is useful as a screening tool for subclinical otitis media suggestive of infection.

Control / treatment. Treatment based on the results of a bacterial culture and sensitivity may give a symptomatic cure, but usually results either in a carrier state or eventual relapse of clinical disease. Enrofloxacin, gentamicin, sulphamethoxazole/trimethoprim or chloramphenicol are generally effective against *Bordetella*. Supportive care should include parenteral fluids, vitamin C, nebulisation therapy and forced-feeding. Dietary and management practices should be reviewed to correct problems, especially vitamin C deficiency.

In cases where guinea pigs are at high risk of exposure to *Bordetella*, IM injection of 0.2 ml of canine or porcine bordetellosis vaccine can be given. A booster should be given 2–3 weeks later followed by semi-annual to annual revaccination. Anecdotally, it has been reported that application of several drops of a canine intranasal vaccine will provide similar protection (Harkness, 1994). Vaccines given by injection must not contain aluminium hydroxide as guinea pigs may have a sensitive reaction. While vaccination will prevent clinical disease, it does not prevent the development of an upper respiratory tract carrier state. In a herd situation, depopulation, disinfection and replacement of stock are recommended.

Chlamydiosis

Agent. Disease caused by *Chlamydia psittaci*, an obligately parasitic coccoid bacterium, is common in many breeding colonies, but is typically confined to guinea pigs aged 2–8 weeks. Adult animals infrequently show clinical signs, although active immunity is inconsistent and usually short-lived. The mode of transmission in guinea pigs is unknown, but inhalation and direct sexual contact are most likely. The incubation period is 2–4 days.

Hosts. Birds are the usual reservoir, but the agent can be enzootic in guinea pig breeding colonies. Guinea pigs have not been shown to be a source of infection for humans.

Clinical signs. In most cases, infection is inapparent, but in rare cases there may be hyperaemia of the lid margins or conjunctivitis with epiphora. Involvement is generally bilateral. In solitary animals, the disease is self-limiting and heals in 3–4 weeks. In colonies, there is a cyclic recurrence of conjunctivitis. Mortality and abortion only occur in conjunction with concomitant bacterial pneumonia or septicaemia.

Diagnosis. Intracytoplasmic chlamydial inclusions can be demonstrated on conjunctival scrapings using immunofluorescent antibodies or Machiavello's or Giemsa stains. Diagnosis by culture is impractical, because *Chlamydia* require specialised cultivation techniques.

Control / treatment. Because the disease is generally self-limiting, treatment is not indicated. Topical tetracycline ophthalmic ointments may be used several times daily.

Viral Diseases

Adenoviral pneumonia

Agent. Adenovirus is a DNA virus, family Adenoviridae, that is distributed worldwide and is transmitted horizontally. The incubation period is 5–10 days, but disease is typically expressed as an inapparent infection with low contagion. Induction of clinical disease is multifactorial and requires a stressor, such as inhalation anaesthesia or immunodeficiency. Additionally, clinical disease does not occur in healthy adult guinea pigs, but rather affects neonates, weanlings and aged animals. Although morbidity is infrequent, the case fatality rate approaches 100%. Unlike most other viruses, adenovirus does not require a bacterial co-pathogen and, acting alone, it can cause acute, fatal disease.

Hosts. Guinea pig adenovirus appears to be species-specific.

Clinical signs. Generally, adenovirus infection is subclinical, but there may be sporadic sudden deaths without prodrome in juveniles. In rare cases, dyspnoea, nasal discharge and depression may be observed prior to death.

Diagnosis. Diagnosis of exposure can be made retrospectively from acute and convalescent titres or, due to the high case fatality rate, at necropsy. Histopathology will show bronchitis/bronchiolitis with typical intranuclear inclusion bodies.

Control / treatment. Treatment is supportive and generally futile due to the unexpected and fulminant nature of the disease, but broad-spectrum antibiotics may be effective in preventing secondary bacterial infection.

Inapparent Respiratory Infections

Several rodent paramyxoviruses, Sendai virus, Simian Virus 5 (SV5) and Pneumonia Virus of Mice (PVM), constitute the most common naturally occurring virus infections of guinea pigs. Virus transmission via aerosol is common in guinea pigs exposed to mice. *Mycoplasma caviae* is distributed worldwide and colonises the nasopharynx and vagina, but does not cause clinical disease and is of unknown pathogenicity. *Pneumocystis carinii* commonly colonises the lungs. Infection with *Mycoplasma* and viruses

is self-limiting and asymptomatic, except for seroconversion, unless complicated by secondary bacterial pneumonia. *P. carinii* only causes disease characterised by wasting and respiratory distress in the face of severe immunosuppression.

Diseases of the Digestive System

Examination of the digestive system should show the intestinal loops and caecum to be free of gas and the anus should be clean and dry. An oral examination is mandatory for animals in poor health, especially those with anorexia, hypersalivation and signs referable to the gastrointestinal system, but requires restraint with light inhalation anaesthesia and the use of a lighted otoscope. The dental arcade should be symmetrical and normal teeth will have smooth occlusal surfaces that are worn evenly on both the mandibular and maxillary arcades and labial and lingual aspects. Sharp edges or points, buccal lacerations, oral discharges or tongue entrapment all indicate malocclusion.

Bacterial Diseases

Clostridiosis

Agent. *Clostridium difficile* (common) and *Clostridium perfringens* Type E (rare), two obligate, anaerobic, spore-forming, toxin-producing Gram-positive bacilli from the family Bacillaceae, cause disease in guinea pigs. Disease most frequently occurs as a consequence of antibiotic administration or other stressors, such as surgery/anaesthesia, corticosteroid administration, fasting or pregnancy, that cause alterations in the protective normal flora of the bowel. Natural infection is thought to be by ingestion of spores from other animals or the spore-contaminated environment by grooming, coprophagy or feeding. However, clostridia can be asymptomatic components of the faecal flora. Once the gastrointestinal tract has been colonised and the protective flora has been breached, the pathogenic clostridia produce cytotoxins and enterotoxins that cause clinical disease.

Hosts. Humans, rabbits, hamsters and guinea pigs are among the species that harbour *C. difficile*, the cause of pseudomembranous colitis in humans. Rats, mice, dogs and cats do not appear to develop clinical disease. *C. perfringens* Type E causes fatal enterotoxaemia in lambs, but does not cause disease in humans.

Clinical signs. Nonspecific signs such as anorexia, lethargy, piloerection and hypothermia precede ileus, caecal bloat and fulminant diarrhoea. In some cases, there may be flaccid hindlimb paralysis (Madden *et al.*, 1970). The clinical course is rapid, with deaths occurring 3–8 days after antibiotics are halted or within 1–3 days of the onset of diarrhoea.

Diagnosis. Because clostridia can be normal inhabitants of the gastrointestinal tract, diagnosis must be based on culture of the organism and demonstration of cytotoxin in the faeces. Diagnosis can be made presumptively based upon a history of antibiotic administration, development of clinical signs and demonstration of abundant Gram-positive bacilli on a faecal Gram-stain.

Control / treatment. Treatment is generally ineffective and the disease is almost always fatal, but long term, systemic administration of either cephalosporins, metronidazole or vancomycin combined with oral cholestyramine (100 mg/ml in the drinking water) and complete daily cage cleaning should be attempted. Faecal cocktails from normal cohorts or live yogurt can be given in an attempt to restore the normal faecal balance.

Colibacillosis

Agent. *Escherichia coli*, a Gram-negative, facultatively anaerobic coccobacillus in the family Enterobacteriaceae, is found most commonly overproliferating in conjunction with clostridiosis. Although *E. coli* is of dubious pathogenicity in the gastrointestinal tract of guinea pigs, fatal enteropathies may be seen following faecal–oral transmission in juvenile animals kept under sub-standard conditions. Following either direct contact or haematogenous spread, *E. coli* may cause mastitis in lactating sows. It may also cause cystitis in adult animals following ascending contamination of the urinary tract.

Hosts. Although widespread in most species, *E. coli* is not normally an inhabitant of the guinea pig gastrointestinal tract.

Clinical signs. Anorexia, weight loss, unkempt appearance, hypothermia and diarrhoea occur over a 4–9 day course, culminating in death. Fulminant fatal mastitis occurs in sows maintained in heavily soiled environments (Kinkler *et al.*, 1976).

Diagnosis. Bacterial culture of faeces, peritoneal fluid, mesenteric lymph nodes, spleen, liver or blood are diagnostic.

Control / treatment. Prevention of disease is through good husbandry techniques. Treatment is generally unsuccessful, but should include fluid and electrolyte replacement therapy and administration of enrofloxacin or chloramphenicol.

Tyzzer's disease

Agent. The causative agent, *Clostridium piliforme*, an unclassified Gram-negative obligate intracellular bacterium having vegetative and spore forms, causes disease most commonly in recent weanlings. Disease is especially common in the face of crowding, poor sanitation or deprivation of food or water. Natural infection is thought to be by ingestion of spore-contaminated food or bedding. Haematogenous vertical transmission may also be a route of infection (Percy and Berthold, 1993). The spores are hardy and can persist in the environment for years. In guinea pigs, the caecum, colon and liver are sites of predilection. Unlike other species, the heart is not involved and, in some cases, the liver may not be affected. The life cycle can be completed entirely in the intestinal tract.

Hosts. *C. piliforme* has been isolated from virtually all species with the exception of humans.

Clinical signs. The disease is highly fatal and is generally preceded by anorexia, debilitation, ascites, dependent subcutaneous inguinal oedema and watery diarrhoea.

Diagnosis. The diagnosis is difficult to establish and is usually based on the postmortem finding of necrotizing hepatitis and enterocolitis with demonstration of the organisms in silver-stained histological sections. Haemorrhagic mesenteric lymphadenitis is common. *C. piliforme* cannot be cultured *in vitro*, but antibodies can be detected serologically.

Control / treatment. There is no effective treatment, although tetracyclines, cephalosporins or chloramphenical are recommended (Harkness and Wagner, 1989; Lindsay *et al.*, 1991). Good sanitation, cleaning with 0.5% sodium hypochlorite and stress-free husbandry practices help prevent disease.

Inapparent gastrointestinal bacterial infections

Guinea pigs can pose a potential health risk to humans as they are presumed to be common, subclinical enteric carriers and shedders of *Listeria monocytogenes* and *Campylobacter* spp.

Viral Diseases

Coronaviral diarrhoea

Agent. Coronaviruses are RNA viruses in the family Coronaviridae that cause disease in weanling animals stressed by shipment or other means. Morbidity is less than 5%, but mortality is approximately 50%.

Hosts. Coronaviruses are ubiquitous in the animal kingdom and affect many domestic and laboratory animals. Interspecies transmission, as a rule, is rare.

Clinical signs. Apparently healthy weanlings will develop acute anorexia with rapid, severe wasting and intermittent, profuse watery diarrhoea. Death occurs in 4–7 days after the onset of clinical signs, but 50% of cases will regain their appetite and recover during the same time interval.

Diagnosis. Diagnosis is based upon clinical signs, the failure to culture pathogenic bacteria from the faeces and demonstration of the virus by transmission electron microscopy of stool specimens. Histopathology shows a necrotising enteritis, often with syncytial cells. Clinical chemistry, haematology and direct faecal examinations are unrewarding.

Control / treatment. The disease is controlled by isolation and quarantine of affected animals while halting new additions to a colony. Treatment consists of supportive care.

Parasitic Diseases

Coccidiosis

Agent. *Eimeria caviae*, is a coccidian in the family Eimeriidae with a worldwide distribution. It occurs sporadically from colony to colony and, in adults, it either resides innocuously in the colon or is eliminated as a consequence of expression of natural immunity. Clinical disease occurs in juveniles, especially recent weanlings, kept under poor conditions or stressed by transportation. The prepatent period for coccidiosis is 6–12 days and transmission is faeco–oral. Following excretion, sporulation, which is required for infectivity, occurs in 2–10 days. The sporulated oocyst contains 4 cysts each containing 2 sporozoites.

Hosts. *E. caviae* is exclusive to the guinea pig. However, guinea pigs can become accidentally infected with intestinal coccidia excreted by rabbits.

Clinical signs. Wasting, weakness and diarrhoea may be seen in heavily parasitised animals 4–8 weeks of age. In severe outbreaks, mortality may approach 40%. Often, infection is subclinical.

Diagnosis. Diagnosis is made by multiple direct examinations of faeces for unsporulated oocysts; however, diarrhoea and fatalities may occur before oocysts are excreted in the faeces.

Control / treatment. Treatment with sulphonamides is highly successful if instituted early in the course of disease and management deficiencies are identified and corrected. Cage sanitation every 2 days will prevent coccidiosis by removing oocysts before they become infective. Feeding and watering should not be done out of open containers.

Cryptosporidiosis

Agent. *Cryptosporidium muris*, a small (2–6 μm) intracellular coccidian protozoan in the family Cryptosporidiidae, is distributed worldwide. It embeds in the the villous epithelium of the ileum. The oocysts are immediately infective and transmission is faeco–oral. Although unreported, in theory, infection can be transmitted from guinea pigs to humans.

Hosts. Cryptosporidiosis is cosmopolitan in the animal kingdom including humans, mice, rats, rabbits, ruminants, birds and snakes.

Clinical signs. Although these parasites infect the intestinal villi, primarily of the ileum, they rarely cause diarrhoea except in recent weanlings (Harkness and Wagner, 1989; Anderson, 1987). In young animals, anorexia, weight loss, weakness, watery diarrhoea, abdominal distension and death, sometimes without prodrome, may be seen.

Diagnosis. Diagnosis of cryptosporidiosis is enhanced by faecal concentration techniques such as Sheather's sugar solution. Sporocysts, each containing 4 sporozoites, may also be seen on direct smear with Giemsa or acid-fast staining of faecal smears.

Control / treatment. There is no effective treatment for cryptosporidiosis beyond supportive care, although treatment with sulphonamides has been recommended (Percy and Barthold, 1993). Oocysts are destroyed by 5% ammonia solution. Stress, particularly at weaning, and contact with other species that may be colonised should be avoided.

Helminthiasis

Agent. Other than *Paraspidodera uncinata*, a rarely pathogenic caecal and colonic heterakid, nematodiasis is uncommon in guinea pigs. *Paraspidodera* is transmitted by faeco–oral ingestion. The life cycle is direct, the eggs require 7–14 days to become infective and the prepatent period is 51–66 days. Enteric cestodiasis has not been reported and trematodiasis is rare. However, cestode infection should be considered a risk for guinea pigs grazed outdoors in areas contaminated by carnivores or other rodents. Trematodiasis requires ingestion of metacercariae encysted on contaminated green vegetation. By the same token, eggs or infected intermediate hosts of nematodes that parasitise wild rodents can be ingested by grazing guinea pigs.

Hosts. Carnivores and wild rodents.

Clinical signs. Intestinal helminthiasis, although rare and generally asymptomatic, should be suspected in cases of diarrhoea, impaction/obstruction, anaemia, or weight loss where animals are overcrowded or kept under insanitary conditions, particularly in the face of poor insect control. *Fasciola hepatica* can cause acute liver failure and *Fasciola gigantica* can cause diffuse abdominal parasitism.

Diagnosis. Diagnosis of intestinal parasitism should be made by faecal flotation and faecal direct smear. The eggs of *Paraspidodera* are oval and thick-shelled, resembling ascarid eggs.

Control / treatment. Nematodiasis can be treated with levamisole, thiabendazole, piperazine or ivermectin given over the course of several days and in combination with cleaning the environment. To prevent accidental infections, fresh greens should not be fed and outdoor grazing should be discouraged. Regular cage sanitation, particularly frequent bedding changes, will remove oocysts before they become infective.

Fungal diseases

Torulopsis pintolopesii, a nonencapsulated candidiform yeast, is a normal inhabitant of the stomach and intestines. While generally non-pathogenic, it can cause opportunistic infections in animals stressed by changes in diet, environment or social group. Clinical signs include anorexia, malodorous diarrhoea and death.

Non-Infectious Diseases

Colorectal impaction

The caecal–colonic orifice may be obstructed with wood shavings, trichobezoars or inspissated faeces leading to fatal caecal bloat. Soft or firm rectal faecoliths can cause impaction in conjunction with many diseases or, most commonly, with age-associated atony.

Clinical signs. Animals with a rectal impaction will show decreased faecal output and may show abdominal enlargement with slow, progressive deterioration. Caecal bloat causes acute abdominal distension and death.

Diagnosis. Rectal impactions are often found during anorectal examination. Caecal impactions are diagnosed by clinical signs and radiography which will show caecal distension or caecal and intestinal distension.

Treatment / control. Impactions of the rectum should be removed with gauze sponges and lubrication. The area should be cleaned regularly with warm water. The owner should check the animal every few days to monitor for recurrence and remove the faecoliths as they occur. The condition may complicate coprophagy and require supplementation with B vitamins and vitamin K. Cases of caecal bloat require surgical intervention. Attempts can be made to treat mild cases with analgesics/tranquillisers, oral dioctyl sodium sulphosuccinate (4–12 mg/kg) and by limiting food intake.

Gastric dilation

Gastric bloat occurs at a low level in the general population of guinea pigs. Predisposing factors appear to be anaesthesia, which may promote aerophagia, or feeding fresh greens, which can induce bloat. Volvulus occurs in many cases. Non-fasted, gravid sows that are anaesthetised appear to be at an increased risk for developing the syndrome (Keith *et al.*, 1992). Changes in the diet, particularly overfeeding of greens and environmental stresses are common causes of maldigestion in guinea pigs.

Clinical signs. Diarrhoea and abdominal enlargement due to gaseous distension of the bowel are the most common clinical signs of maldigestion. Guinea pigs with gastric dilation will show tachycardia, dyspnoea, cyanosis and marked abdominal distension. Death results from a combination of respiratory embarrassment secondary to compromised diaphragmatic excursion and impairment of cardiac venous return.

Diagnosis. The diagnosis is made by correlating the clinical signs with the history and ruling out infectious agents. Radiography is useful in determining the site (i.e. stomach, bowel or caecum) of involvement.

Treatment / control. For mild or recurrent cases, easily corrected management problems should be ruled out before instituting relatively costly diagnostic and treatment measures. Mild cases of maldigestion, which usually show some degree of bloat with diarrhoea, can be managed through dietary correction and administration of analgesics. Decompression by gastric intubation is usually not successful because the tube either becomes blocked with stomach contents or, in the case of torsion, cannot pass through the cardia. Consequently, surgical intervention is required to correct volvulus or relieve distension that does not respond rapidly to medical therapy.

Although effective treatments have not been developed, mild cases can be treated with 1–3 ml of vegetable oil or a surfactant, such as dioctyl sodium sulphosuccinate (4 mg/ml), given when gastric intubation has been done. The guinea pig should then be observed closely. While anaesthetised, unfasted, pregnant sows may be at a higher risk for developing gastric dilation/volvulus, withholding food preoperatively is not recommended because it may cause pregnancy toxaemia. Instead, anaesthesia of pregnant sows should only be done when absolutely required. In these cases, the sows should be closely watched for signs of abdominal distension and, where positioning must be adjusted, the cranial abdomen should be supported to prevent rotation of the stomach (Keith *et al.*, 1992). Maldigestion is prevented by avoiding environmental stresses and dietary changes including the feeding of fresh greens.

Malocclusion

Although herbivores naturally salivate profusely, drooling is most commonly a consequence of malocclusion from congenital defects, ageing, trauma or tooth loss, as a consequence of a poor nutritional plane, especially hypovitaminosis C or fluorosis. The incisors and cheek teeth of guinea pigs are open rooted and grow continuously and the premolars are most commonly overgrown.

Clinical signs. Excessive salivation, presenting as moist skin around the oral cavity and ventral neck, is the most common sign of malocclusion. Anorexia and weight loss are accompanying manifestations, although affected animals may appear hungry and may eat softened foods.

Diagnosis. A thorough oral examination using an otoscope or arthroscope is essential to diagnose malocclusion. The limited range of extension of the mandible and the abundant buccal skin obscure visualisation of the cheek teeth and necessitate examination under anaesthesia. Cases of malocclusion will show mandibular premolars/molars overgrown in the lingual direction and maxillary premolars/molars overgrown labially. Incisors most often overgrow secondarily to malocclusion of the cheek teeth. Tongue entrapment and buccal mucosal ulceration are common sequelae.

Treatment / control. Following induction of anaesthesia with isoflurane, the guinea pig should be placed in sternal recumbency and the mouth should be opened with gauze loops around the maxillary and mandibular incisors. The premolar and molar arcades are viewed by abducting the cheeks using a small vaginal speculum with a light source. After retraction of the tongue, careful use of a dental bur is ideal for correcting malocclusion, but a small rongeur will also work well. Jagged edges left after rongeuring should be gently sanded taking care not to cut the lip or tongue. Overgrown incisors should be cut to the level of the lips. Unless a pair is specifically dedicated to the purpose, pet toenail clippers should not be used on incisors as they dull and can cause microfractures in enamel. Malocclusion tends to recur and treatment must be repeated every 1–2 weeks for primary malocclusion of the incisors and every 3–5 months for cheek teeth. Vitamin C supplementation should be given unless the diet is proven to be of consistently high quality.

Trauma and Congenital Defects

Hernias through the thin diaphragmatic wall commonly occur in animals that are dropped or hugged overzealously. Hepatic laceration with life-threatening haemorrhage occurs in guinea pigs that are either dropped or handled improperly by suspension from one hand without a supporting hand under the hindquarters. Congenital imperforate anus or umbilical hernia rarely occur.

Clinical signs. Diaphragmatic hernias typically present as cases of dyspnoea, while umbilical hernias, unless there is strangulation, present as clinically silent focal swellings at the umbilicus. Imperforate anus presents as abdominal distension, tenesmus and anorexia shortly after the pup begins nursing. Guinea pigs with internal haemorrhage will have weakness, pallor and respiratory distress.

Diagnosis. Radiographs, evaluated in the context of the presentation and history, are diagnostic. Paracentesis yielding blood is suggestive of intra-abdominal haemorrhage secondary to hepatic laceration.

Treatment / control. These conditions require surgical intervention.

Diseases of the Genitourinary System

Examination of the genitourinary system should show the external genitalia to be clean, dry and free of adhered foreign material. The penis should be withdrawn within the prepuce and, when manually extruded, should have two prongs of equal length at the tip. If one or both are missing, the boar will be infertile. Urinalysis of a normal guinea pig will show alkaluria and often calcium carbonate or phosphate crystalluria. Urine contains negligible protein and ketones. Mild glycosuria may be masked by ascorbic acid excretion.

Bacterial Diseases

Bacterial cystitis

Agent. The most common pathogens involved are faecal coliforms, staphylococci and *Streptococcus pyogenes*. Cystitis occurs most commonly as a clinically silent, chronic disease and is most common in sows over 2 years of age. It is found at a frequency of less than 1% and occurs most frequently without uroliths (Peng *et al.*, 1990; Wood, 1981). Cystitis is rare in males, but it may occur as a sequel to occlusion of the penile urethra with coagulated seminal vesicle secretions or calculi. Post-renal obstruction of the urethra with proteinaceous concretions is a not uncommon cause of death of aged males. Immunosuppression from metabolic disease, nutritional deficiency or environmental conditions predispose to bacterial cystitis (Quesenberry, 1994). Mechanical irritation of the urinary bladder through pooling of urine may occur as a consequence of cystic herniation through the abdominal wall. This occurs most commonly in sows as a consequence of parturition (Wood, 1981).

Given the common hypercalciuria of guinea pigs, urinary calculi are not uncommon. Uroliths are most frequently composed of calcium carbonate, magnesium ammonium phosphate, calcium phosphate or calcium oxalate. Unilateral or bilateral ureteral calculi can occur in aged guinea pigs. Predisposing factors include reduced water intake or availability, nutritional imbalances, heritable anatomic defects and pre-existing bacterial infection. Aged females are the most commonly afflicted.

Clinical signs. Cystitis is manifested as either a clinically silent, chronic disease or as acute ulcerative inflammation. In older sows, cystitis is mild and chronic. In sows with symptomatic disease, the presenting complaint is most often blood spots in the cage or blood on the vulva. If they show clinical signs, boars will show dysuria. Anuria, anorexia and listlessness will occur in acute cases. Urolithiasis may be clinically silent or present with signs consistent with cystitis or acute urinary obstruction such as dysuria, stranguria and haematuria. Urolithiasis should be suspected in any case of chronic haematuria that is not responsive to antibiotic therapy. However, haematuria or haemoglobinuria may also be caused by septicaemia unrelated to urinary tract disease. With obstruction or herniation of the abdominal wall, there may be pendulous swelling of the lower abdomen.

Diagnosis. The diagnosis of urinary tract disease is based on clinical signs, urinalysis (including sediment examination) and urine bacterial culture and sensitivity testing; urine is preferably obtained by cystocentesis. Abdominal palpation and radiography should be done in cases of suspected urolithiasis. Obstructive post-renal disease may be confirmed by elevations in serum creatinine and blood urea nitrogen. It is important to rule out hypervitaminosis D and hyperparathyroidism as contributing factors.

Treatment / control. The treatment for bacterial cystitis should be based on urinary culture and bacterial sensitivity. Mild, uncomplicated cases generally respond to antibiotic therapy. Nitrofurantoin, trimethoprim/sulphonamide and enrofloxacin can be used empirically. Cystic calculi must be removed surgically by cystotomy, because passage of a urethral catheter for flushing purposes is difficult. Urethral foreign bodies usually must be flushed antegrade from a cystotomy entrance site. Ureteral calculi should be gently advanced manually to the bladder. Calculi should be chemically analysed and urine cultures should be collected at surgery, if this has not been done previously. The prognosis following immediate surgical correction is good for healthy animals, but recurrence is high. Preventive measures for recurrence are largely empirical. Magnesium ammonium phosphate (struvite) uroliths are formed as a consequence of bacterial infection. Struvite formation may be preventable by urinary acidification through daily high-dose vitamin C therapy. There is no preventive medical treatment for calcium oxalate crys-

talluria other than to avoid greens, many of which contain oxalates. Forages, such as alfalfa, clover and some hays, as well as many fresh fruits, vegetables and greens have high concentrations of calcium and should be avoided or gradually eliminated from the diet. The calcium requirement of 4 mg/kg/day will be met by feeding a pelleted diet. Daily oral supplementation with magnesium hydroxide (4 mg/kg) may also be protective against calcium uroliths (Johansson *et al.*, 1982). Animals with a history of urolithiasis should always have plenty of fresh water available.

Erysipelas

Erysipelothrix rhusiopathiae has been documented in a solitary case report to cause vulvar bleeding, abortion and sudden death of gravid sows (Okewole *et al.*, 1989).

Parasitic Diseases

Parasitic nephritis

Klossiella cobayae (*caviae*), a coccidian of worldwide distribution with a direct life cycle, proliferates in the renal capillary and tubular epithelium and is excreted in the urine. Although frequently referred to in older texts, the incidence of disease is low and infection is asymptomatic.

Non-Infectious Diseases

Balanoposthitis
The most common cause of preputial disease is irritation from bedding particles lodged in the preputial folds usually following copulation. Aged boars may develop a chronic, irreversible paraphimosis. A foreign body reaction to the entrapped particles is common.

Clinical signs. Presenting complaints include bedding caked on the genitalia, infertility or a chronic penile prolapse.

Diagnosis. The diagnosis is based upon clinical signs.

Treatment / control. Treatment should consist of removing offending foreign bodies under anaesthesia, cleansing the area with saline and replacing the bedding with a larger particle substrate. Topical treatment with zinc oxide ointment or combination antibiotic–steroid creams should be used in the face of severe inflammation. Chronic paraphimosis requires daily penile cleaning.

Vaginitis

Vaginal inflammation occurs most commonly from entrapment of bedding in the vagina. Treatment involves washing the area and changing the bedding. Antibiotics should be considered in severe cases.

Diseases of the Nervous System

Viral Diseases

Lymphocytic choriomeningitis (LCM)

Guinea pigs are rarely infected with this agent, an RNA virus in the family Arenaviridae. Most cases of infection are asymptomatic, but clinical signs may include progressive flaccid paralysis, meningitis or pneumonia.

Diseases of the Special Senses

Bacterial Diseases

Otitis media / interna

Agent. *Streptococcus equi*, *Bordetella bronchiseptica*, *Streptococcus pneumoniae* and coliforms (including *Klebsiella* and *Pseudomonas*) are the most common causes of otitis. Coagulase-positive staphylococci are less common invaders. Agents in the *Pasteurella–Actinobacillus* group, including *Pasteurella multocida*, *P. pneumotrop-ica*, *Actinobacillus ligniersi* and *A. equuli*, are normal inhabitants of the nasopharynx with unclarified roles as pathogens of the middle and inner ear.

Infection of the middle ear is commonly associated with pneumonia or silent colonisation from the nasopharynx. The vast majority of cases are affected bilaterally. In some cases, different bacterial species may colonise each bulla. While the incidence of middle ear infection is approximately 15%, less than 1% of these cases affect the inner ear and show clinical signs.

Clinical signs. Otitis media, without pneumonia, is usually clinically silent, but extension into the inner ear may cause circling, torticollis, ataxia and rolling.

Diagnosis. Radiology is superior to all other diagnostic techniques, including otoscopy which is made difficult due to the long, narrow and tortuous auditory canal. Radiographically, the osseous bulla will show radiopacity induced by osteosclerosis and bony lysis. However, early, mild or primarily serous inflammation may not be detectable. In some cases, direct otoscopy of the tympanic membrane will show thickening and opacity with or without suppurative exudate. Assessment of the auditory reflex by exposing guinea pigs to a sharp sound, to which they should normally cock the pinna of the ear, may show deafness.

Control / treatment. Treatment, short of drainage of the bullae which has never been described in the guinea pig, is uniformly unsuccessful.

Non-Infectious Diseases

Cataracts are most commonly a consequence of diabetes mellitus, protein deficiency or consumption of cow's milk (Manning *et al.*, 1984; Richardson, 1992; Elward, 1980; Lang and Munger, 1976).

Diseases of the Integument and Musculoskeletal System

Examination of the integumentary and musculoskeletal systems should show the feet to be free of swelling, callouses and ulcerations. Excessively long claws should be clipped at the time of examination. Torn ears and skin abrasions and ulcerations are common fight-related lesions. Abscesses and swollen lymph nodes are usually the consequence of infectious diseases. However, hypovitaminosis C should be suspected as contributory to any abnormal skin condition. Polyuria may be manifested as a contact dermatitis from urine-scalding.

Bacterial Diseases

Mastitis

Agent. *E. coli* or, less frequently, *Klebsiella*, *Proteus*, coagulase-positive staphylococci, *Streptococcus equi*, or alpha-haemolytic streptococci cause opportunistic infection of the mammary gland. Coliforms may also, in rare cases, be opportunistic invaders and cause fatal septicaemia, peritonitis, pleural effusion or pneumonia in animals kept under suboptimal conditions. Infection occurs by entrance of bacteria through the teat canal in the face of unsanitary conditions. Abrasive bedding or cageing, biting by the animal's offspring and mammary impaction following premature weaning are predisposing factors. Mastitis is most often encountered during lactation when the milk makes an excellent medium for bacterial growth. The case incidence rate during lactation is approximately 2%. Inbreeding increases the susceptibility to infection.

Clinical signs. Mastitis may occur as a local disease or have systemic manifestations. In the former, the gland may be slightly increased in size, but without other signs or lesions. With the latter, sows will show fever, inappetence, depression, oligodipsia, dehydration, weight loss, agalactia and litter desertion. The mammary glands are swollen, indurated, warm, painful and discoloured. There may be accompanying ulcera-

tion. The milk is often thick or clotted and blood-tinged. The sow usually dies from sepsis or endotoxaemia within a few days.

Diagnosis. The diagnosis is based on clinical signs and cytological evaluation of tissue aspirates. Leucopenia is common with endotoxaemia.

Control / treatment. Mastitis should be treated with broad-spectrum antibiotics and warm compresses for 7–10 days. Chloramphenicol or sulpha-trimethoprim are empiric agents of choice. Complicating ulceration should be treated with topical cleansing agents. The environment should be disinfected with sodium hypochlorite solution and the level of hygiene improved.

Staphylococcosis

Agent. *Staphylococcus aureus* and *S. epidermidis*, Gram-positive, coagulase-positive bacterial cocci in the family Micrococcaceae, are transmitted by direct contact and require a break in the physical host defences to cause dermatitis. Pododermatitis, the classical disease presentation, is predisposed by obesity and rusted, abrasive or soiled wire flooring. Affected stock are generally aged 1 year or over. Vitamin C deficiency is also a contributory factor.

Hosts. Staphylococci are normal inhabitants of the skin and nasopharynx with a cosmopolitan species distribution.

Clinical signs. The classical presentation is of swollen feet that, depending on the progression of the disease, may be acutely erythematous have ulcerations or proliferative callouses. The forefeet are affected more commonly than the hindfeet and the nails are often distorted. Periods of healing are often followed by recrudescence. Lymphadenopathy and inflammation may occur in draining lymph nodes. The morphological abnormalities of nail distortion and foot swelling persist indefinitely and chronic inflammation leads to osteoarthritis, tendonitis and amyloidosis of kidney, liver, spleen, adrenal glands and pancreatic islets. Less frequently, staphylococci may cause cheilitis, conjunctivitis, mastitis, cystitis, haematogenous osteomyelitis and sudden death from pneumonia or septicaemia. Exfoliative staphylococcal dermatitis can occur in young animals, particularly those born to dams with a history of the disease (Percy and Barthold, 1993). Affected animals show erythema, alopecia and exfoliation of the abdominal epidermis. Skin lesions begin resolving spontaneously within 2 weeks, although mortality can be high.

Diagnosis. The diagnosis is based upon the clinical signs and culture of the organism from affected sites.

Control / treatment. Prompt treatment is vital to provide comfort and halt the continuous immunostimulation that will lead to amyloidosis and organ failure. Treatment must be directed at ameliorating lesions and causative factors. Mild cases of pododermatitis should be treated by applying warm chlorhexidine soaks, bag balm (0.3% 8-hydroxyquinoline) or dimethyl sulphoxide (DMSO) containing a topical antibiotic. For severe cases, gentamicin, chloramphenicol, trimethoprim/sulphonamides or enrofloxacin and dexamethasone should be given systemically and the feet should be treated with topical antibacterial ointment, such as povidone-iodine, and bandaged. Wound dressings that promote epithelialisation are particularly helpful for treating ulcers. Distorted nails will required regular clipping. The use of wire flooring must be halted and affected animals should be kept on 5–7 cm of soft bedding on a smooth surface. Soiled bedding should be removed daily until ulcers are healed. Amputation at the sacrohumeral joint should be considered in cases that are not amenable to treatment to prevent the progression to amyloid formation. The husbandry procedures should be reviewed and any deficiencies corrected and, for obese animals, a gradual weight loss programme should be instituted. Simple cases of dermatitis can be

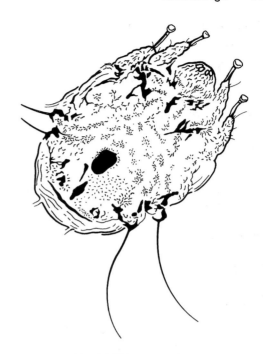

FIG. 4.4 *Trixacarus caviae.*

treated with regular cleaning and application of topical antibiotics.

Parasitic Diseases

Acariasis

Agent. The sarcoptid mites, *Trixacarus caviae* (Fig. 4.4), *Sarcoptes muris* (rare) and *Notoedres muris* (rare), as well as *Chirodiscoides caviae* (Fig. 4.5) and *Myocoptes musculinus*, are in the suborder Astigmata. *Demodex caviae* (rare) is in the suborder Prostigmata.

Acariasis is most severe in debilitated, aged, or chronically diseased adults, immature animals and animals kept in unsanitary conditions. *Chirodiscoides* is found on the skin surface, while *Trixacarus* is a burrowing mite with zoonotic implications. *D. caviae* can colonise the skin, but is almost invariably subclinical. Although the life cycles are not well characterised, transmissions can be by direct or indirect contact. The life cycle of *Trixacarus* takes 14 days, pruritus may

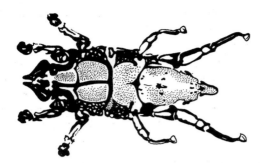

FIG. 4.5 *Chirodiscoides caviae*, male.

be seen within 8 days of exposure and alopecia may be evident within 2 weeks. Nursing pups may be clinically affected. Show animals, because they are often stressed and exposed to animals from multiple sources and of dubious health status, are at high risk for developing infestations. Low temperature and high humidity favour survival of mites (Harkness and Wagner, 1989).

Hosts. *Trixacarus, Chirodiscoides* and *D. caviae* are unique to guinea pigs, but infestation is generally uncommon. *S. muris, M. musculinus* and *N. muris* are common to other rodents, but only found on guinea pigs aberrantly following direct contact with host species.

Clinical signs. Trixacariasis will cause inflammation and hyperkeratosis with variable alopecia and inconsistent pruritus. Lesions of trixacariasis are found most commonly on the neck and shoulders and less commonly on the abdomen and inner thighs. *Chirodiscoides* is distributed on the rump, flanks and abdomen. Pruritus, when present, is intense and may be complicated by self-mutilation, convulsions, dementia, debilitation, and, in the case of pregnant sows, abortion. Severely parasitised animals may die as a consequence of the infestation. Anorexia may be a secondary complication of impaction of the oral cavity with depilated hair. *C. caviae*, while generally considered to be harmless, infrequently may cause pruritus and alopecia localised primarily to the caudodorsal area of the trunk. Demodico-

sis rarely causes clinical signs, but may cause alopecia of the face, particularly the eyelids and forelimbs.

Diagnosis. In cases of suspected acariasis, diagnostic procedures should include a close examination of the fur for the 0.4 mm long *Chirodiscoides* mites and their ellipsoidal 0.25 mm × 0.07 mm eggs. *Chirodiscoides* mites are often collected and observed as noncopulating pairs of adult males and nymphal females, but are often overlooked due to small size and paucity of lesions. Several skin scrapings should be done to detect trixacariasis. Acariasis should not be ruled out on the basis of a single negative skin scraping. In difficult cases, multiple biopsies of the skin may be necessary to diagnose trixacariasis. Eosinophilia is common in cases of ectoparasitism.

Control / treatment. Ectoparasites should be treated every 7 days with either ivermectin (500 µg/kg) given by injection for 3 treatments, lime sulphur (1:40) applied for 6 treatments, or 1% lindane solution for 3 treatments. *Chirodiscoides* will respond to the treatments as described for trixacariasis as well as weekly treatments with bromocyclen, 5% methylcarbamate, 0.5% carbaryl, 0.15% trichlorfon or permethrin dusting powders or acaricidal shampoos that are approved for use in cats. Whatever the treatment plan, adults, weanlings, other contacts and the environment should be included in the strategy. Malathion should not be used, because safer effective compounds are available. Tranquillisation with diazepam may be useful in reducing self-mutilation induced by acariasis or the hind feet can be bandaged. Lesions will resolve completely within a month of completion of successful treatment.

Pediculosis

Agent. *Gliricola porcelli* (Fig. 4.6) and *Gyropus ovalis* (Fig. 4.7) are mallophagan lice from the family Gyropidae and *Trimenopon hispidum* is a sucking louse from the family Trimenoponidae.

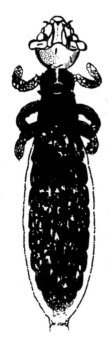

FIG. 4.6 *Gliricola porcelli.*

All louse species infesting guinea pigs are distributed worldwide. The life cycle of these species is poorly understood, but eggs are cemented to hairs and all life stages are found on the skin. Louse transmission is by direct contact. *T. hispidum* is rarely encountered.

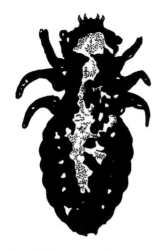

FIG. 4.7 *Gyropus ovalis,* immature.

Lice are highly species-specific and are not transmitted from guinea pigs to humans.

Clinical signs. Louse infestations are usually asymptomatic, but large numbers of parasites, especially in young animals stressed by poor care, may cause dermatitis with alopecia, unthriftiness, roughened hair and pruritus.

Diagnosis. Diagnosis is usually made by direct observation of the adults and the black or white nits on hair shafts with a hand lens during physical examination. Grooming of the coat with a toothbrush can be used as a concentration method for obtaining lice and nits. *Gliricola porcelli*, seen most commonly, is a slender 1.0–1.5 mm by 0.3–0.4 mm louse, while *Gyropus ovalis* is oval and 1.0–1.2 mm × 0.5 mm. *Trimenopon* is similar in size and morphology to *G. ovalis*, but has only five abdominal segments, compared to eight.

Control / treatment. Infested animals should be treated with topical 1% lindane baths, 0.5% lindane dusts or 0.2% pyrethrins. Alternatively, ivermectin injections can be given. Treatment should be repeated 3 times at weekly intervals. Cages, bedding and equipment should be discarded or properly cleaned and sanitised at the same time. Wild rodents should be excluded.

Fungal Diseases

Cryptococcosis

Cryptococcus neoformans, a yeast with worldwide distribution, can cause locally progressive ulcerative dermatitis, particularly of the nose. Direct contact with bird droppings or pigeon nests are common sources of exposure to the infectious yeast.

Dermatophytosis

Agent. *Trichophyton mentagrophytes, Microsporum audouinii, Microsporum canis* (rare) and

Microsporum gypseum (rare) are saprophytic, aerobic fungi and the most common fungal pathogens of guinea pigs. The carriage rate for dermatophytes in apparently normal guinea pigs ranges from 6 to 14%. Dermatophytes are transmitted by direct contact with spores on hair, bedding, soil or fomites. The vast majority of cases are caused by *T. mentagrophytes*. Dermatophytosis is a common, often epizootic, disease of young guinea pigs kept under marginal conditions or on a low nutritional plane. The stress of parturition can also induce disease. Secondary bacterial dermatitis and delayed type hypersensitivities are common complications.

Hosts. Dermatophytes can be harboured by numerous species and transmitted to humans.

Clinical signs. Dermatophytosis is often asymptomatic, but may cause oval to patchy areas of alopecia and dermatitis with easily epilated hair, with or without hyperkeratotis and seborrhoea. Lesions are seen most commonly on the nose but may spread to involve the face, ears, eyelids, pectoral limbs and trunk. Infection can be fatal in neonatal animals. Lesions often regress spontaneously as juveniles approach adulthood.

Diagnosis. Diagnostic procedures must include a 10% KOH digest of hair and a provisional diagnosis should be supported by fungal cultures. Culture material can be obtained by grooming the hair coat with a sterile toothbrush and inoculated onto dermatophyte growth medium. Methenamine silver or PAS stains are best for observing the fungi in biopsy materials.

Control / treatment. Dermatophytosis should be treated with topical 1.5% griseofulvin in DMSO for 5–7 days or a topical antimycotic, such as 7.5% povidone–iodine or 1% tolnaftate, applied twice daily for 2–4 weeks. Oral griseofulvin appears to be toxic for immature and foetal guinea pigs and should only be given to nonpregnant adults. Adults can be treated at a dose of 15–25 mg/kg given orally once daily in a liquid fatty acid supplement or 0.75 mg/kg in the feed for 14–28 days. Antifungal shampoos, left with 1–2 h contact time, are effective for cases with seborrhoea. In large colonies, culling and euthanasia may be the most effective control method.

Non-Infectious Diseases

Alopecia

Most cases of alopecia without inflammation are either of endocrine origin or caused by behavioural or environmental abnormalities. Barbering and stress-induced alopecia are particularly a problem in nervous or overcrowded animals. Hair loss in all age groups is predisposed by wire flooring and has been associated with the late stages of gestation and multiple parities.

Clinical signs. In all cases of uncomplicated alopecia, the skin will not be inflamed and will not be pruritic. Multiparous sows often show diffuse hair loss over the flanks and back such that sows that are intensively bred using the postpartum oestrus may appear almost bald. This condition may be complicated by hair-plucking by the young. Hair loss is particularly common in weanlings from large or poorly nourished litters. Weanlings will also develop a transient thinning of the hair coat as the neonatal fur is replaced by the mature coat. Hair loss in pups may also be due to overzealous grooming by the sow.

Barbering is easily identified by patches of unevenly chopped hair in a stepwise pattern. Lesions are usually distributed over the dorsal lumbar area and flanks, progressing to the head or thorax. Cases of self-inflicted barbering are typically a consequence of boredom and will show the head and neck to be uninfected. Animals barbered by others will have a distinctive pattern of well demarcated hair loss, often involving the head. Boars may barber subordinates, especially pups.

Diagnosis. These diagnoses are based on the history to identify susceptible age groups, reproductive and environmental factors, and behavioural abnormalities. Examinations and cultures for ectoparasites and dermatophytes will be negative. Serum clinical chemistries and hormonal assessments are useful for identifying endocrine abnormalities.

Control / treatment. Barbering can be reduced or prevented by enriching the environment and protecting pups from boars. Hair loss associated with intensive breeding is believed to be related to decreased anabolism of maternal skin, but generally reverses following parturition if rebreeding is not done. In this case, the hair coat is usually restored within 3–4 weeks.

Circumanal Sebaceous Secretions

Excessive accumulation of sebaceous secretions occurs in the folds of the circumanal glands and genitalia of mature boars. The folds should be cleaned periodically to preclude infections and odours.

Fractures

Fractures can be caused by wire flooring or the guinea pig being stepped-on, dropped or crushed. Long bone fractures are rare in adult animals, but occur most commonly in the rear legs of immature animals. The tibia is the most common bone fractured. Wherever possible, fractures should be managed nonsurgically, with a lightweight splint or cage confinement, to permit healing and minimise stress.

Neoplasia

The skin is one of the most common sites of neoplasia for guinea pigs, while bone and to an even lesser extent, muscle are seldom involved.

Clinical signs. The most common skin neoplasm is the trichofolliculoma. It is a benign neoplasm derived from basal cells and occurring as a rounded, firm nodule most commonly in the lumbosacral area. Trichofolliculomas can be found in animals as young as 6 months of age. Epidermoid cysts, derived from hair follicles and possessing a thick, keratinised exudate, are found most commonly on the back. Fibrosarcomas, sebaceous adenomas and lipomas occur less frequently. Recurrence in many cases is common. Mammary tumours can occur in either sex and are primarily benign fibroadenomas. Approximately 30% are malignant adenocarcinomas, but metastases are rare.

Diagnosis. Nodule resection or biopsy with histopathology is diagnostic.

Control / treatment. The treatment for cutaneous nodules is surgical excision. Mammary tumours should be removed with wide excision, but presurgical thoracic radiographs should be done to rule out pulmonary metastases. The local lymph nodes should be resected for histopathology to rule out metastases.

Nutritional Muscular Dystrophy (Hypovitaminosis E)

Clinical signs. Affected animals will present with spontaneous hindlimb weakness, lameness, or paralysis and depression. Conjunctivitis may also be seen. Death typically occurs within 1 week of the onset of clinical signs. Infertility and teratogenesis will be seen in breeding animals.

Diagnosis. The diagnosis is suggested by consideration of the clinical signs in conjunction with elevations of serum CPK. Definitive diagnosis is made by analysis of the diet for vitamin E. Necropsy will show marked pallor of affected muscles and analysis of the liver will show it to be deficient in vitamin E.

Control / treatment. Treatment of clinical cases should consist of daily administrations of vitamin E (5–10 mg/kg). For normal health and reproduction and prevention of disease, the diet should be fortified with 50 mg/kg vitamin E and stored in a cool, dry place.

Osteoarthritis

Idiopathic cartilage degeneration, synovitis, subchondral bone sclerosis, cyst formation and osteophytosis occur commonly in the stifle and, less frequently and less severely, in the elbow and shoulder. Degenerative lesions begin at 3 months of age and focus primarily on the medial tibial plateau. Mechanical stress from obesity is an important risk factor. Neither cage flooring nor gender are influential in the pathogenesis.

Clinical signs. Lameness and weight loss develop in animals over 9 months of age.

Diagnosis. The diagnosis is based on the clinical signs, absence of systemic disease, presence of radiographic lesions and synovial fluid analysis.

Control / treatment. Treatment should be focused on weight control and pain abatement. Unfortunately, dosages have not been established for nonsteroidal anti-inflammatory agents, but treatment with acetaminophen or flunixin meglumine may be effective and should be attempted.

Ulcerative Dermatitis

Numerous non-infectious factors can cause skin ulcers, including physical trauma from cage surfaces, roughened implements or fighting, dietary deficiencies, pregnancy and parturition.

Clinical signs. Localised skin abscesses, ulcers and abrasions are most often a consequence of rubbing against damaged food containers, water bowls and roughened cage sides or fighting. Dominant boars will bite, lacerate and notch the ears of juvenile males. Young males approaching sexual maturity may be attacked and bitten on the back and neck by dominant males. The spinal cord may be traumatised in these attacks, resulting in hindlimb paralysis and requiring euthanasia. Solitary areas of hair loss progressing to ulcers can occur in association with pregnancy or parturition, exhibition, overheating, protein deficiency, mineral deficiency or feeding barley, flaked maize or rabbit chow. Perineal contact dermatitis is most often caused by irritation from urine-scalding, soiled bedding or, in sows that have had a difficult and exhaustive labour, ungroomed parturient fluids.

Diagnosis. The diagnosis is based on the observation of abraded or ulcerated skin with a history of trauma, pregnancy or parturition. Infectious causes must be ruled out.

Control / treatment. Management changes should be instituted to eliminate sources of trauma and lesions should be treated accordingly. Ear biting, for example, is exacerbated by overcrowding and the stress of forming new cohort groups. Ear biting can be reduced by providing multiple feed and water sites in a pen, niches for seclusion and adequate space. Young boars should be removed from mature boars at weaning and breeding groups should have only a solitary boar per pen.

Abscesses should be lanced, drained and cleaned and packed with topical antibiotics. Ulcerative lesions should be gently cleaned and calamine lotion or zinc oxide can be applied to weeping lesions (Richardson, 1992). Treatment of idiopathic ulcerations should be with polyunsaturated oils, vitamins A and E and the B complex (Richardson, 1992).

Systemic Diseases

Bacterial Diseases

Salmonellosis

Agent. *Salmonella typhimurium*, *Salmonella enteriditis* and *Salmonella dublin*, Gram-negative, anaerobic bacilli of the family Enterobacteriaceae, are distributed worldwide and, historically, have been common pathogens of guinea pigs. Contamination of foodstuffs, bedding or drinking water by wild rodents and direct contact with carriers are the most common sources of infection. Following a 5–7-day incubation period, Salmonellae in guinea pigs are most commonly localised to the conjunctiva, cervical lymph nodes and upper respiratory tract. The mesenteric lymph nodes and uterus may be infected variably. The most common route of transmission is by direct contact with the ocular secretions of infectious and often asymptomatic animals, while oral ingestion is less reliable (Iijima *et al.*, 1987). Although all age groups and sexes may be affected, weanlings, postpartum sows and aged animals are at greatest risk of developing clinical disease. Clinical disease occurs most commonly during periods of dramatic weather fluctuations or as a sequela of vitamin C deficiency. The development of a carrier state following exposure is inconsistent.

Hosts. A wide range of species may be hosts for *Salmonella*, including humans, livestock, fowl and rodents.

Clinical signs. In enzootic infections, most animals are chronic carriers and do not exhibit signs of disease unless stressed or infected with a highly virulent serotype. Animals that become stressed die of septicaemia without exhibiting clinical signs or develop an ostensibly fatal syndrome lasting less than a week and characterised nonspecifically by unthriftiness, anorexia, fever, lethargy and wasting. In a colony situation, the first clinical sign is sporadic unexpected mortality. In the face of an outbreak, colony mortality may range from 5 to 90%. Infected animals rarely show diarrhoea, but conjunctivitis is a common sign. Hepatosplenomegaly and mesenteric lymphadenopathy may be evident on abdominal palpation. In rare cases, cervical lymphadenopathy may be seen. Pregnant sows usually abort, but may survive infection.

Diagnosis. Bacterial culture using selective media of the blood of moribund animals, the spleen or cervical lymph nodes of dead guinea pigs or the ocular secretions of animals with conjunctivitis is diagnostic. Faecal cultures are unreliable. Postmortem lesions, with the exception of splenomegaly, may be absent in acute and peracute cases. Chronic cases may show disseminated granulomatous disease.

Control / treatment. Treatment with antibiotics may give a symptomatic cure, but recovered animals will become intermittent and unpredictable shedders. Consequently, affected animals and their contacts should be destroyed and the premises disinfected. Proper husbandry, isolation and screening of new arrivals, exclusion of wild rodents and avoidance of contaminated foodstuffs is preventive.

Streptobacillosis

Agent. *Streptobacillus moniliformis*, a Gram-negative, facultatively anaerobic bacterium in the family Pasteurellaceae, is distributed worldwide, but is an uncommon cause of disease in guinea pigs and is of low contagion. Transmission occurs through bites, aerosols and fomites.

Hosts. Rats are the usual reservoir for *S. moniliformis*, however, evidence suggests that guinea pig isolates are species-specific. The guinea pig is a potential reservoir for human infection.

Clinical signs. The disease is manifested generally as bilateral submandibular swelling. Infected nodes may frequently rupture and discharge pus or, less frequently, regress. Less commonly, the agent may cause pneumonia. Deaths are rare, but may occur from septicaemia or pneumonia.

Diagnosis. Clinical signs and culture of affected sites form the basis of the diagnosis.

Control / treatment. Surgical drainage and abscess removal can be done but carries the risk of sepsis. A carrier state does exist. Affected animals should be euthanased.

Streptococcal lymphadenitis / septicaemia

Agent. There are two organisms that classically cause this clinical syndrome in guinea pigs, *Streptococcus equi* ss *zooepidemicus* and *Streptococcus equi* ss *equisimilis*. *Streptococcus equi* is a Gram-positive, facultatively anaerobic coccus classified as Lancefield Group C and in the family Streptococcaceae. Infection occurs worldwide and in all ages and sexes, but there is a predilection for disease in females. Although the degree of contagion is low, *S. equi* is the most common cause of cervical lymphadenopathy in guinea pigs. The organisms are commonly found on the tonsils, pharynx or conjunctiva of apparently healthy animals and gain entrance to the body through mucocutaneous abrasions secondary to the trauma of eating coarse feeds such as hay or oats. Fighting enhances transmission and dissemination via aerosol or sexual contact is also possible. The incubation period is 1–2 weeks.

Hosts. Horses, wild rodents, dogs and humans may be carriers of pathogenic streptococci. The public health significance of *S. equi* in guinea pigs is not known.

Clinical signs. *S. equi* ss *zooepidemicus* is manifested generally as bilateral submandibular swellings known classically as cervical lymphadenitis. Infected nodes rupture recurringly and discharge a non-odourous, thick, yellowish-white, purulent exudate. In most cases, infection is typically confined to the submandibular nodes and otherwise the animal remains in good health. Rarely, the mesenteric or retro-orbital lymph nodes may be involved. Sudden deaths may occur from septicaemia or pneumonia. Otitis media/interna, peritonitis, suppurative hepatitis, metritis, mastitis, panophthalmitis, pleuritis, hydrothorax, cellulitis, arthritis and pericarditis may be sequelae. Young animals often rapidly succumb to sepsis, while adults may show a more chronic course of infection with progressive wasting. *S. equi* ss *equisimilis* has a rapid clinical course with a sudden onset and rapid death. It causes marked haemorrhage from the nose, mouth and vagina.

Diagnosis. Many pathogens, in addition to *S. equi*, can cause cervical lymphadenopathy. Consequently, the diagnosis must be based on bacterial culture and isolation. Gram-stains of purulent exudates, lymph node aspirates or tissue impression smears are helpful in establishing diagnoses. Infection with *S. equi* ss *equisimilis* is fulminant and diagnosis is often made at necropsy where haemorrhagic pleural effusion, pneumonia and gastroenteritis will be seen.

Control / treatment. The treatment of choice is complete surgical resection of affected lymph nodes. Otherwise, incision, surgical drainage and multiple daily flushings of abscesses should be done. Surgical intervention carries the risk of inducing sepsis. Consequently, administration of a cephalosporin or other antibiotic should be considered. Recurrence is possible, because the animal invariably becomes a carrier. Avoiding feeding coarse feedstuffs is largely preventive, but strict control is only achieved by killing affected animals and their contacts and disinfecting the premises.

Streptococcal pneumonia / septicaemia

Agent. *Streptococcus pneumoniae* and *Streptococcus pyogenes*, Gram-positive bacterial cocci, are the most important members of the family Streptococcaceae causing fulminant systemic disease in guinea pigs. *S. pneumoniae* (pneumococcus, diplococcus) capsular polysaccharide types 3, 4 and 19 are pathogenic for guinea pigs. *S. pneumoniae* does not have a Lancefield designation, but *S. pyogenes* is placed in Lancefield Group A. Both of these organisms can be harboured subclinically in the nasopharynx. *S. pneumoniae* may also be a subclinical inhabitant of the female genital tract. Transmission of *S. pneumoniae* is primarily by aerosol, while biting insects represent an important route of transmission for *S. pyogenes*. Streptococci usually cause disease opportunistically in animals stressed by pregnancy, vitamin C deficiency, environmental fluctuations, suboptimal care or pre-existing bordetellosis. Immature animals and pregnant sows are at greatest risk of infection.

Hosts. Humans are the main natural hosts for both of these species. *S. pneumoniae* causes disease in mice, rats and nonhuman primates. Group A streptococci can cause sepsis and polyarthritis in foals and calves.

Clinical signs. Infection may be manifested as acute death without premonitory signs, chronic illness with nonspecific signs, or multisystemic clinical disease including dyspnoea, sneezing, coughing, purulent or haemorrhagic rhinorrhoea, localised abscesses, septic arthritis, anorexia, weight loss, hunched posture, conjunctivitis, otitis media and haematuria. Sows may develop metritis and, if pregnant, will abort or deliver stillborn pups. Chronic cases commonly develop pleuritis, haemopericardium, pleural effusion, pericarditis, peritonitis and meningitis. There may be palpable hepatosplenomegaly.

Diagnosis. Diagnosis is based upon bacterial culture and isolation from blood, transtracheal washes, nasal or conjunctival swabs, or tissues taken at necropsy. Gram-stains of clinical materials, including impression smears of lung, will show characteristic organisms and are helpful in establishing a preliminary diagnosis.

Control / treatment. While infection is highly fatal, treatment based on the results of a bacterial culture and sensitivity may give a symptomatic cure. Chloramphenicol is the treatment of choice. Trimethoprim/sulphonamides can also be used empirically. However, treatment usually results in a carrier state. The disease is rare in well cared for colonies. It is prevented by maintaining 'closed' colonies of pathogen-free stock and, for fanciers, permanently and effectively isolating show animals from breeders.

Yersiniosis

Agent. *Yersinia pseudotuberculosis* is a Gram-negative, anaerobic bacterium in the family Enterobacteriaceae. Infection is transmitted through consuming contaminated food, through skin lacerations resulting from fighting or from contact with exudates from abscesses. All ages and both sexes are affected equally. Disease is most common in the winter months. Wild rodents and birds, particularly pigeons, are sources of infection. However, indirect transmission through contaminated foodstuffs is most important for pets.

Hosts. In addition to guinea pigs, susceptible animals include rabbits, mice, horses, sheep, swine, goats, nonhuman primates, humans, poultry and other birds. The agent is ubiquitous in nature and found in dust, soil, water, fodder and milk.

Clinical signs. There are three categories of disease: acute, fatal septicaemia, chronic wasting and submandibular lymphadenopathy. In addition, infection may be harboured subclinically in carriers. Palpable mesenteric lymphadenopathy and disseminated granulomas occur in animals with chronic, systemic disease. Young animals tend to die of sepsis, while adults tend to show either submandibular lymphadenopathy or progressive wasting. Diarrhoea is an inconsistent sign.

Diagnosis. Selective media and cold enrichment are necessary for culture and isolation of the organism from abscesses, blood or affected sites. At necropsy, the principal findings are lymphadenopathy and necrotising hepatitis and splenitis.

Control / treatment. Because of zoonotic implications and the likelihood of post-treatment carriers, rigid culling of affected animals and their progeny and contacts is the only method of control. Wild birds and rodents must be excluded from the premises, including feed storage areas. Regular abdominal palpation of mesenteric lymph nodes is helpful for detecting carriers.

Other bacterial pathogens

In rare cases, opportunistic infections may be caused by a number of bacteria including *Citro-*

bacter freundii, *Pseudomonas aeruginosa*, *Corynebacterium kutscheri* and *Corynebacterium pyogenes*. Citrobacteriosis causes dyspnoea, anorexia, adipsia, gastric ulcers and diarrhoea. The mortality rate averages 10%. *Pseudomonas* and the corynebacterial infections cause sudden deaths secondary to septicaemia.

Viral Diseases

Herpesviruses

Agent. Caviid herpesvirus type 1 (cytomegalovirus, CMV), type 2 (Epstein–Barr-like virus) and type 3 are DNA viruses in the family Herpesviridae. Cytomegalovirus is sialotropic and subclinical. Persistent infection is suspected to be widespread. Caviid herpesviruses types 2 and 3 cause subclinical infections and are most common in older inbred research animals. Herpesvirus type 2 is pantropic and causes lifelong viraemia, while types 1 and 3 show only transient viraemia following infection. In rare cases, such as following the stress of intermixing animals, herpesvirus type 2 may be associated with foetal wastage and neonatal unthriftiness. The transmission of all three herpesviruses occurs transplacentally, via sexual contact and may occur in the saliva and urine. Type 2 herpesvirus has also been transmitted horizontally through contaminated water bottles and sipper tubes.

Hosts. All three herpesviruses are specific to guinea pigs.

Clinical signs. Infection is chronic and subclinical, except in immunosuppressed animals or pregnant sows where acute infection in late gestation will cause abortion. Histopathology of salivary ductal epithelium containing herpesvirus type 1 shows cells enlarged 3–4 times with intranuclear and intracytoplasmic inclusions.

Diagnosis. The diagnosis is based upon histopathological demonstration of the characteristic lesions in salivary gland, kidney and liver. Herpesvirus types 2 and 3 do not show inclusion bodies, but type 2 can be demonstrated by virus isolation from the spleen or oropharynx onto special transport media. Antibodies to all three viruses can be shown serologically.

Control / treatment. Infection is prevented by maintaining a closed colony of virus-free animals. Transmission within a colony is prevented through daily replacement of water bottles and cessation of breeding.

Parasitic Diseases

The protozoans *Encephalitozoon cuniculi* and *Toxoplasma gondii* both cause inapparent infections. Encephalitozoonosis is transmitted via the urine and causes renal and, less commonly, cerebral infections. *Toxoplasma gondii* is spread by faecal–oral transmission but transmission between guinea pigs can occur horizontally by cannibalism or vertically through the placenta. Acute toxoplasmosis can cause vulval bleeding and abortion in pregnant sows. Viable tissue cysts can persist for years in muscle, heart, eye and other organs including brain.

Fungal Diseases

Histoplasma capsulatum is a rare cause of chronic, progressive emaciation and hind limb lameness. Immature animals develop conjunctivitis and diarrhoea and die in 2–4 weeks. Classically, infection is acquired by inhalation of spores, however, infections in guinea pigs have been presumed to be from ingestion of spores from contaminated food or bedding.

Non-Infectious Diseases

Anorexia

Inappetence is a common, early, nonspecific sign of illness and can be caused by almost any problem. It is a life-threatening condition that necessitates aggressive supportive care during the course of diagnostics and treatment. If sufficient nutritional support is not given, hepatic lipidosis and death will be the consequences.

Clinical signs. Dramatic reduction in appetite or failure to eat any food offered.

Control / treatment. Particularly disconcerting in the treatment of guinea pigs is their propensity to surrender when ill, refuse to eat, deteriorate and perish. Consequently, forced feeding must be done with repeated orogastric intubation or by inserting and maintaining a nasogastric tube. A paediatric infant feeding tube, lubricated with lignocaine gel, can be inserted into the nares of a depressed or sedated animal, secured to the skin with suture and protected with an Elizabethan collar. Pharyngostomy technique has not been described for the guinea pig but could be attempted. Short-term nutritional support can be done with isotonic liquid nutritional supplements fortified with high caloric supplements. Puréed baby vegetables or cereals can also be given. Blended pelleted diet should be provided if forced feeding is done for more than 1–2 days and vitamin C should always be supplemented. Yogurt supplementation may be useful in reconstituting the normal gastrointestinal flora (Anderson, 1987). In all cases, vitamin C supplementation must be given and administration of B vitamins and anabolic steroids may be useful (Harkness and Wagner, 1989).

Scurvy

Absolute and marginal dietary deficiencies of vitamin C (ascorbic acid) are a significant cause of clinical and subclinical disease in guinea pigs. **The importance of vitamin C in maintaining normal health cannot be over-emphasised.** Failure to provide adequate vitamin C causes scurvy and contributes to increased susceptibility to infectious diseases, malocclusion and other maladies.

Clinical signs. Overt signs of deficiency are manifested within 11–14 days in animals fed a deficient diet, but are often vague, particularly in mature animals. Lethargy, weakness, anorexia and unexpected deaths are consistent early signs of a marginal or absolute deficiency. Rapidly growing weanlings and pregnant sows are affected first. Weight loss and dehydration occur secondarily. Other nonspecific signs associated with deficiency include a roughened hair coat, abortion/stillbirths, ocular and nasal discharges, hypersalivation and delayed wound healing. Voluminous, malodorous soft stools or diarrhoea are secondary to maldigestion caused by bile acid deficiency and pyogranulomatous enteritis. The faeces are frequently positive for occult blood. In some cases, a shuffling gait with short strides may be manifested. The classical lesions of scurvy, including painful, enlarged joints and costochondral junctions, pathological fractures, osteopetrosis, dentine abnormalities, gingivitis, loose teeth, epiphyseal and long bone malformations, and blood vessel friability leading to widespread haemorrhages of subcutaneous tissues, bone and joints are most commonly manifested in young animals. Scurvy may also cause impairments in the blood clotting cascade, anaemia and immunosuppression. If untreated, scorbutic guinea pigs will die within 2 weeks of the onset of clinical signs usually from starvation or secondary infection.

Diagnosis. The diagnosis should be based on the dietary history and clinical signs. Radiography may be useful in demonstrating lesions. The faeces of animals with diarrhoea should be checked for occult blood indicative of internal bleeding. Dietary deficiency can be confirmed by ration analysis, while tissue depletion can be verified by postmortem splenic assay. Vitamin C deficiency should be suspected in any presentation with anorexia, lethargy, weakness or diarrhoea, and empiric vitamin C therapy should be instituted. Often response to empiric treatment is diagnostic.

Control / prevention. Guinea pigs suffering from deficiency will respond dramatically to daily tissue saturation doses (50–100 mg/kg) of vitamin C given either by injection in the hospital or orally at home. Oral multivitamin drops carry the risk of overdosage of other vitamins and must be avoided. Complete clinical resolution of signs takes approximately 7 days. Because vitamin C is retained in the tissues for a maximum of 4 days, anorexia from any cause carries the risk of contributory scurvy and the stress of illness will also increase the metabolic demand for vitamin C. Consequently, all ill animals should receive vitamin C supplementation. Scurvy is entirely preventable by feeding fresh, commercially milled, properly stored guinea pig diet.

Diseases of the Haematopoietic System

Bacterial Diseases

Haemobartonella caviae, a Gram-negative bacterium in the order Rickettsiales of the family Anaplasmataceae, may be observed in vacuoles or in indentations on the surface of erythrocytes in smears of the peripheral blood. It can cause anaemia, haemoglobinuria, hypoproteinaemia, reticulocytosis, increased clotting time. Dyspnoea and weight loss occur in immunosuppressed or splenectomised animals with active infection.

Viral Diseases

Leukaemia / lymphosarcoma

Agent. An endogenous Type C, RNA Oncornavirus in the family Retroviridae causes haematopoietic malignancy. Disease is relatively rare in a general population of non-inbred animals, but may occur in approximately 2% of aged animals. Historically, lymphosarcoma of B cell origin has been the most common reported malignancy of guinea pigs. Lymphoproliferative neoplasia occurs more commonly in females than males and the age of onset is typically over 2 years of age.

Hosts. Guinea pigs.

Clinical signs. The disease is expressed most commonly as leukaemia, but may also present as aleukaemic lymphoma. Leukaemic guinea pigs will have a peripheral white cell count typically exceeding $25,000/mm^3$ and often reaching $180,000/mm^3$ or more. Initial signs are vague and non-specific. As the disease progresses, affected animals develop generalised lymphadenopathy, palpable hepatosplenomegaly, anaemia, thrombocytopenia and loss of the righting reflex. The condition may present initially strictly as cervical lymphadenopathy. Many tissues can be infiltrated with neoplastic lymphocytes although infiltration of the bone marrow or thymus is uncommon. Signs consistent with liver or kidney failure may be evident if the organs are infiltrated. In many cases, body weight and general well being are preserved until late in the course of disease. For instance, there are reports of sows successfully weaning litters and then succumbing to leukaemia within 3 weeks. After the onset of clinical signs, the clinical course is rapid with death occurring within 7 days.

Diagnosis. The diagnosis is made by observing clinical signs in conjunction with demonstration of neoplasia by lymph node or liver biopsy. Leukaemia will show a dramatic lymphocytosis in the peripheral blood.

Control / treatment. Because cases have a silent clinical progression and invariably present with extensive systemic involvement, euthanasia is usually the only recourse. However, single administrations of cyclophosphamide have been reported to be curative. Relapses may occur after 10–30 days. If the disease is refractory to treatment, death is typically caused by infiltrative meningitis. Other agents, such as vincristine, methotrexate and prednisolone, are ineffective.

Diseases of Metabolic Origin

Diabetes Mellitus

Spontaneous diabetes mellitus is a rarely reported condition with no sex predilection.

An uncharacterised infectious agent has been reported to induce diabetes mellitus in Abyssinians (Lang and Munger, 1976). Congenital manganese deficiency may cause juvenile-onset disease (Bell *et al.*, 1978). Clinical disease usually occurs in animals over 5 months of age. Diabetes mellitus enhances the severity of idiopathic glomerulopathy and glycosuria predisposes to cystitis.

Clinical signs. Disease is characterised by pronounced glycosuria with rare ketoacidosis. In the minority of cases, animals present with polyuria, polydipsia, cataracts and weight loss. Infertility, stillbirths and foetal mortality are common manifestations in breeding colonies.

Diagnosis. In most cases, the animals are not obviously ill and blood glucose levels are inconsistently elevated. However, hyperlipidaemia is common and oral glucose tolerance tests are abnormal. Following an 18 h fast and after an oral glucose challenge of 1.75 g/kg body weight, the glucose values 4 h post-dosing will be at least double the fasted baseline level in diabetics (Lang and Munger, 1976). In normal animals, the 4 h post-administration glucose level rarely exceeds 1.5 times the baseline.

Treatment / control. Exogenous insulin is not required for survival and spontaneous remissions are common.

Eclampsia

Eclampsia occurs due to acute calcium deficiency as a consequence of parturition and lactation.

Clinical signs. Postparturient sows will present with depression, muscle spasms and convulsions.

Diagnosis. The diagnosis is based upon the history and clinical signs.

Treatment / control. Hypocalcaemic sows should be treated with calcium gluconate. Eclampsia is prevented by feeding a high quality commercial diet. For sows on a dubious plane of nutrition, dietary calcium supplementation during pregnancy aids prevention.

Heat Stress

Guinea pigs are particularly susceptible to heat stroke and risk overheating in the face of ambient temperatures in excess of 27°C. High relative humidity, thick hair coat, obesity, direct sunlight, crowding, poor ventilation and warm or insufficient water enhance susceptibility.

Clinical signs. Affected animals will have hyperaemia of peripheral vessels, rapid respiration, profuse salivation (as a cooling mechanism) and hyperthermia with a rectal temperature above 41°C. Acute cases will rapidly proceed to cyanosis, prostration and death. The diagnosis is based on the clinical signs and a history of excessive heat exposure. Ketosis, intoxications and other conditions may need to be ruled out. Mental retardation is a risk in pups exposed *in utero* to high temperatures.

Diagnosis. The diagnosis is based on the history and clinical signs.

Treatment / control. Affected animals should be carefully cooled with sprayed water, a cool water bath or alcohol sprays. As with other pets, supportive care, including parenteral fluids and corticosteroids, may be useful. Preventive practices include providing adequate shade, temperature control and air circulation.

Ketosis (Pregnancy Toxaemia)

This poorly characterised condition is most common in nulliparous or primiparous sows and occurs as two syndromes, a metabolic (fasting) form and a toxic (circulatory) form. Sows are affected 7–10 days prior to parturition and the first 7 days postpartum.

The toxic syndrome is seen in obese pregnant sows where massive foetal displacement of the abdominal viscera may cause aortic compression and impaired blood flow through the uterine arteries leading to uterine ischaemia, foetal death and disseminated intravascular coagulation. Obese sows carrying three or more foetuses are at greatest risk. Some sows may develop the syndrome because of heritable hypoplasia of uterine vessels.

The metabolic form is predisposed by obesity combined with fasting or stress such as that caused by transportation, changes in diet or alterations in housing. Pregnancy is an important, but not necessary predisposing factor. Obese boars and virgin sows can also be affected.

Overt and subclinical ketosis is responsible for maternal death and foetal wastage in many colonies. Natural hypoglycaemia, occurring in late pregnancy, is easily aggravated by minor stressors and is probably contributory.

Clinical signs. Regardless of the form, the onset of clinical signs is abrupt and death may occur without premonitory signs. Affected animals may show lethargy, weakness, anorexia, adipsia, profuse salivation and inco-ordination leading to hyperexcitability, muscle spasms, respiratory distress, convulsions, coma and death. Pregnant sows may abort. Hepatic lipidosis is a common sequela. The clinical course is rapid with death occurring within 2–5 days after the appearance of clinical signs. Gastric ulceration is a common complication.

Diagnosis. The diagnosis is made by the history and clinical signs. Ketones may be detectable on the breath. Urinalysis will show aciduria, proteinuria and inconsistent ketonuria. The urine of the herbivorous guinea pig is normally cloudy and alkaluric, but it becomes clear and acidotic in toxaemic animals. Biochemical complications may include many of the following: hypoglycaemia, hyperlipidaemia, hyperkalaemia, hyponatraemia and hypochloraemia. Haematology shows anaemia and thrombocytopenia. Necropsy lesions include hepatic lipidosis, adrenomegaly and an empty stomach. Infarction, haemorrhage and necrosis of the placenta are common.

Treatment / control. Treatment is rarely successful, although parenteral administration of dextrose-containing fluids, calcium gluconate and corticosteroids is recommended. Magnesium sulphate solution has been recommended to promote arteriolar dilatation and uterine perfusion. Overfeeding of adult animals, particularly breeding and pregnant sows, must be avoided. Weight loss through gradual dietary reduction and exercise should be instituted in obese boars and sows. Minimising stresses, such as visits to the veterinary clinic, handling and weighing, should be avoided late in gestation. Prevention is achieved through weight control, ensuring that pregnant sows are not stressed, providing ample fresh food, avoiding dietary changes and supplementing with calcium.

Diseases of Ageing

Cystic Ovarian Disease

Cystic ovaries are a common senescent change in ageing guinea pigs. The aetiology is unknown, although oestrogenic substances in mouldy hay have been incriminated in some cases.

Clinical signs. Sows with cystic ovarian disease may be asymptomatic or present with a history of progressive, bilaterally symmetrical, nonpruritic alopecia over the flanks and ventrum, abdominal enlargement and infertility.

Diagnosis. The cysts are typically bilateral, may range up to 7 cm in diameter and are often palpable at physical examination as discrete, large, rounded, mid-abdominal masses. Diagnosis is based on demonstration of the cysts by ultrasound or laparotomy.

Treatment / control. The treatment of choice is ovariohysterectomy, but, in some cases, temporary resolution can be achieved with HCG (human chorionic gonadotropin) given every 7 days for 1–3 weeks. Cystic endometrial hyperplasia, mucometra, endometritis and leiomyomas often occur in concert with cystic ovaries.

Metastatic Calcification

Metastatic calcification of internal organs, including the kidneys, heart, stomach wall, aorta, distal colonic flexure and cornea, may be prevalent in aged guinea pigs and is secondary to alterations in the complex relationship between calcium, phosphorus, magnesium and potassium (Manning *et al.*, 1984; Anderson, 1987; Wagner, 1979; Bauck, 1989; Sparschu and Christie, 1968; Benirschke *et al.*, 1978). Lethal metastatic mineralisation is induced by diets high in phosphorus and deficient in magnesium and potassium. Guinea pigs have a relatively high requirement for potassium to offset an inability to conserve fixed base (Bell *et al.*, 1978).

Clinical signs. Unexpected death is the most common presentation, but organ-specific failure, most particularly renal failure or weight loss secondary to maldigestion, may be evident clinically. Dietary-induced hypokalaemia or copper deficiency has been associated with bleeding disorders including epistaxis and postpartum uterine haemorrhage.

Diagnosis. The diagnosis is typically made at necropsy.

Treatment / control. The diet should contain 0.9–1.1% calcium, 0.6–0.7% phosphorus, 0.3–0.4% magnesium and 0.4–1.4% potassium. The ratio of dietary calcium to phosphorus should be 1.5:1.0. Potassium supplementation daily with 0.5–1.0 mg/kg by oral administration is curative for hypokalaemia.

Neoplasia

With the exception of skin tumours and malignancies of the haematopoietic system, neoplasia is virtually nonexistent in animals less than 4–5 years of age. However, in a geriatric population of guinea pigs, the incidence of cancer exceeds 15%. The distribution and incidence of various neoplasms in pet guinea pigs is imprecise and can only be speculative. Surveys of tumours on non-inbred, aged guinea pigs have been few and based on small numbers of observations.

Bronchogenic and alveologenic papillary adenomas are among the most common non-lymphatic proliferative disorders and may occur in up to 30% of animals over 3 years of age. Primary malignant pulmonary tumours are rare. Foreign body inhalation probably plays a role in the pathogenesis of these lesions which typically are solitary and peripheral but locally proliferative. Aged animals with such lesions may present with signs suggestive of pneumonia. Radiography is necessary to establish a diagnosis.

Neoplastic disease of the reproductive tract accounts for approximately 25% of tumours in guinea pigs, but is confined almost exclusively to females over 3 years of age. Approximately 60% of all reproductive tract cancers are benign uterine leiomyomas, ovarian teratomas or ovarian cystadenomas. Ovarian and parovarian cysts are common in aged breeding females. Teratomas and embryonal placentomas may be found within the ovaries of young sows. Ovarian teratomas arise from parthenogenic oocytes and occur unilaterally as palpable abdominal masses. They may reach a diameter of 10 cm and consist of a mixture of structures including glandular and connective tissue. Some portions may implant on the abdominal peritoneum. Radiography is helpful in displaying large tumours or those containing bone or teeth. Diagnosis is based on clinical findings. Surgical excision is recommended, but intraperitoneal haemorrhage is a life-threatening complication. Another third of neoplasms occur in the uterus. The vast majority of these are benign leiomyomas, fibromas, or fibromyomas. Malignancies account for less than 20% of these cases. There have been solitary reports of cancer of the testes and Fallopian tube.

Reports of gastrointestinal, hepatic, biliary and peritoneal neoplasia are rare, comprising less than 5% of all cases. Benign connective tissue neoplasms, such as leiomyomas and fibromyomas, may occur on the greater curvature of the stomach near the pylorus, but have not been shown to cause functional obstruction or significant pathology. Malignancies occur in less than 20% of cases.

Tumours of the cardiovascular system also constitute approximately 5% of reported cases. Mesenchymomas of the right atrium, often detected electrocardiographically, and cardiac fibrosarcomas have been reported.

Endocrine neoplasms are among the rarest reported in guinea pigs. However, hormonally non-functional, benign tumours have been reported in the adrenal cortex, thyroid and pancreatic islets.

Osteosarcomas comprise approximately 1% of all reported cases and occur in animals as young as 1 year of age. Disease is typified by acute onset of swelling and pain.

The urinary bladder, kidneys, brain and peripheral nerves are the least likely organs to be affected by neoplasia.

Renal Disease

Hydronephrosis occurs spontaneously in guinea pigs over 4 years of age and chronic segmental nephrosclerosis is a common, but poorly understood, incidental ageing lesion. Chronic renal failure from idiopathic glomerulonephropathy or hypertensive nephrosclerosis is a common cause of wasting and death in aged animals. Nephrosclerosis is predisposed by a dietary calcium:phosphorus imbalance. Renal amyloidosis may occur as a consequence of chronic immunostimulation such as that associated with staphylococcal pododermatitis.

Clinical signs. Guinea pigs in renal failure will be depressed and dehydrated and may show oliguria or polyuria. Unexpected death may be the only presenting sign.

Diagnosis. Serum biochemistry will show elevations of blood urea nitrogen and creatinine. Urinalysis will show isosthenuria and proteinuria. Radiography shows that the kidneys are decreased in size. Confirmation can be made by renal biopsy or at necropsy.

References

Anderson, L. C. (1987) Guinea pig husbandry and medicine. *Veterinary Clinics of North America: Small Animal Practice* **17**, 1045–1060.

Bauck, L. (1989) Ophthalmic conditions in pet rabbits and rodents. *Compendium on Continuing Education for the Practising Veterinarian* **11**, 258–266.

Bell, J. M., Benevenga, N. J., Farmer, F. A. *et al.* (1978) *Nutrient Requirements of Laboratory Animals*, 3rd revised edn, pp. 59–69, National Research Council, Washington.

Benirschke, K., Garner, F. M., Jones, T. C. (eds) (1978) *Pathology of Laboratory Animals*, Vols 1 and 2, Springer Verlag, New York.

Carraway, J. H. and Gray, L. D. (1989) Blood collection and intravenous injection in the guinea pig via the medial saphenous vein. *Laboratory Animal Science* **39**(6), 623–624.

Collins, B. R. (1994) Common diseases and medical management of rodents and lagomorphs. *Veterinary Clinics of North America: Small Animal Practice* **24**, 261–316.

Debout, C., Caillez, D. and Izard, J. (1987) A spontaneous lymphoblastic lymphoma in a guinea pig. *Pathology Biology* **35**, 1249–52.

Ediger, R. D. (1976) Care and management. In: *The Biology of the Guinea Pig*, pp. 5–12, Wagner, J. E. and Manning, P. J. (eds). Academic Press, Orlando.

Elward, M. (1980) *Encyclopedia of Guinea Pigs*. T.F.H. Publications, Inc., Neptune.

Flecknell, P. A. (1991) Guinea pigs. In: *Manual of Exotic Pets*, pp. 51–62, Beynon, P. H. and Cooper, J. E. (eds). British Small Animal Veterinary Association, Gloucestershire.

George, L. W. (1984) Antimicrobial agent-associated colitis and diarrhoea: Historical background and clinical aspects. *Review of Infectious Diseases* **6** (1), S208–S213.

Green, C. J. (1982) *Animal Anaesthesia*. Laboratory Animals Ltd, London.

Harkness, J. E. (1994) *Guinea Pig Biology and Medicine*. North American Veterinary Conference. Orlando.

Harkness, J. E. and Wagner, J. E. (1989) *The Biology and Medicine of Rabbits and Rodents*, 3rd edn. Lea and Febiger, Philadelphia.

Harper, L. V. (1976) Behaviour. In: *The Biology of the Guinea Pig*, pp. 31–51, Wagner, J. E. and Manning, P. J. (eds). Academic Press, Orlando.

Hintz, H. F. (1969) Effect of coprophagy on digestion and mineral excretion in the guinea pig. *Journal of Nutrition* **99**, 357–358.

Howell, J. M. and Buxton, P. H. (1975) Alpha-tocopherol responsive muscular dystrophy in guinea pigs. *Neuropathology and Applied Neurobiology* **1**, 49–58.

Iijima, O. T., Saito, M., Nakayama, K. *et al.* (1987) Epizootiological studies of *Salmonella typhimurium* infection in guinea pigs. *Experimental Animal* **36**, 39–49.

Johansson, G., Backman, U., Danielson, B. G. *et al.* (1982) Effects of magnesium hydroxide in renal stone disease. *Journal of American College of Nutrition* **1**, 179–185.

Keith, Jr, J. C., Bowles, T. K. *et al.* (1992) Correspondence. *Laboratory Animal Science* **42**(4), 331–332.

Kinkler, Jr, R. J., Wagner, J. E., Doyle, R. E. and Owens, D. R. (1976) Bacterial mastitis in guinea pigs. *Laboratory Animal Science* **26**, 214–7.

Lang, C. M. and Munger, B. L. (1976) Diabetes mellitus in the guinea pig. *Diabetes* **25**, 434–443.

Lindsey, J. R., Boorman, G. A., Collins, M. J. *et al.* (1991) *Infectious Diseases of Rats and Mice*, p. 131. National Research Council, National Academy Press, Washington.

Madden, D. L., Horton, R. E. and McCullough, N. B. (1970) Spontaneous infection in ex-germfree guinea pigs due to *Clostridium perfringens*. *Laboratory Animal Science* **20**, 454–5.

Manning, P. J. (1976) Neoplastic diseases. In: *The Biology of the Guinea Pig*, pp. 211–25, Wagner, J. E. and Manning, P. J. (eds). Academic Press, Orlando.

Manning, P. J., Wagner, J. E. and Harkness, J. E. (1984) Biology and diseases of guinea pigs. In: *Laboratory Animal Medicine*, pp. 149–81, Fox, J. G., Cohen, B. J. and Loew, F. M. (eds). Academic Press, Orlando.

Muir, W. W. and Hubbell, J. E. (1989) *Handbook of Veterinary Anaesthesia*. The C. V. Mosby Co., St. Louis.

Okewole, P. A., Odeyemi, P. S., Oyetunde, I. L. *et al.* (1989) Abortion in guinea pigs. *Veterinary Record* **124**, 245.

Peng, X., Griffith, J. W. and Lang, C. M. (1990) Cystitis, urolithiasis and cystic calculi in ageing guinea pigs. *Laboratory Animals* **24**, 159–63.

Percy, D. (1984) Guinea pigs. *Guide to the Care and Use of Experimental Animals*, Vol. 2, pp. 103–112. Canadian Council on Animal Care, Ottawa.

Percy, D. H. and Barthold, S. W. (1993). *Pathology of Laboratory Rodents and Rabbits*, pp. 146–78. Iowa State University Press, Ames.

Quesenberry, K. E. (1994) Guinea pigs. *Veterinary Clinics of North America: Small Animal Practice* **24**, 67–87.

Quillec, M., Debout, C. and Izard, J. (1977) Red cell and white cell counts in adult female guinea pigs. *Pathology and Biology* **25**, 443–446.

Richardson, V. C. G. (1992) *Diseases of Domestic Guinea Pigs*. Blackwell Scientific Publications, Oxford.

Sirois, M. (1989) The pet guinea pig. *Vet Technician* **10**, 50–55.

Sisk, D. B. (1976) Physiology. In: *The Biology of the Guinea Pig*, pp. 63–98, Wagner, J. E. and Manning, P. J. (eds). Academic Press, Orlando.

Sparschu, G. L. and Christie, R. J. (1968) Metastatic calcification in a guinea pig colony: a pathological survey. *Laboratory Animal Care* **18**(5), 520–526

Sutherland, S. D. and Festing, M. F. W. (1987) The guinea-pig. In: *The UFAW Handbook on the Care and Management of Laboratory Animals*, 6th edn, pp. 393–410, Poole, T. B. (ed.). Longman Scientific and Technical, Essex.

Townsend, G. H. (1975) The guinea pig: General husbandry and nutrition. *Veterinary Record* **96**, 451–454.

Wagner, J. E. (1979) Guinea pigs. In: *Handbook of Diseases of Laboratory Animals*, pp. 137–62, Hime, J. M. and O'Donoghue, P. N. (eds). Heineman Veterinary Books, London.

Wood, M. (1981) Cystitis in female guinea pigs. *Laboratory Animals* **15**, 141–43.

Wriston, Jr, J. C. and Yellin, T. O. (1973) L-Asparaginase: A review. *Advances in Enzymology* **39**, 185–248.

Further Reading

Bielfeld, H. (1983) *Guinea Pigs: A Complete Pet Owner's Manual*. Barrons. Woodbury.

Hawk, C. T. and Leary, S. L. (1995) *Drug Information and Formulary for Laboratory Animals*, Iowa State University Press, Ames.

Schuchman, S. M. (1989) Individual care and treatment of rabbits, mice, rats, guinea pigs, hamsters and gerbils. In: *Current Veterinary Therapy (i.e.*

Current Veterinary Therapy X: Small Animal Practice), pp. 738–65, Kirk, R. W. (ed.), WB Saunders Co., Philadelphia.

Wagner, J. E. and Manning, P. J. (eds) (1976) *The Biology of the Guinea Pig*. Academic Press, Orlando.

(Data Tables follow).

Data Tables

COMMON DISEASES—GUINEA PIGS						
Disease	Aetiology	Diagnosis	Clinical signs and history	Treatment and control	Zoonotic potential	Comments
Respiratory system						
Bordetellosis	*Bordetella bronchiseptica*	Culture of respiratory secretions	Respiratory distress Weight loss Sudden death	Enrofloxacin 10 mg/kg Gentamicin 5 mg/kg or Trimethoprim/ Sulphamethoxazole 30 mg/kg Supportive care	No	
Chlamydiosis	*Chlamydia psittaci*	Clinical signs Conjunctival scrapings	Conjunctivitis	None	Unknown	Self-limiting disease
Klebsiella pneumonia	*Klebsiella pneumoniae*	Culture blood or respiratory secretions	Respiratory distress Sudden death	Gentamicin 5 mg/kg Tobramycin 30 mg/kg Enrofloxacin 10 mg/kg	No	
Adenoviral pneumonia	Adenovirus	Serology Necropsy	Respiratory distress Sudden death	Supportive care	No	Often subclinical
Pneumonitis	Aspiration/ inhalation	History/ clinical signs Necropsy	Acute respiratory distress	Oxygen administration Airway suctioning	No	Often asymp-tomatic
Gastrointestinal system						
Aflatoxicosis	*Aspergillus flavus* *A. fumigatus*	History of feeding mouldy hay	Stillbirth Abdominal bloat/pain Sudden death	Gastric intubation Gastrotomy Correct diet	No	
Clostridiosis	*Clostridium difficile* *Clostridium perfringens* Type E	Faecal culture Faecal cytoxin assay Faecal Gram stain	Diarrhoea Anorexia	Cholestyramine 100 mg/ml in drinking water Cephalexin 15 mg/kg Decontaminate environment	No	Almost always fatal
Colibacillosis	*Escherichia coli*	Faecal culture	Diarrhoea Anorexia	Enrofloxacin 10 mg/kg Chloramphenicol 50 mg/kg Supportive care	No	

Fig. 4.8—continued

COMMON DISEASES—GUINEA PIGS						
Disease	Aetiology	Diagnosis	Clinical signs and history	Treatment and control	Zoonotic potential	Comments
Tyzzer's disease	*Clostridium piliforme*	Necropsy	Diarrhoea	Decontaminate environment	No	Formerly *Bacillus piliformis*
Viral diarrhoea	Coronavirus	Faecal electron microscopy	Diarrhoea Anorexia	Supportive care	No	Diagnosis of exclusion
Coccidiosis	*Eimeria caviae*	Faecal direct smear	Diarrhoea in juveniles	Sulphaquinoxaline 1% in drinking water	No	
Crypto-sporidiosis	*Cryptosporidium muris*	Faecal examin-ation following concentrations in Sheather's sugar solution	Diarrhoea Bloat	Supportive care Decontaminate environment	Unknown	
Helminthiasis	*Paraspidodera uncinata*	Faecal flotation	Diarrhoea	Ivermectin 500 μg/kg Decontaminate environment	No	
Candidiasis	*Torulopsis pintolopesii*	Faecal examination	Diarrhoea Sudden death	None known	No	
Gastric dilatation	Anaesthesia Feeding greens Stress	History Clinical signs Radiography	Abdominal distension	Gastric intubation Gastrotomy Correct diet Eliminate stress	No	
Colorectal impaction	Foreign body Senescence	Clinical signs Radiography Anorectal examination	Abdominal distension	Laparotomy Removal of rectal faecoliths	No	
Malocclusion	Ageing Scurvy Fluorosis Inadequate diet Congenital defect	Oral examination	Slobbering Weight loss Anorexia	Bur teeth	No	

Fig. 4.8—continued

COMMON DISEASES—GUINEA PIGS						
Disease	Aetiology	Diagnosis	Clinical signs and history	Treatment and control	Zoonotic potential	Comments
Genitourinary system						
Cystitis	Coliforms (*Staphylococcus* spp.) (*Streptococcus pyogenes*)	Urinalysis Urine culture Urolith analysis	Haematuria Dysuria	Nitrofurantoin 50 mg/kg Enrofloxacin 10 mg/kg	No	Treatment started empirically should be modified based on the results of a urine culture owing to the many pathogens that could be involved and the prospect of antibiotic resistance
Erysipelas	*Erysipelothrix rhusiopathiae*	Bacterial culture from sites of haemor-rhage	Abortion Vaginal haemorrhage Sudden death	Chloramphenicol 50 mg/kg Cephalexin 15 mg/kg	No	
Balanoposthitis	Irritation from bedding Ageing	Clinical signs	Penile prolapse Infertility	Penile cleaning	No	
Vaginitis	Irritation from bedding	Clinical signs	Vulval/vaginal inflammation	Daily cleaning	No	
Nervous system						
Lymphocytic chorio-meningitis	Arenavirus	Clinical signs Histopathology Serology	Flaccid paralysis Respiratory distress CNS signs	No treatment Exclude vermin	Yes	
Polio	Enterovirus	Clinical signs	Flaccid paralysis Histopathology Weight loss	None	No	Rare incidence

Fig. 4.8—continued

COMMON DISEASES—GUINEA PIGS						
Disease	Aetiology	Diagnosis	Clinical signs and history	Treatment and control	Zoonotic potential	Comments
Sensory organs						
Otitis	*Streptococcus equi* *Bordetella bronchiseptica* *Streptococcus pneumoniae* Coliforms *Pasteurella* spp. *Actinobacillus* spp.	Radiography	CNS signs	None	No	Usually clinically silent
Cataracts	Diabetes mellitus Protein deficiency	Ocular examination	Lenticular opacity	None	No	
Integument and musculoskeletal system						
Mastitis	Coliforms *Staphylococcus* spp. *Streptococcus equi*	Clinical signs Cytology	Swollen mammary glands Agalactia Depression Weight loss	Chloramphenicol 50 mg/kg Trimethoprim/ sulpha 30 mg/kg Improve sanitation	No	Usually a conse- quence of poor hygiene
Staphy- lococcosis	*Staphylococcus aureus* *Staphylococcus epidermidis*	Clinical signs Bacterial culture	Pododermatitis Dermatitis Mastitis	Antibiotics Replace wire flooring Topical bag balm or chlorhexidine	No	Gentamicin 5 mg/kg, Enrofloxacin 10 mg/kg, Chloram- phenicol 50 mg/kg, or Trimethoprim sulpha 30 mg/kg are good empiric choices

Fig. 4.8—continued

COMMON DISEASES—GUINEA PIGS						
Disease	Aetiology	Diagnosis	Clinical signs and history	Treatment and control	Zoonotic potential	Comments
Acariasis	*Trixacarus caviae* *Sarcoptes muris* *Notoedres muris* *Myocoptes musculinus* *Demodex caviae*	Clinical signs Skin scrapings Pelage examination Skin biopsy	Alopecia Dermatitis Pruritus	Ivermectin 500 μg/kg	No	
Pediculosis	*Gliricola porcelli* *Gyropus ovalis* *Trimenopon hispidum*	Clinical signs Pelage examination	Alopecia Dermatitis Pruritus	Ivermectin 500 μg/kg Lindane (1%) dips	No	Often asymptomatic
Cryptococcosis	*Cryptococcus neoformans*	Skin biopsy	Ulcerative dermatitis	Euthanasia	No	
Dermatophytosis	*Trichophyton mentagrophytes* *Microsporum* spp.	Clinical signs 10% KOH digest of hair Fungal culture	Alopecia	Tolnaftate (1% topical) Povidone–iodine (7.5% topical) Griseofulvin (25 mg/kg PO)	Yes	
Alopecia, non-infectious	Cystic ovarian disease Wire flooring Barbering Weanling transitional hair Parturition/ lactation	History Clinical signs	Alopecia	Environmental enrichment Eliminate wire flooring Halt reproduction House singly	No	Usually a diagnosis of exclusion
Neoplasia	Trichofolliculoma Epidermoid cyst Mammary fibroadenoma Others	Biopsy with histopathology	Cutaneous or subcutaneous nodule(s)	Surgical resection	No	Thoracic radiographs should be done to rule out metastases

Fig. 4.8—continued

COMMON DISEASES—GUINEA PIGS						
Disease	Aetiology	Diagnosis	Clinical signs and history	Treatment and control	Zoonotic potential	Comments
Osteoarthritis	Cartilage degeneration	Clinical signs Radiography Synovial fluid analysis	Lameness Weight loss	Weight control Flunixin meglumine Acetaminophen	No	
Ulcerative dermatitis	Trauma Pregnancy/ parturition Nutritional deficiency	History Clinical signs	Skin ulcers, abscesses or abrasions Ear lacerations	Prevent fighting Correct sources of environmental trauma	No	
Systemic diseases						
Cervical lymphadenitis	*Streptococcus equi* ss *zoo-epidemicus Streptococcus equi* ss *equisimilis Streptobacillus moniliformis*	Clinical signs Bacterial culture	Lymphadenopathy Sudden death (rare)	Lymphadenectomy Euthanasia	No	Carrier state common
Citro-bacteriosis	*Citrobacter freundii*	Clinical signs Faecal bacterial culture Blood bacterial culture	Respiratory distress Diarrhoea	Chloramphenicol (50 mg/kg) Gentamicin (5 mg/kg) Tobramycin (30 mg/kg)	No	
Coryne-bacteriosis	*Cornye-bacterium kutscheri Cornye-bacterium pyogenes*	Blood culture	Sudden death	Chloramphenicol (50 mg/kg)	No	Carrier state possible
Pseudomoniasis	*Pseudomonas aeruginosa*	Blood culture	Cutaneous abscesses (rare) Sudden death	Gentamicin (5 mg/kg) Tobramycin (30 mg/kg)	No	Often transmitted in drinking water
Salmonellosis	*Salmonella typhimurium Salmonella enteritidis*	Blood culture Conjunctival culture	Abortion Sudden death Conjunctivitis	Euthanasia	Yes	Carrier state common

Fig. 4.8—continued

COMMON DISEASES—GUINEA PIGS						
Disease	Aetiology	Diagnosis	Clinical signs and history	Treatment and control	Zoonotic potential	Comments
Streptococcal pneumonia	*Streptococcus pneumoniae* *Streptococcus pyogenes*	Gram stain Bacterial culture	Chronic weight loss Respiratory signs Abortion Arthritis Sudden death	Chloramphenicol (50 mg/kg) Trimethoprim sulpha (30 mg/kg)	No	Carrier state common
Yersiniosis	*Yersinia pseudo-tuberculosis*	Bacterial culture	Submandibular swelling Chronic weight loss Sudden death	Euthanasia	Yes	Carrier state common
Herpes	Caviid herpesvirus 1,2,3	Histopathology (salivary gland)	Abortion	None	No	
Encephalito-zoonosis	*Encephalito-zoon cuniculi*	Necropsy Serology	Asymptomatic	None	No	Toxo-plasmosis differential
Toxo-plasmosis	*Toxoplasma gondii*	Necropsy Serology	Abortion Sudden death	None	No	Felids are the definitive host
Histo-plasmosis	*Histoplasma capsulatum*	Fungal culture	Weight loss CNS signs	None	No	
Mucormycosis	*Absidia ramosa A. corymbifera*	Lymph node aspirate	Lymphadenopathy	None	No	Infection is nonfatal and self-limiting
Anorexia	Varies	Clinical signs	Appetite reduction Weight loss	Forced feeding Vitamin C (50–100 mg/kg)	No	Nonspecific sign of illness requiring aggressive nutritional support
Scurvy	Vitamin C deficiency	Clinical signs	Weight loss Unthriftiness Abortion Hypersalivation Diarrhoea Reluctance to move Sudden death	Vitamin C (50–100 mg/kg)	No	The most common preventable disease of guinea pigs

Fig. 4.8—continued

COMMON DISEASES—GUINEA PIGS						
Disease	Aetiology	Diagnosis	Clinical signs and history	Treatment and control	Zoonotic potential	Comments
Haematopoietic system						
Leukaemia/ Lympho- sarcoma	Oncornavirus	Clinical signs Lymph node or liver biopsy Haematology	Lymphadenopathy Hepatosplenomegaly Anaemia Lymphocytosis	Cyclophos- phamide (300 mg/kg)	No	
Haemo- bartonellosis	*Haemobartonella caviae*	Haematology Urinalysis	Dyspnoea Weight loss Splenomegaly Anaemia Haemoglobinuria		No	Disease is expressed in immuno- suppressed animals
Other systems						
Diabetes mellitus	Spontaneous	Clinical signs Oral glucose tolerance test	Glycosuria Polyuria Polydipsia Cataracts Weight loss Reproductive problems	None usually needed	No	Often self-limiting
Eclampsia	Calcium deficiency	History Clinical signs	Postpartum depression Muscle spasms Convulsions	Calcium gluconate (1 mg/kg)	No	
Heat stress	Ambient temperature above 27 °C	History Clinical signs	Hyperaemia Hyperthermia (> 41 °C) Cyanosis Prostration	Topical cooling Prednisone (2 mg/kg) Fluid therapy	No	Predisposed by thick hair coat, direct sunlight, obesity, crowding, poor ventilation, inadequate water, high relative humidity
Ketosis	Obesity and stress Pregnancy	History Clinical signs Urinalysis Serum chemistry	Respiratory signs CNS signs Reproductive problems	Dextrose fluid therapy Calcium gluconate (1 mg/kg) Prednisone (2 mg/kg)	No	Treatment is rarely successful

Fig. 4.8—continued

COMMON DISEASES—GUINEA PIGS						
Disease	Aetiology	Diagnosis	Clinical signs and history	Treatment and control	Zoonotic potential	Comments
Ageing						
Cystic ovaries	Senescence Mouldy hay	Abdominal palpation Ultrasound Laparotomy	Alopecia Abdominal enlargement Infertility	Ovario-hysterectomy HCG 1000 units	No	
Metastatic calcification	Calcium, phosphorus, magnesium and potassium imbalance	Clinical signs Necropsy	Weight loss Corneal calcification Sudden death	Correct diet	No	Lesions are irreversible
Renal disease	Senescence Toxicity	Clinical signs Serum chemistry Urinalysis	Polyuria Polydipsia Weight loss	None	No	

FIG. 4.8 Common diseases—guinea pigs.

CLINICAL SIGNS AND DIFFERENTIAL DIAGNOSES—GUINEA PIGS

Abdominal distension
Abdominal hernia
Ascites
  Clostridium piliforme
  Hepatic failure
Bloat
  Aflatoxicosis
    (intussusception)
  Clostridiosis
  Cryptosporidiosis
  Gastric volvulus
  Maldigestion
Rectal impaction
Cystic ovarian disease
Neoplasia
Urinary tract
  obstruction

Abortion/Stillbirth
Dystocia/asphyxiation
Environmental stress
  Food restriction
  Heat stress
  Loud noises
  Predators
  Social destabilisation
High protein diet
Infectious agents
  Bordetellosis
  Erysipelas
    rhusiopathiae
  Herpesvirus
  Salmonellosis
  Streptococcus
    pneumoniae
  Toxoplasmosis
  Trixacariasis
Intoxication
  Organophosphate
  Aflatoxicosis
  Oestrogen in feed
Ketosis
Vitamin C deficiency

Agalactia
Exhaustive parturition
Mastitis
Water restriction

Alopecia
Infectious causes
  Acariasis
  Dermatophytosis
  Pediculosis
Noninfectious causes
  Barbering
  Cystic ovarian disease
  Mechanical abrasion
  Parturition/lactation
  Pregnancy
  Protein deficiency
  Transitional hair
    coat (weanling)
  Vitamin B deficiency
  Vitamin C deficiency

Anorexia
Infectious causes
  Acariasis
  Clostridium piliforme
  Bordetellosis
  Colibacillosis
  Coronavirus
  Cryptosporidiosis
Noninfectious causes
  Behavioural submission
  Cage relocation
  Environmental stress
  Food spoilage
  Loss of olfaction
  Malocclusion
  Neoplasia
  Pain
  Renal failure
  Staphylococcosis
  Trichobezoar
  Unpalatable/novel diet
  Vitamin B deficiency
  Vitamin C deficiency
  Vitamin E deficiency

Bone/Joint Swelling
Osteoarthritis
Osteomyelitis
Septic arthritis
Staphylococcosis
Vitamin C deficiency
Vitamin D deficiency

**Conjunctivitis/
ocular discharge**
Infectious causes
  Bordetellosis
  Candida
    albicans (rare)
  Chlamydia psittaci
  Histoplasmosis
  Salmonellosis
  Staphylococcus
  Streptococcus
    pneumoniae
Noninfectious causes
  Ammonia vapours
  Cigarette smoke
  Foreign body
  Trauma
  Vitamin A deficiency
  Vitamin C deficiency
  Vitamin E deficiency

**Cutaneous or
Subcutaneous swelling**
Abscess
Cryptococcosis (rare)
Cystitis
Foreign Body
Lymphadenopathy
  Lymphosaracoma
  Mucormycosis (rare)
  Pseudomoniasis
  Salmonellosis (rare)
  Staphylococcosis
  Streptobacillus
    moniliformis (rare)
  Streptococcus equi
  Yersinia
    pseudotuberculosis
Mastitis
Neoplasia
Trauma

**Death, Unexpected,
Adult**
Infectious causes
  Adenovirus
  Aflatoxicosis
  Bordetellosis
  Clostridiosis
  Corynebacteriosis
    (rare)

  Erysipelas
    rhusiopathiae
  Klebsiella
    pneumoniae
  Pseudomoniasis
  Salmonellosis
  Staphylococcosis
    (rare)
  Streptococcus
    equi (rare)
  Streptococcus
    pneumoniae
  Streptococcus
    pyogenes
  Torulopsis
    pintolopesii
  Toxoplasmosis
Noninfectious causes
  Chilling
  Dehydration
  Dystocia
  Gastric/caecal
    torsion
  Heat stress
  Ketosis
  Vitamin C deficiency

**Death, Sudden,
Neonate/Juvenile**
Infectious causes
  Clostridium piliforme
  Colibacillosis
  Cryptosporidiosis
  Yersinia
    pseudotuberculosis
Noninfectious causes
  Aflatoxicosis
    (maternal)
  Agalactia (maternal)
  Anoxia
  Chilling
  Environmental
    disturbances
    (maternal)
  Ketosis (maternal)
  Maternal inexperience
  Mastitis
  Small pups
  Vitamin K deficiency

Fig. 4.9—continued

CLINICAL SIGNS AND DIFFERENTIAL DIAGNOSES—GUINEA PIGS

Dermatitis
Infectious causes
Acariasis
Cryptococcosis
Dermatophytosis
Fleas
Myiasis
Pediculosis
Pseudomoniasis
Staphylococcosis
Noninfectious causes
Anal fold dermatitis
Chronic liver failure
Fatty acid deficiency
Fighting
Postpartum mineral/
protein deficiency
Scent gland dermatitis
Stress
Sunburn
Urine scald
Vitamin A deficiency
Vitamin C deficiency

Diarrhoea
Infectious causes
Absidia
Aflatoxicosis
Clostridium piliforme
Citrobacter freundii
Coccidiosis
Colibacillosis
Coronavirus
Clostridiosis
Cryptosporidiosis
Helminthiasis (rare)
Histoplasmosis
Salmonellosis (rare)
Torulopsis pintolopesii
Yersinia
pseudotuberculosis
Noninfectious causes
Chronic liver failure
Chronic renal failure
Environmental
stresses
Folic acid deficiency

Maldigestion
Vitamin B deficiency
Vitamin C deficiency

Dyspnoea
Infectious causes
Adenovirus (rare)
Bordetellosis
Citrobacter freundii
(rare)
Klebsiella
pneumoniae (rare)
Pulmonary papillary
adenoma (rare)
Staphylococcosis (rare)
Streptobacillus
monilformis
Streptococcus equi
Streptococcus
pneumoniae
Noninfectious causes
Allergy (rare)
Diaphraghmatic hernia
Dust (food, hay,
bedding)
Gastric torsion
Heat stress
Ketosis
Psychological distress
'Short-nosed'
phenotype

Dystocia
Excessively large young
Fused pubic symphysis
Maternal immaturity
Obesity

Haemorrhage
Copper deficiency
Erysipelas
rhusiopathiae
Haematuria/vaginal
bleeding
Abortion
Cystitis
Neoplasia

Urolithiasis
Vaginitis
Potassium deficiency
Streptococcal
septicaemia
Vitamin C deficiency
Vitamin K deficiency

Ileus/Constipation/
Obstipation
Clostridiosis
Gastrointestinal
mineralisation
Gastrointestinal
torsion/
intussusception
Rectal impaction

Incoordination/
Convulsions
Aflatoxicosis
Clostridiosis
Eclampsia
Hepatic failure
Idiopathic epilepsy
Ketosis
Perinatal anoxia
Toxoplasmosis
Trixacariasis
Vitamin B deficiency
Vitamin E deficiency

Infertility
Bedding adhered
to genitalia
Crowding
Cystic ovarian disease
Diabetes mellitus
Environmental stress
Oestrogens in feed
Metritis
Obesity
Penile malformation
Senescence
Vitamin E deficiency
Wire flooring

Nasal discharge
Infectious disease
Adenovirus
Bordetellosis
Citrobacter freundii
(rare)
Klebsiella
pneumoniae (rare)
Pseudomoniasis (rare)
Staphyloccosis (rare)
Streptobacillus
moniliformis (rare)
Streptococcus equi
Streptococcus
pneumoniae
Noninfectious causes
Allergy/irritation
Heat stress
Ketosis
Vitamin C deficiency

Ocular Opacity
Cataracts
Corneal oedema
Entropion
Foreign body
Trauma
Corneal mineralisation

Otitis Media/Interna
Actinobacillosis (rare)
Bordetellosis
Encephalitozoonosis
(rare)
Pasteurella
multocida (rare)
Pseudomoniasis
Streptococcus equi
Streptococcus
pneumoniae

Fig. 4.9—continued

CLINICAL SIGNS AND DIFFERENTIAL DIAGNOSES—GUINEA PIGS			
Paralysis/Reluctance to move	Trauma (fracture/luxation)	Heat stress	**Weight loss/ poor growth**
Infectious causes	Vitamin B deficiency	Ketosis	Aflatoxicosis
Bordetellosis	Vitamin C deficiency	Malocclusion	Chronic renal disease
Clostridiosis	Vitamin E deficiency	Ageing	Diabetes mellitus
Histoplasmosis (rare)		Congenital	Ectoparasitism
	Pododermatitis	Trauma	Endoparasitism
Lymphocytic choriomeningitis (rare)	Obesity	Vitamin D deficiency	Folic acid deficiency
	Poor sanitation	Oral foreign body	Inability to access feed/water
	Pregnancy	Vitamin C deficiency	
Poliomyelitis virus (rare)	Staphylococcosis		Infectious bacterial disease(nonspecific)
	Wire flooring	**Rough hair coat/seborrhoea**	
Salmonellosis		Abyssinian genetics	Malocclusion
Streptobacillus moniliformis	**Polyuria/polydipsia**	Acariasis	Metastatic calcification
	Chronic liver disease	Aggressive behaviour	Neophobia toward feed/feeders
Staphylococcosis	Dandelion ingestion	Chronic liver disease	
Streptococcus equi	Diabetes mellitus	Dermatophytosis	Neoplasia
Streptococcus pneumoniae	Lactation (polydipsia only)	Heat stress	Pododermatitis
		Infectious disease (nonspecific)	Protein deficiency
Toxoplasmosis	Pregnancy		Vitamin A deficiency
Noninfectious causes	Psychogenic	Moist cage	Vitamin B deficiency
Eclampsia	Renal failure	Vitamin C deficiency	Vitamin C deficiency
Fluorosis			Wire flooring
Hypervitaminosis D	**Ptyalism**	**Torticollis**	
Metastatic calcification	Adrenocortical insufficiency	Congenital disease	
		Encephalitozoonosis	
Osteoarthritis	Fluorosis	Otitis interna	
Osteosarcoma	Folic acid deficiency	Trauma	
Pregnancy			

FIG. 4.9 Clinical signs and differential diagnoses—guinea pigs.

PHYSIOLOGICAL DATA—GUINEA PIGS	
Adult body weight, male	700–1200 g
Adult body weight, female	600–900 g
Life span	3–4 years;
	6–8 years (max.)
Water consumption	80–100 ml/kg/day
Temperature (rectal)	37.2–39.5 °C
Food consumption	50–60 g/kg/day
Heart rate	230–380/min
Respiratory rate	42–150/min
Urine production (ml/adult day)	20–25
Systolic arterial blood pressure (mmHg)	77–94
Diastolic arterial blood pressure (mmHg)	47–58
Tidal volume (ml/kg)	2.3–5.3
Data taken from Harkness and Wagner (1989), Manning *et al.* (1984), Richardson (1992), Flecknell (1991), Sutherland and Festing (1987), Green (1982), Hong *et al.* (1977), Muir and Hubbell (1989) and Sirois (1989).	

FIG. 4.10 Physiological data–guinea pigs.

HAEMATOLOGICAL VALUES—GUINEA PIGS	
PCV %	35–49
Haemoglobin g/dl	12–16
RBC × 10^6/mm^3	4.3–6.6
Reticulocytes %	0–4
WBC × 10^3/mm^3	6.2–16.5
Neutrophils	1.9–8.1 (26–42 %)
Mononuclear cells (lymphocytes/monocytes)	3.3–9.1 (39–74 %)
Eosinophils	0.1–0.8 (1–5 %)
Basophils	0.0–0.5 (0–3 %)
Foa–Kurloff cells	0.0–0.8 (0–4 %)
Platelets 10^3/mm^3	250–850
MCV μM^3	75–93
MCH pg	25
MCHC %	28–33
Blood volume	60–75 ml/kg
Data taken from Harkness and Wagner (1989), Manning *et al.* (1984), Richardson (1992), Flecknell (1991), Percy (1984), Green (1982), Quesenberry (1994), Benirschke *et al.* (1978) and Quillec *et al.* (1977).	

FIG. 4.11 Haematological values—guinea pigs.

CLINICAL CHEMISTRY VALUES—GUINEA PIGS	
Calcium mg/dl	5.3–12.0
Phosphorus mg/dl	3.0–7.6
Sodium mEq/l	120–152
Chloride mEq/l	90–115
Potassium mEq/l	3.8–8.9
Glucose mg/dl	60–180
BUN mg/dl	9–32
Creatinine mg/dl	0.6–2.2
Total bilbirubin mg/dl	0.3–0.9
Total protein g/dl	4.7–6.4
Albumin g/dl	2.1–3.9
Globulin g/dl	1.7–2.6
Cholesterol mg/dl	16–43
Triglycerides mg/dl	0–145
Alkaline phosphatase IU/l	55–108
SGOT IU/l	27–68
SGPT IU/l	25–59
CPK IU/l	76–646
Serum lipids mg/dl	95–240
Phospholipids mg/dl	25–75
Bicarbonate mEq/l	13–30
Magnesium mEq/l	1.8–3.0
Data taken from Harkness and Wagner (1989), Manning *et al.* (1984), Percy (1984), Quesenbery (1994) and Howell and Buxton (1975).	

FIG. 4.12 Clinical chemistry values—guinea pigs.

REPRODUCTIVE DATA—GUINEA PIGS	
Breeding age, male	3–4 months (550–700 g)
Breeding age, female	2–3 months (350–450 g)
Oestrous cycle	Polyoestrous
Duration of oestrous cycle	15–19 days
Gestation	59–72 days
Average litter size	1–6
Birth weight	60–115 g
Eyes open	at birth
Wean	14–21 days (150–200 g)
Postpartum oestrus	2–15 h
Number of mammae	2
Breeding duration	18–24 months
Oestrous period	1–15 h
Data taken from Harkness and Wagner (1989), Manning *et al.* (1984), Richardson (1992), Flecknell (1991) and Sutherland and Festing (1987).	

FIG. 4.13 Reproductive data—guinea pigs.

5

Chinchillas

JAMES G. STRAKE, LAURA A. DAVIS, MARIE LaREGINA and KENNETH R. BOSCHERT

Introduction

Chinchillas are hystricomorph rodents closely related to the domestic guinea pig. They were originally found high in the Andes mountains of South America where the temperature is cool and the humidity low. In their natural habitat, chinchillas live in groups of 14–100 individuals in rock crevices or burrows, but do not hibernate (Hoefer, 1994). Several years ago, chinchillas were hunted nearly to extinction for their soft, silky fur, considered among the most valuable in the world. Today breeding farms supply the majority of chinchillas needed for pelts. Chinchillas are also useful animal models of human diseases, such as cholera, diabetes, oxalate nephrosis and acoustic trauma. Chinchilla vestibulo-ocular reflexes and corpus luteum functions closely mimic their human counterparts (Peiffer and Johnson, 1980). The chinchilla's friendly nature has made them popular as pets. *Chinchilla laniger*, the long-tailed chinchilla (Fig. 5.1) and *Chinchilla brevicaudata*, the main short-tailed chinchilla, are the two main recognised species (Webb *et al.*, 1991).

Unique Biology

Newborn chinchillas, like guinea pigs, are fully furred, able to walk and have open eyes. Newborn chinchillas weigh 30–60 g; adults weigh 400–600 g. Teeth are present at birth. The dental formula of chinchillas is $2(I\frac{1}{1} \ C\frac{0}{0} \ P\frac{1}{1} \ M\frac{3}{3})$. The teeth are open-rooted and grow continuously throughout life. The incisors are yellow and grow 4–6 cm per year (Hoefer, 1994).

Like most other herbivores, the chinchilla's gastrointestinal tract has evolved the necessary adaptations to accommodate a plant diet. The large stomach and caecum and long intestinal tract allow a longer time for digestion of plant material. The chinchilla's renal system is able to resist dehydration in a similar way to desert rodents, although chinchillas are not native to desert regions (McManus, 1971). The chinchilla's thymus is located entirely intrathoracically (Cartell, 1979).

Chinchilla's ears are large, thin and often referred to as 'bat-like'. The auditory bullae of chinchillas are also large and well developed, making them useful animal models for auditory research. Chinchillas are nocturnal but can be active during the day (Hoefer, 1994). Chinchilla's corneas are large, a common characteristic of other nocturnal species (Peiffer, 1980). Normal physiological, haematological and clinical chemistry values are found at the end of the chapter.

Reproduction

The most reliable way to determine the sex of a chinchilla is by observing the anogenital distance, the length between the anus and the external genitalia. This distance is roughly twice as long in the male chinchilla (Fig. 5.2) compared with the female. In females, the large cone-shaped clitoris located ventral to the vagina is often mistaken for a penis. The vagina can be identified as a transverse slit between the anus and the clitoral papilla (Fig. 5.2) (Bickel, 1987). Female chinchillas are usually slightly larger than the males. The female reproductive tract consists of two uterine horns, each with separate openings into a single cervix. A vaginal mem-

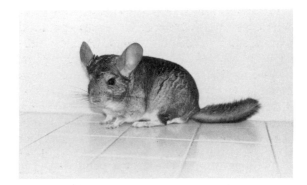

FIG. 5.1 The long-tailed chinchilla, *Chinchilla laniger*.

brane is present and opens during oestrus and parturition. Females have four mammary nipples with one pair located in the inguinal area and one on each lateral rib cage.

The male's penis can be exposed by gentle downward pressure. The chinchilla's penis is supported by a small bone called a baculum (Bickel, 1987). A true scrotum is not present. The testicles are located just below the skin in the area of the inguinal canal. The testicles are approximately 20 mm in length and oblong in shape. If a male chinchilla is in the vicinity of a female in oestrus, the usually undetectable testicles become swollen and are easily observed. Castrated male chinchillas have thicker hair coats and are more compatible cage mates (Bickel, 1987). When castrating a chinchilla, the inguinal

canals should be closed. For the operative technique, please refer to *Chapter 8*.

Mating

The chinchilla's oestrous cycle lasts 24–40 days. Postpartum oestrus will occur 12 h following parturition and lasts approximately 48 h (Kennedy, 1970). Females in oestrus can usually be identified by an open, reddened vagina. Gentle pressure to the genital papilla will usually open the vagina. If the animal is not in oestrus, vaginal opening will not be possible (Bickel, 1987). A reddening of the nipples and restless behaviour is occasionally seen in oestrus females (Bickel, 1987; Kennedy, 1970). Vaginal cytology can be used to determine the stage of the oestrous cycle with 70% accuracy (Jarosz, 1973).

Sunlight or fluorescent lighting is especially important for breeding animals. Increasing exposure to light may have a beneficial effect on breeding success by simulating the onset of spring and summer. A relatively quiet environment is important because chinchillas do not breed well if constantly disturbed by loud noises (Bickel, 1987).

Wax-like oestrus plugs measuring 2.5–3 cm are normally ejected from the female at the onset of oestrus. Occasionally a plug gets stuck and a small amount of lubricating ointment must be applied to expel it. The significance of the

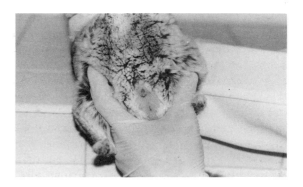
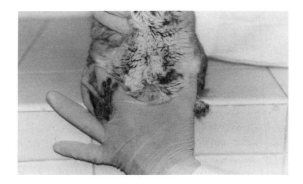

FIG. 5.2 The length between the anus and the external genitalia is twice as long in the male chinchilla (left) as in the female (right). The vagina can be identified as a transverse slit between the anus and the clitoral papilla.

oestrus plug is unknown. Similar copulatory or fertilisation plugs, commonly referred to as 'stoppers', are formed by the mixing of the male and female reproductive fluids. These plugs are found in the female's vagina after mating and are thought to prevent loss of semen. The plugs, measuring up to 3.75 cm in length, remain in place for several hours, then fall out. Copulatory plugs can be confused with oestrus plugs, but the latter are usually seen at the onset of oestrus. Since chinchillas normally mate at night, the best time to check for copulatory plugs is the morning following mating (Bickel, 1987). Plugs can be found at the bottom of the cage or nest box. Like other hystricomorphs, chinchillas have extremely long gestation periods. The gestation of 111 days is due to the slow rate of foetal growth, especially in the early stages (Roberts, 1971).

Introducing potential mates before the female enters oestrus can reduce fighting and increase compatibility. A refuge box should be provided for the male, especially when first introduced to the female. Allowing intended mates to use the same sand bath prior to exposure to one another also increases the likelihood of acceptance. Non-oestrus female chinchillas can aggressively attack males attempting to mate with them. In this situation some males will lose their desire to mate. The female can be fitted with a muzzle to prevent her from biting the male or she may have a collar attached that would prevent her from aggressively chasing the male. Muzzles should be made from soft, thin glove leather and must be wide enough to hold the animal's mouth shut. The conical end is positioned over the animal's face and attached around the neck by a small buckle. The collar can be made from light-weight rubber. It should be 10 cm wide at the bottom, rounded off along the top and 15 cm high in the centre. A circular hole approximately 3–4 cm in diameter is cut in the upper third so the collar can be pulled over the head of the aggressive female. The collar will prevent her from chasing the male when she steps on the rubber. Males will fight one another in the presence of a female in oestrus (Bickel, 1987).

Economic pressures have changed the once common method of breeding animals in pairs to a polygamous breeding system (Bickel, 1987). Chinchillas used for polygamous breeding are housed so that a single male is able to service multiple females. There are several types of housing arrangements that allow polygamous mating. The first arrangement is a single large cage with multiple boxes to allow the male and subordinate females to escape from the dominant females. Escape cages can be simple metal boxes or metal cans with one open end, or open plastic drainage pipes (Bickel, 1987).

An alternative housing arrangement known as a harem system permits each female to reside in her own individual cage, connected to other females' cages by a small tunnel passageway. Females are restricted to their own individual cage by a flat, lightweight metal disc attached around their neck. This disc prevents passage through the connecting tunnel because its circumference is larger than the tunnel opening. Segregation of females eliminates the possibility of fighting (Jenkins, 1992) and since males are not fitted with collars, they are able to pass freely between connecting cages. The harem system permits males to escape to the safety of the tunnel and avoid female aggression. Some breeders remove collars from females after they become pregnant and close the tunnel, denying access to the male. Others transfer females to maternity/delivery cages (Bickel, 1987). In a polygamous mating system, one male is normally used to mate with 4–5 females (Zeinert, 1983).

A third type of polygamous breeding system consists of a male's cage surrounded by several cages for females. Although the layouts of the design vary, there is a common principle behind each housing arrangement. The male should have easy, unrestricted access to each of the females and there should be an area that will allow him to escape. This design also utilises collars for the females. An empty cage serves as a resting place for the male. As many as 20% of female chinchillas refuse to breed with a particular male, necessitating the use of an alternative male. The harm that a male can experience when co-housed with an incompatible female is not limited to physical injury. Repeated aggression elicits a conditioned avoidance response in the male, making him an unsatisfactory breeder (Bickel, 1987).

Some breeders use a colonial breeding system in which a group of male and female chinchillas are housed in a single large enclosure. The purpose of this breeding arrangement is to mimic the natural setting and allow for natural selection. The drawbacks associated with this method include fighting and the additional expense of maintaining a larger population of males.

Gestation and Birth

When chinchillas near parturition, they may become inactive and anorectic. Increased aggression toward a previously compatible mate is another sign of impending parturition. In addition to weight gain and behaviour changes, a near-term chinchilla's vagina begins to open and take on a bluish hue. Once parturition begins, the interval between successive births varies from several minutes to several hours (Bickel, 1987). Generally all kits are born within a 4 h period (Zeinert, 1983) and during delivery the dam will actively pull the young from the birth canal (Bickel, 1987). An unusual and currently unexplained phenomenon is the larger ratio of males to females born, 119:100 (Galton, 1968). *C. laniger* normally produce larger litters than *C. brevicaudata* (Bickel, 1987).

Chinchilla dams normally will not build a nest at parturition. In the absence of a nesting box the dam will deliver kits directly on either solid or wire mesh floors (Hoefer, 1994). Nesting boxes are not absolutely necessary, however they may help decrease neonatal mortality caused by cold stress. Nesting boxes should be designed to prevent actively moving young from leaving the box. If urine collects inside the nesting box, remove the bottom of the box, so that urine simply falls to the collecting pan below.

Neonatal chinchillas are particularly sensitive to draughts and cold temperatures and a significant number of neonatal deaths have been linked to hypothermia (Bickel, 1987). Nest boxes should be free from draughts. A kit accidentally separated from its mother can become chilled and moribund. Steps to revive hypothermic kits must be instituted quickly. Brisk rubbing, thorough drying of fur and placement on a heating pad or into an incubator will help restore normal temperatures. Once recovered, they can be returned to the nest box to be cared for by the mother. Small heating pads can be used as a source of supplemental heat for newborn kits, but care should be taken to avoid overheating (Zeinert, 1983). Warm water heating blankets are preferred over electric types due to decreased risk of thermal burns.

Most captive-bred chinchillas deliver their young with no difficulty and interference with delivery is not advisable. The female normally eats the foetal membranes following parturition and the vagina remains open 3–4 days before the vaginal membrane reforms (Bickel, 1987).

Following parturition, some dams become intolerant to the presence of males. If this occurs, remove the male from the cage until the kits are weaned. Alternatively, a refuge box can be placed in the cage to provide the male with a safe area to hide (Kennedy, 1970). Reproductive information is summarised in Fig. 5.10 found at the end of the chapter.

Husbandry

Housing

To keep chinchillas in good health, their housing environment should be dry, draught-free and moderately cool. The preferred temperature range for chinchillas housed indoors is 10.0–15.6°C (50–60°F) (Zeinert, 1983). Temperatures outside the recommended range, or rapidly fluctuating temperatures, can lead to stress and increase susceptibility to disease. Chinchillas are prone to heat stroke in hot, humid environments (Jenkins, 1992; Dieterich, 1979). They start to become uncomfortable at 21.1°C (70°F) and can die if exposed to temperatures above 32.2°C (90°F) (Dieterich, 1979). High humidity levels may also have untoward effects on breeding. Chinchillas kept dry and housed in a draught-free area can withstand temperatures below 0°C (32°F) if adapted to a cooler environment gradually. Cold temperatures stimulate the production of a thick hair coat allowing the animal to thrive. It is not uncommon to have decreased breeding behaviour during the cooler months of the year (Bickel, 1987).

There are many types of caging systems available for housing chinchillas. Wire mesh cages, 1 m × 1.5 m, 30–40 cm high, are superior to wooden cages because of the chinchilla's gnawing habits (Hoefer, 1994; Nickelson, 1993). Wire mesh cages also allow urine and faeces to fall below the cage, protecting the animal and making cleaning relatively easy. To prevent potential problems with limb injuries, the size of the mesh openings should not exceed 15 mm × 15 mm (Hoefer, 1994). Neonatal cold stress is a potential problem that can be alleviated by placement of a nesting box.

When solid-bottomed cages are used as an alternative, bedding choice becomes important to prevent parasitic contamination, fur staining and skin drying. Solid flooring can reduce the incidence of limb injuries. Soft wood shavings are often used as cage bedding material, but resinous woods, woods high in tannic acid and woods that have been treated, dyed or polished should be avoided due to their potentially toxic effects. Fuller's earth or cat litter are other types of satisfactory bedding materials. They keep animals dry without creating excessive skin dryness, eliminate the need for sand baths and need to be replaced only once every 10 days (Kline, 1979). As a form of environmental enrichment, chinchillas can be housed in multilevel cages and when given the opportunity, they actively move between the various levels (Jenkins, 1992).

Dust baths consist of mixtures of silver sand and Fuller's earth (9:1) and may be offered to the chinchillas for approximately 10 min each day (Zeinert, 1983; Jenkins, 1992). Commercial brands of dust bath filler are also available. The dust bath helps satisfy the chinchilla's desire to groom. Dust bath pans should not remain in the cage over long periods since they will become soiled with faeces and food debris. Providing chinchillas with dust baths on a regular basis helps keep the fur clean and well groomed (Webb, 1991). Dust bath pans must be large enough to allow the chinchilla to roll over. The pan should contain 4–6 cm of the dust bath mixture (Zeinert, 1994). Chinchillas will occasionally develop conjunctivitis secondary to dust irritation. If this occurs, remove the dust bath until the condition has completely cleared and treat the eyes with an antibiotic ophthalmic ointment. Dust baths must not be provided to near-term dams or to mothers with young, because neonates may accumulate dust in their mouth and eyes.

Nutrition

Chinchillas should be provided with feeders that attach to the outside of the cage or heavily weighted crock bowls. This will minimise waste caused by overturned food and water dishes. Feeders and waterers maintained outside the cage are easily refilled without opening the cage and disturbing the animals. Placing hay in elevated feeders permits chinchillas to pull through individual pieces and decreases soilage.

In the wild, chinchillas eat a high fibre diet (Kennedy, 1970). Exact nutritional requirements for chinchillas have not been determined, creating disagreement about the best feeding practices. Poor nutrition may result in higher mortality rates and developmental abnormalities in young and decreased milk production in lactating females. Inadequate diets can upset normal gut flora. Overfeeding leads to the development of soft stools or diarrhoea. Normally chinchilla faeces should be somewhat dry (Bickel, 1987). Coprophagy is normal in chinchillas (Ebino, 1993).

Feeding chinchillas twice daily rather than once a day can be psychologically stimulating and provide additional opportunities to observe the animal's health. Breeding animals are generally fed a restricted ration, depending on their body condition and stage of gestation. Animals produced for pelt production and lactating dams are usually fed *ad libitum*. Weighing the animals on a regular basis will help determine if they are receiving an appropriate amount of food (Bickel, 1987).

Chinchillas living in the wild rarely drink water, since they are able to maintain their hydration by licking dew drops and eating plants. Chinchillas in captivity can adapt to drinking water from either valved waterers or water bottles with sipper tubes. Watering systems should be cleaned regularly or contamination may lead to disease outbreaks such as septicaemia caused by *Pseudomonas aeruginosa*.

Commercial pelleted diets for either chinchillas or guinea pigs may be used with satisfactory results. Adult chinchillas should receive 1–2 tablespoons of pellets daily. Pelleted food can be used exclusively or supplemented with small amounts of either fresh or dried produce. Supplementing the diet with hay contributes a source of roughage and can provide environmental enrichment. New diets should be introduced gradually by mixing portions of the old diet with the new. Increasing the percentage of new diet over a period of days will decrease the likelihood of enteric disorders related to shipping stress and diet change.

Many modern day forages, including timothy, orchard grass, blue grass and common prairie grass, have been used as ingredients in chinchilla feed, however alfalfa is the most popular feed source. The recommended amount of plant protein for chinchillas is between 14.0 and 16.0%. Alfalfa averages about 14% protein. Ladino or white clover may cause bloating and is therefore not recommended. Alsike and white Dutch clover are unpalatable and of questionable nutritional value (Kennedy, 1970).

Since chinchillas are not able to regurgitate, they cannot quickly eliminate contaminated or spoiled foods that upset the gastrointestinal tract (Zeinert, 1983). Hay exposed to high humidity can quickly mould, making it unsuitable for food and potentially deadly. Hazardous toxins can result if hays are permitted to ferment. Soiled and leftover hay should be discarded and replaced daily. Hay fed to chinchillas should be stored in a well ventilated, dry area.

If necessary, vitamin supplements are useful, but grains should be avoided to prevent disturbing the dietary balance (Kennedy, 1970). Proponents of feeding fresh produce claim this improves fertility and serves as a source of trace minerals. Others claim feeding fresh produce is laborious and contributes to a variety of problems such as death in young animals, poor lactation, miscarriages, stillbirths and infertility. Nuts should be avoided because of their high fat content. Salt licks containing trace minerals and edible chalk can be offered to chinchillas (Bickel, 1987).

Orphaned chinchilla kits can be cross-fostered on to other lactating females or if necessary, on to guinea pigs. It is better for orphaned animals to nurse from a foster mother than to be hand-fed (Webb, 1991; Kennedy, 1970). If a foster mother is not available, then it is necessary to hand-feed the kits for 2–3 weeks until they are able to feed themselves. Young chinchillas can learn to nurse artificial milk from an eyedropper, syringe or small nursing bottle (Webb, 1991). A suitable milk formula consists of 1 part water to 2 parts of condensed milk. When full, a baby chinchilla will usually attempt to push the dropper or syringe away. When hand-feeding orphaned kits, it is better to slightly underfeed than to overfeed (Kennedy, 1970). Orphaned kits should be hand-fed every 2–3 h (Zeinert, 1983; Kennedy, 1970). The quantity fed depends on age, size and whether the feedings are supplementary to the mother's milk. The frequency of the feedings can be decreased as the animal gets older. Eventually the orphan can be taught to drink from a small dish. Within the first week of life, newborn kits will be able to eat small amounts of solid food.

The dam's diet can be supplemented during the last month of pregnancy with vitamins derived from vegetables or commercially available vitamin drops. As the gravid uterus occupies an increasing space within the abdomen, its pressure on the intestinal tract can cause constipation. Lush greens should be avoided during the later stages of pregnancy due to the gaseous intestinal distension caused by fermentation (Kennedy, 1970).

Handling, Injection, Specimen Collection

Handling

Chinchillas are relatively easy to handle but it should be done calmly and gently and minimised as much as possible (Thompson, 1980). Most chinchillas are non-aggressive but others can bite or scratch and require extra precautions, like leather gloves (Bickel, 1987) when handling. There are several ways a chinchilla can be safely removed from its cage. Like rabbits, chinchillas should not be lifted by their ears. Follow the chinchilla about its cage until it can be firmly grasped by the base of the tail. The animal can then be removed from the cage by lifting the tail base while using the opposite hand to support the body (Fig. 5.3 (top)) (Hoefer, 1994). The chinchilla can also be placed on the opposite forearm where it will usually sit quietly (Fig. 5.3 (middle)). This is the handling method of choice for relatively docile chinchillas. Chinchillas should not be suspended by their tails for extended periods and pregnant dams should never be lifted in this fashion.

Improper handling often results in a phenomenon known as 'fur slip'. This is when an animal releases a patch of fur leaving only clean, smooth skin. Fur slip is a protective mechanism that chinchillas in the wild use to escape an attacker. Anything that overexcites chinchillas can trigger the fur slip response, including improper restraint, chasing about the cage, or even bumping into the cage wall. Fur regrowth can take several months and will frequently grow back a slightly different shade (Thompson, 1980).

If a chinchilla cannot be caught quickly, it should be guided into its nesting box or a catching cage, which is a small enclosure with one open end. The chinchilla is coaxed into the box and a hand is placed over the opening of the box as it is lifted from the cage. This will provide restraint with minimal stress to both handler and animal. When a chinchilla must be restrained for longer periods, for treatment or close examination, a squeezable restraining device can be used. This allows one person to do routine clinical

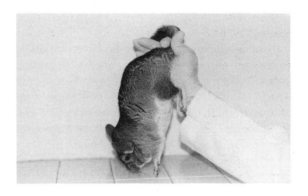

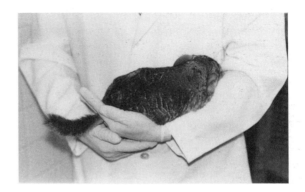

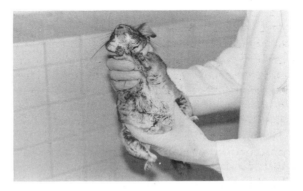

Fig. 5.3 (top) Chinchillas can be removed from their cages by gently lifting from the base of the tail while using the opposite hand to support the body. (middle) Chinchillas will sit quietly on a forearm once removed from their cage. (bottom) If restraint is necessary, smaller chinchillas can be grasped gently around the thorax taking care not to impede respiration.

procedures with minimal risk of personal injury (Strout, 1976).

Smaller chinchillas should be grasped gently around the thorax in a manner so that breathing is not restricted (Fig. 5.3 (bottom)). A small net should be available to catch chinchillas that escape from their cages. Routine restraint can be accomplished by wrapping a towel or other large piece of fabric around the body.

Generally, pregnant females should be left alone and human intervention minimised as much as possible (Bickel, 1987). Frequent attempts to detect pregnancy are not recommended due to the potential for damage to the foetuses and undue stress on the dam. Pregnancy can be detected by palpation at 90 days gestation. Experienced personnel can detect pregnancy as early as 60 days gestation (Kennedy, 1970). At approximately 2 months gestation the female's breasts and teats begin to swell. The nipples aquire a red colour and there is a doughy distension of the abdomen. These changes become more pronounced as pregnancy progresses. Individual foetuses can be palpated in late stages of gestation. It is possible to determine the number of foetuses, but this requires extensive experience. Pregnancy determination can also be accomplished by regular weighing. Weight gain in pregnant chinchillas will be minimal during the first 6 weeks and increases rapidly thereafter (Bickel, 1987).

Improper handling of a pregnant chinchilla may result in abortion or absorption of the foetuses. These losses can go unnoticed and cost time and money in a breeding operation. Other factors causing abortion in chinchillas include poor housing conditions and severe stress (Thompson, 1980).

Oral administration of medications or other fluids can be performed with a small syringe or eyedropper positioned at the diastema. Chinchillas can bite the syringe or eyedropper, therefore glass or easily broken materials should not be used. Care must be taken to avoid positioning the tip of the dropper or syringe too deeply in the animal's mouth since this can result in aspiration. When the animal is able to eat, medica-

tion can be mixed in with food or water. Drugs or fluids can be directly deposited into the stomach via a stomach tube. A speculum should be used to prevent the animal from biting through the tube. Personal preference will determine what type of speculum to use. A simple wooden rod can be positioned on one side of the mouth and permit passage of the stomach tube. When doing this, hold the chinchilla's mouth firmly closed on the speculum to prevent its release. If necessary, medication can be administered rectally.

Injection

For drug or therapeutic administration in chinchillas, oral, subcutaneous (SC), intramuscular (IM), intravenous (IV) and intraperitoneal (IP) routes are used. The flank and interscapular region are common sites for SC injections. SC injections can be given in the inner thigh area to minimise potential damage to the pelt. The large thigh muscles (semitendinosus and quadriceps femoris) are preferred sites for IM injections (Fig. 5.4). The amount of material injected per site IM should be limited to 0.3 ml. A 23 gauge needle or smaller is preferred .

Several peripheral veins are accessible for intravenous administration (Tappa *et al.*, 1989). The femoral, cephalic, lateral saphenous (Tappa

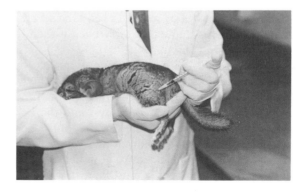

FIG. 5.4 Intramuscular injections can be given in the posterior thigh muscles while the chinchilla is restrained between the arm and the body of the handler.

et al., 1989), jugular (Hoefer, 1994), auricular (Fig. 5.5), dorsal penile, lateral abdominal and tail veins can be used in unanaesthetised chinchillas. The most commonly used sites include the femoral, cephalic and lateral saphenous veins. A 25 gauge or smaller needle should be used for venepuncture.

Specimen Collection

Only very small amounts of blood may be collected from most peripheral vessels. Ear vessels should not be lacerated in attempting to collect blood. If large amounts of blood are needed, the jugular vein or orbital sinus may be used. Under anaesthesia, 1–3 ml of venous blood can be collected from the orbital sinus, which is entered via the medial canthus using a similar technique to that commonly performed in rats or mice. Repeated collections by this method can cause ocular damage or haemorrhage and lead to difficulty in future collections (Brookshyser et al., 1977). Blood collection from the transverse sinus is used when repeated samples are needed (Hoefer, 1994; Boettcher et al., 1990). These techniques are not recommended for inexperienced personnel (Boettcher et al., 1990).

Diseases—An Introduction

Diseases affecting the gastrointestinal tract, respiratory system and integument are commonly seen in pet chinchillas. Published reports refer to diseases affecting multiple chinchillas in

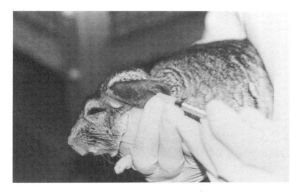

FIG. 5.5 The auricular vessel can be used for intravenous injections using a 25 gauge needle.

production colonies. Refer to Fig. 5.6 for a summary of the primary diseases that affect chinchillas.

Diseases of the Respiratory System

Infectious Diseases

Inadequate housing conditions such as high humidity, poor ventilation and overcrowding contribute to an increased incidence of respiratory disease in chinchillas. Neonatal chinchillas are particularly prone to pneumonia when exposed to cold drafts. To minimise this problem, nest boxes with solid bottoms should be utilised. Cageboards or other absorbent material can be placed in nest boxes to facilitate cleaning (Balows et al., 1991).

Upper respiratory infections

Upper airway infections involving nasal sinuses and nasal mucous membranes occur frequently as secondary disease conditions. Damp and cool conditions can precipitate outbreaks of respiratory symptoms in young or debilitated chinchillas.

Agent. Bacteria that have been specifically isolated in kits include *Streptococcus* spp., *Pseudomonas aeruginosa*, *Pasteurella* spp. and *Bordetella* spp. (Hoefer, 1994). It is not known if these organisms are primary pathogens or simply opportunistic invaders.

Hosts. Although transmission from humans to chinchillas has not been proven, it has been suggested. People with respiratory symptoms should avoid contact with chinchillas.

Clinical signs. Upper respiratory infections present with varying degrees of severity. The most common clinical indication of upper respiratory disease in adult chinchillas is an inflamed, reddened nose without nasal discharge. Gross lesions include purulent debris in the sinus cavities and partial necrosis of the nasal septum with occasional extension into the brain. Occasionally, chinchillas are found dead with no previous clinical signs of disease. Kits often present sneezing and shivering, burrowing into the dam's fur in an effort to stay warm. A serous oculonasal discharge is noted in kits and thickens as the disease progresses, making breathing difficult and matting the eyelids closed. If left untreated, upper respiratory infections often progress to pneumonia.

Diagnosis. Definitive diagnosis is obtained through bacterial culture and isolation.

Treatment. Antibiotic therapy based on culture and sensitivity is of limited value due to the severity of disease by the time the condition is clinically apparent. Treatment of affected kits consists of gently soaking the nose and eyes with warm water and removing any crusts. Once the eyes are open, an antibiotic ointment may be applied.

Pneumonia

Agents. Pneumonia is characterised by inflammation of the lung parenchyma and associated airways. Bacterial agents are often isolated from chinchillas with lowered host resistance from housing in cold, damp environments. Such bacteria include *Bordetella* spp., *Streptococcus* spp. and *Pasteurella* spp., often seen as concurrent infections.

Clinical signs. Clinical signs can rapidly progress from nonspecific lethargy to laboured, shallow breathing and a marked febrile response of 40.0–40.6°C (104–105°F). In advanced stages of the disease, chinchillas will assume a hunched posture and be reluctant to move. Auscultation reveals wheezing sounds across the entire lung field. Grossly, lesions may range from a focal bronchopneumonia involving only a small area of one lobe to complete consolidation. Often, small amounts of purulent debris can be expressed from the cut surface of the lung bronchioles.

Treatment. Treatment is usually unsuccessful if large areas of consolidation of the lungs are present, but antibiotics may be helpful with a focal bronchopneumonia. Drug therapy should be complemented with supportive care, minimal stress and warm, dry housing. Prophylactic treatment of other clinically unaffected chinchillas can minimise further spread of the disease.

Non-Infectious Diseases

Choke

This condition is occasionally seen in chinchillas due to occlusion of the entrance of the trachea by a large piece of food or other foreign body. In addition to occlusion, aspiration of minute particles from the foreign body can irritate the lower respiratory tract and precipitate an oedematous response.

Clinical signs

When choke occurs, the chinchilla initially appears startled and soon begins coughing and struggling in an attempt to dislodge the foreign body. The animal's condition deteriorates rapidly and death due to suffocation often occurs (Kennedy, 1970).

Miscellaneous

Occasionally on post-mortem examination, chinchillas housed in dusty conditions will present with multiple, pin-point, flat, dark foci scattered over the surface of the lungs. The clinical significance of this finding is unknown but is thought to be reflective of poor air quality (Kennedy, 1970).

Diseases of the Gastrointestinal System

Most gastrointestinal disorders in chinchillas present with similar clinical signs that are nonspecific and representative of many different aetiologies. Some of the more common gastrotestinal conditions include gastric tympany, gastric ulcers, intestinal obstruction and gastroenterocolitis while single reports of less frequent problems include intestinal volvulus and torsion and diaphragmatic hernia (Kennedy, 1976; Dall, 1967). An affected chinchilla presents with lethargy, anorexia, roughened haircoat and dull eyes. This can be accompanied by significant weight loss, clinical dehydration, fever or hypothermia, pain on abdominal palpation, flatulence and diarrhoea or constipation. Diarrhoea is usually hypersecretory and may range from haemorrhagic to mucoid in nature. Perineal staining is evident and rectal prolapse will frequently occur in response to abdominal straining. A differential diagnosis for diarrhoea includes nutritional, bacterial, protozoal and parasitic aetiologies. It is also seen as a stress-induced response, for example, with overcrowding. The principles for diarrhoea therapy are the same regardless of the aetiology. Any disturbance of the the gastrointestinal tract requires a diet of roughage, decreasing the amount of grains and concentrates fed. Feeding *Lactobacillus* sp., in the form of yogurt with active cultures, will often help re-establish normal bacterial flora within the digestive tract (Ellett and Moellering, 1974). Antibiotics should be used cautiously, since they can further disrupt the bacterial flora of the gastrointestinal tract and exacerbate the diarrhoea. Supportive care is important and hydration must be maintained.

Constipation is another non-specific sign occasionally seen as a sequel to intestinal obstruction. As with any small mammal, increasing the fibre in the diet, by supplementing with alfalfa cubes, or adding mineral oil to the feed may relieve constipation. If there is no response to these measures, repeated soapy, warm water enemas are indicated. Constipation due to a persistent intestinal blockage may require surgical intervention. Intussusception often accompanies gastrointestinal hypermotility caused by a primary disorder (Kennedy, 1970).

Infectious Diseases

Gastroenteritis can be an acute or chronic condition. Acutely, the animal is found dead without previous clinical signs. In the chronic condition, diarrhoea is the primary clinical sign. Aetiologies for gastroenteritis include bacterial, protozoal and parasitic diseases. Each of these three groups is discussed in detail below.

Bacterial gastroenteritis

Bacterial enteritis can result from alterations in nutrition or the misuse of certain antibiotics. The chinchilla's intestinal flora is primarily composed of Gram-positive bacteria including *Bifidobacterium* sp., *Bacteroides* sp., *Eubacterium* sp. and aerobic *Lactobacillus* sp. The β-lactam antibiotics erythromycin, clindamycin and lincomycin will alter normal bacterial flora by eliminating the Gram-positive bacteria and allowing overgrowth of Gram-negative bacteria such as *Escherichia coli*, *Proteus* sp., *Salmonella typhimurium*, *Salmonella arizona* (Mountain, 1989) and *Yersinia* sp. or Gram-positive bacteria such as *Clostridium* sp. (Kennedy, 1976; Jenkins, 1992).

Clostridial enterotoxaemia

Clostridial enterotoxaemia is the most common bacterial enteritis encountered.

Agents. *Clostridium perfringens* Type D is typically isolated, but *Clostridium perfringens* Type A has also been identified.

Clinical signs. Death usually occurs 24–48 h post-infection. Hepatomegaly and splenomegaly are also present.

Diagnosis. Serological tests and identification of the toxin in gastric contents help confirm the diagnosis.

Treatment. Vaccination of chinchillas with clostridial toxoid decreases morbidity and mortality in affected colonies (Webb, 1991; Bartoszcze *et al.*, 1990; Moore and Greenlee, 1975).

Corynebacterial enteritis

Agent. *Corynebacterium* sp. has been isolated in chinchillas. Modes of transmission include direct and indirect contact and ingestion of contaminated feed.

Clinical signs. Chinchillas exhibit signs of diarrhoea, abdominal pain, progressive hindlimb paralysis and death. Pathological findings include enteritis, intestinal abscessation and peritonitis with intestinal adhesions.

Diagnosis. Bacterial culture of the intestinal tract and isolation of the organism constitutes definitive diagnosis.

Treatment. Antibiotic therapy using sulphonamides is reported to have variable success against active infection (Kennedy, 1970). The use of penicillin in chinchillas has not been reported but it is effective against corynebacterial infections in other species (Fraser *et al.*, 1978). Inoculation of bacterins is effective in preventing the spread of disease (Kennedy, 1970).

Protozoal enteritis

Giardia sp. are motile flagellate protozoans commonly found in the small intestine when clinical diarrhoea is not present. *Trichomonas* sp., a flagellate protozoan, commonly infects the caecum causing a haemorrhagic typhlitis, while *Balantidium* sp., a ciliated protozoan, is commonly associated with a haemorrhagic colitis. *Trichomonas* and *Balantidium* are occasionally present in clinically normal chinchillas. Increased numbers of these protozoans in the faeces in the presence of diarrhoea often indicate an underlying disease problem (Kennedy, 1970; Moreland, 1967). *Cryptosporidium* has been reported in an 8-month-old chinchilla with severe diarrhoea. Gross pathology findings included enteritis, mesenteric lymphadenopathy and hepatitis (Yamini and Raju, 1986). There also is one report of clinical coccidiosis in chinchillas. *Eimeria chinchillae* was isolated and found to be transmissible to other rodents. Intestinal protozoans are diagnosed by direct faecal smear and should be treated with appropriate antiprotozoal drugs (DeVos, 1970).

Parasitic enteritis

A number of trematodes, nematodes and cestodes have been identified in the chinchilla. Frequently, they are diagnosed on routine faecal flotation but are not associated with clinical diarrhoea unless the animals have severe infestations. *Physaloptera* sp. (Kennedy, 1970), *Hymenolepis* sp. (Fox *et al.*, 1984) and *Haemonchus contortus* (Boisvenue and Hendrix, 1968) have been reported in the chinchilla. Parasitic enterocolitis should be treated with the appropriate anthelmintic.

Non-Infectious Diseases

Malocclusion

Abnormalities involving the teeth are common in chinchillas. Chinchillas can be affected by malocclusion when they are as young as 6 months of age. It is important to avoid breeding these chinchillas as the condition tends to be inherited. Females nursing their first litter are often affected with abnormalities of the teeth due to a nutritional mineral imbalance.

Clinical signs. Clinically, a chinchilla with malocclusion has general loss of condition, rough haircoat, weight loss and anorexia. Partially chewed food can be observed on the cage floor. The primary clinical sign is hypersalivation resulting in inflammation and alopecia of the skin on the chin and ventral neck. If the malocclusion is not corrected, a secondary infection develops as a result of penetration of the hard palate by the overgrown teeth. Affected animals develop a mucopurulent oculonasal discharge. As the condition progresses, the chinchilla becomes severely malnourished. Severe hypoglycaemic episodes can result leading to seizures, paralysis, coma and death.

Diagnosis. To determine the exact nature and severity of the problem, a thorough examination of the mouth is necessary. Effective restraint of the chinchilla is essential. If this cannot be accomplished manually, chemical sedation is required. Maximal visualisation is important and can be accomplished using a small vaginal speculum or an otoscope. Alternatively, gauze strips can be wrapped around the incisors to open the mouth. Sufficient light is important.

When examining the mouth, observe for areas of tooth decay. These will appear as spots or patches of brown on the lingual surfaces of the teeth. Check the teeth to see if any are broken, have ridges or sharp points, or are loose in their sockets. Note the angles and length of the molars and incisors as well as the incisor pigmentation. The normally orange pigment of the incisors will fade with dental disease. With malocclusion, the upper and lower incisors will overgrow and curl inwards. If left untreated, they will penetrate the respective palates. The lower molars often angle towards the tongue and in severe cases, entrap the tongue. Overgrowth of the upper molars often results in lateral angulation of the teeth. Check behind the molars and in any spaces between the teeth for impactions of food or foreign bodies. Examine the oral mucosa for any ulcerations or nodules that may have developed. Dental radiographs are helpful in monitoring the position of the teeth and detecting overgrowth of the roots. With malocclusion, the roots of the lower molars can extend deep into the mandible while the roots of the upper molars can extend into the orbit and potentially interfere with lacrimation. Overgrowth of the roots will appear as bulging or lytic areas on radiographic examination.

Treatment. Prophylactic care of chinchillas with malocclusion is critical. Usually, this is a chronic condition for the life of the chinchilla. After initial diagnosis, treatment involves trimming and filing the teeth with a small bone rongeur or dental drill. Remove any food impactions and clean any mucosal ulcerations that are apparent. Place a ground pumice stone in the chinchillas's cage and supplement the diet with vitamins A and B complex, dicalcium phosphate and trace minerals. Examine teeth frequently and monitor body weight to prevent further problems (Webb,

1991; Hoefer, 1994; Kennedy, 1970; Moreland, 1967; Heyden, 1968; Kline and Kline, 1978).

Nutritional gastroenteritis

Gastroenteritis often develops in response to alterations in the animal's diet. This might be due to feeding an increased amount of fruits and greens, resulting in increased consumption of cellulose and fibre. A decrease in peristalsis occurs, permitting bacteria to invade the gastroenteric mucosa. Additionally, a diet higher in carbohydrates, fats and protein and lower in fibre will alter fermentation within the caecum, disrupting normal pH and motility and resulting in typhlitis. Feed can also be contaminated by moulds or chemicals. Deficiencies of vitamins A, B complex, or C, also may result in gastroenteritis. Commonly, kits develop diarrhoea in response to stressors such as inadequate milk or the use of milk replacers (Kennedy, 1970).

Gastric tympany

Gastric tympany, or bloat, is frequently related to a change in diet and results from gastrointestinal stasis allowing the accumulation of gas produced by bacterial flora.

Clinical signs. Gastric tympany has an acute onset that usually occurs 2–4 h post-prandially. The chinchilla has a distended, painful abdomen and dyspnoea. Generally, affected animals are seen rolling or stretching in an attempt to relieve the discomfort. Grossly, the stomach often contains doughy ingesta and a large accumulation of gas. The duodenum is usually gas-filled, the caecum is packed with doughy ingesta and the colon contains small hard faeces.

Treatment. Gastric tympany is considered an emergency and is treated by passing a stomach tube or performing paracentesis to relieve gas build-up (Webb, 1991; Kennedy, 1970; Ellett and Moellering, 1974).

Gastric ulcers

Gastric ulcers are common and are frequently observed when feeding coarse, fibrous roughage or mouldy feeds. Yearling chinchillas are most often affected.

Clinical signs. Often, gastric ulcers are observed only on postmortem examination when a black, thickened fluid covering the gastric mucosa with underlying gastric ulcers and erosions is revealed. Clinically, an affected chinchilla appears anorectic and regurgitates often.

Treatment. Treatment includes gastric protectorants and feeding more easily digestible feeds (Kennedy, 1970).

Intestinal obstruction

Factors which often result in intestinal obstruction include adhesions constricting the intestinal lumen, tumours, abscesses, food or faecal impactions, or foreign bodies.

Clinical signs. Constipation is often indicative of intestinal obstruction. Abdominal palpation reveals the presence of a firm mass within the intestinal tract. Segmental enteritis and congestion are often present. Failure to diagnose and treat the impaction can result in intestinal perforation and peritonitis.

Diagnosis. Contrast radiography aids in identifying impactions.

Treatment. Conservative therapy consists of warm soapy water enemas to soften food or faecal impactions. Surgical intervention is often necessary and involves enterotomy and intestinal anastomosis (Kennedy, 1970).

'Tympanites'

A condition called 'tympanites' is seen in lactating females, usually 2–3 weeks post-partum and is characterised by gastrointestinal stasis resulting in gaseous distension of the stomach and intestines. Hindlimb paralysis may also be evident and treatment of affected chinchillas with calcium gluconate has been reported to diminish clinical signs (Kennedy, 1970). A specific dose for calcium gluconate in chinchillas is not re-

ported but the small animal dose of 94–140 mg/kg IV or IP slowly to effect is suggested (Plumb, 1991). This condition bears strong similarities to ruminant milk fever caused by acute hypocalcaemia.

Diseases of the Genitourinary System

Infertility

The causes of infertility are numerous, including genetic factors, inadequate nutrition, sperm abnormalities, hormone imbalances, infectious agents, metritis, lack of breeding experience and animals in poor breeding condition. The most common causes are infections of the reproductive tract and poor conditioning secondary to improper diet or overzealous breeding. Both underweight and overweight chinchillas are poor breeders. Obese, pregnant females often deliver small litters. Breeding stock should be carefully selected. Examine all animals prior to breeding for inherited physical anomalies or any conditions that may impede breeding success (Kennedy, 1970).

Abortions

Abortions may be caused by several conditions, including interruption of the uterine blood supply, poor nutrition, septicaemia, fever and trauma. In late pregnancy, simply startling a female can induce an abortion.

Clinical signs. The aborted kits are often unnoticed due to the female ingesting them immediately after abortion. Abortion should be suspected in any female that suddenly loses weight. A recently aborted female will often have a bloody vaginal discharge that stains the perineum.

Treatment. If an abortion occurs, flush the reproductive tract gently with an antiseptic solution and begin treatment with parenteral antibiotics (Kennedy, 1970).

Retained Foetus

Foetuses that die later in gestation can be delivered at parturition along with live young, retained within the uterus, or they can become mummified.

Clinical signs. If a dead foetus is retained, the dam will often neglect her live young and become increasingly depressed as toxicity develops.

Diagnosis. Ideally, all dams should be examined shortly after parturition to determine if there are retained foetuses. Identifying retained kits by abdominal palpation can be difficult, making it necessary to use radiography.

Treatment. If the mother is unable to pass a retained foetus, surgery may be necessary. The surgical approach and technique is comparable to other caesarian sections. To minimise complications, surgery should be performed without delay in order to avoid the development of toxicity in the dam.

Foetal Mummification

Foetuses that die early in gestation are usually resorbed without complication but can become mummified. Mummification of the foetus occurs from loss of foetal fluids. The mummified foetus can remain within the uterus for extended periods and prevent further pregnancies. It is not uncommon to discover a mummified foetus during a post-mortem examination of a female thought to be sterile. The exact aetiology of mummified foetuses is unknown, but many of the same conditions that cause abortions may be involved. Many complications associated with parturition can be avoided if breeding females are of sufficient size and age and in good physical condition (Kennedy, 1970).

Dystocia

Chinchilla dystocias are rare (Bickel, 1987). They are often caused by malpositioned or abnormally large foetuses (Jones, 1990). Additionally, thin, poorly conditioned females can develop a primary uterine inertia or simply lack sufficient strength to deliver the kit (Bickel, 1987).

Treatment. Intervention may be necessary if labour continues for greater than 4 h (Kennedy, 1970). An injection of oxytocin aids in expulsion of the foetus. An alternative treatment is to administer 0.5 ml of 20% calcium solution IM (Prior, 1986). If these have no effect, then it will be necessary to remove the foetus by caesarian section. Caesarian sections are performed by a similar approach to those in dogs or cats via a ventral abdominal incision.

Metritis

Metritis occurs in acute and chronic forms. Acute metritis is generally more serious.

Agents. A variety of bacterial agents have been incriminated as potential causes. Acute metritis results from bacterial contamination of a retained placenta or a foetus lodged within the birth canal. Either condition could cause the cervix to remain patent and provide an entrance for bacteria and a suitable media for proliferation. Overzealous manipulation with surgical instruments during a dystocia can also damage the reproductive tract and initiate metritis.

Clinical signs. Clinically, a foul smelling, purulent vaginal discharge is present. Early in the disease, the chinchilla is febrile with temperatures of 40–41.1°C and has a reddened, swollen vulva. The vulva can turn nearly black as the disease progresses. Anorexia and a stilted gait are evident and lactation often ceases. The young can contract the infection by close contact with their mother, accidentally ingesting infected discharge while attempting to suckle.

Treatment. Mild cases of metritis can be treated by irrigating the reproductive tract with an antiseptic solution such as 2% boric acid and administering systemic antibiotics such as crystalline penicillin or neomycin. Oxytocin aids uterine contraction and expulsion of debris (Kennedy, 1970).

Pyometra

Pyometra, an accumulation of purulent debris within the uterus, occasionally follows an episode of acute metritis or normal parturition. After the clinical signs of acute metritis have dissipated, small numbers of bacteria may remain within the uterus and eventually develop into a purulent exudate. Alternatively, small remnants of placenta may be retained post-partum and cause a slowly developing pyometra. It can also be seen in unbred animals.

Clinical signs. The affected female loses weight and the coat is of poor condition. The vulva is open and can have a purulent discharge that stains the perivulvar areas. Insertion of a blunt rod a short distance into the vagina can reveal the discharge in cases where it is not readily apparent.

Treatment. A chinchilla with pyometra is no longer a suitable breeder. Medical management of pyometras is unrewarding with ovariohysterectomies constituting the best option (Kennedy, 1970).

Puerperal Septicaemia

Puerperal septicaemia is a septicaemic condition that occurs in the dam following parturition.

Agents. The aetiology remains unclear. Either a primary pathogenic micro-organism is involved or a commensal organism proliferates because of reduced host resistance.

Clinical signs. When this condition occurs, the dam becomes acutely depressed, anorectic and febrile within 12–24 h of parturition. There is usually a brown uterine discharge and as in metritis, milk production will decrease. In later stages of the disease, the animal becomes hypothermic and recumbent.

Treatment. It is extremely important to begin treatment early in the disease process. Therapy includes parenteral antibiotics such as crystalline penicillin or neomycin injected SC or IP. A documented treatment regime includes uterine irrigation with normal saline, followed by sulphathiazole in mineral oil. A small rubber catheter or a small syringe can be used to pass the material into the uterus. Alternatively, penicillin, bacitracin, or neomycin solutions or ointments may be placed in the uterus following irrigation. The animal should also be supported with fluids, good nutrition and a comfortable environment (Kennedy, 1970).

Cannibalism

Chinchillas occasionally cannibalise their kits, especially if the young appear weak or malformed. This also can occur in association with hormonal disturbances, inadequate lactation, or dystocia. Some easily excitable or frequently disturbed dams will kill their young (Kennedy, 1970). Once the young are freely moving about the cage, it is imperative that they do not enter another female's cage via the transport tunnels, since the strange female will probably kill them (Bickel, 1987). Often the only indication that cannibalism has occurred is missing kits. Other than providing a balanced ration and avoiding the rebreeding of affected animals, little can be done to prevent this occurring (Kennedy, 1970).

Agalactia

Lactational problems are usually noted during the first several weeks following birth. Agalactia can be inherited, nutritional, infectious, or caused by breeding animals that are too young or too old.

Clinical signs. Examine the female's teats soon after parturition for adequate milk production. If the nipples are difficult to locate, the mammary glands are inadequately developed. High mortality rates in kits are often a result of inadequate milk production (Volcani *et al.*, 1973). Kits from agalactic dams are restless, cry often and lose weight.

Treatment. Females that are initially agalactic will often increase milk production 12–72 h post-partum. If this does not occur, administer oxytocin to stimulate milk letdown. In unresponsive cases, all of the young must either be hand-raised or cross-fostered with compatible females or guinea pigs. The scent of unrelated kits can be masked by applying cologne to the kits (Kennedy, 1970).

Miscellaneous Lactational Problems

Often, a female will give birth to a large litter and be unable to supply sufficient milk to support all the young. To complicate matters further, litters of seven or more are often already weak and do not survive (Bickel, 1987). Cross-fostering some of the kits will ensure an adequate supply of milk and also prevent the extreme loss of condition seen in dams nursing large litters.

Female chinchillas will often bite and possibly kill kits in response to painful suckling (Kennedy, 1970). The teats of a lactating dam should be frequently observed for damage caused by the nursing kit's sharp teeth. Relatively superficial lesions can be treated by a light application of antibiotic ointment and warm compresses. More severe damage requires cross-fostering or hand-raising the young.

Hair Rings

Male chinchillas sometimes develop a ring of hair around the penis just inside the prepuce that can lead to a secondary paraphimosis (Hoefer, 1994), oliguria, or dysuria (Kennedy, 1970). Hair rings often occur after copulation, therefore it is prudent to check the male at this time. Lubricating the penis or mildly sedating the animal will facilitate gentle removal of the fur ring (Hoefer, 1994).

Diseases of the Nervous System

Infectious Diseases

Cerebral nematodiasis

Agent. Cerebral nematodiasis occurs in chin-

chillas infected with the raccoon roundworm, *Baylisascaris procyonis*. Transmission often occurs by feed contaminated with raccoon faeces.

Hosts. *Baylisascaris* infections are common in the Mid Western and North Eastern USA and are potentially zoonotic, causing a fatal encephalopathy in humans.

Clinical signs. Infected chinchillas exhibit progressive clinical signs of ataxia, torticollis, incoordination, tumbling, paralysis, recumbency, coma and death. Pathological findings include meningitis and necrotic foci. Ascarid larvae are also found in the midbrain, medulla and cerebellar peduncles.

Diagnosis. Diagnosis is confirmed with histological stains.

Treatment. Treatment with various anthelmintics has proven ineffective (Kennedy, 1970; Sanford, 1991).

Lymphocytic choriomeningitis

Lymphocytic choriomeningitis, a zoonotic disease, has been reported in chinchillas. Clinical signs include conjunctivitis, tremors and convulsions (Hoefer, 1994).

Non-Infectious Diseases

Thiamine deficiency

Thiamine or vitamin B1 is required for carbohydrate metabolism and protein synthesis and its deficiency causes reversible damage to the peripheral motor nerves.

Clinical signs. Pre-prandial trembling, paralysis, circling and convulsions are suggestive of thiamine deficiency.

Treatment. For immediate treatment, IM injections of thiamine or B complex vitamins are useful. A source of thiamine should be added to the diet (1 mg thiamine/kg feed). Other dietary sources of thiamine include leafy vegetables, good quality hay and wheat germ meal.

Diseases of the Sensory Organs

Infectious Diseases

Otitis media

Otitis media occurs frequently in young chinchillas as a sequel to trauma. As healing of the ear progresses, scar tissue encloses the ear canal trapping cerumen and debris inside. Accumulation of debris causes significant inflammation with tissue thickening and potential spread to deeper tissues and development of otitis interna.

Treatment. Treatment of this condition is difficult due to the proliferation of tissues and risk to the large, fragile tympanic bulla and involves surgical reopening of the closed ear canal. Cauterizing the ear canal edges may aid in preventing reclosure. Regular cleanings, as well as topical and systemic antibiotics, will help insure the ear canal remains patent until healing is complete (Kennedy, 1970).

Otitis interna

Inner ear infections are uncommon, but have been reported in chinchillas.

Clinical signs. Clinically, the animal will tilt its head to the side of the affected ear. Examining the ear canal is not likely to reveal any abnormalities, although at post-mortem, purulent debris is present in the tympanic bulla. Occasionally, infections extend into the brain resulting in meningitis.

Treatment. Treatment with systemic antibiotics has variable success (Kennedy, 1970).

Conjunctivitis

Conjunctivitis is often reported in young chinchillas.

Agents. Catarrhal or mechanical conjunctivitis is typically caused by introduction of a foreign body into the eye. Purulent conjunctivitis can be caused by bacterial infection of the eye secondary to mechanical conjunctivitis, or in kits, due to direct contact with vaginitis in the dam. *Staphylococcus* sp. and *Pseudomonas aeruginosa* are often isolated.

Clinical signs. Affected eyes often exhibit conjunctival hyperaemia, palpebral oedema and a serous or purulent ocular discharge.

Treatment. These infections are usually resolved after flushing the affected eye with topical antibiotic drops. Occasionally, systemic antibiotics are warranted (Kennedy, 1970).

Non-Infectious Diseases

Ear trauma

Chinchillas have large, relatively delicate ear pinnae that may be subject to traumatic injury. Bite wounds are the most common cause of ear injuries, often involving only the edges of the ear pinnae.

Treatment. Traumatised areas should be cleaned with an antiseptic solution and treated with antibiotic ointment. Suturing large lacerations is not effective and should be discouraged. Severe damage of the ear requires extensive debridement or partial surgical removal. Open lesions should be treated with systemic antibiotics to minimise potential for sepsis.

Frostbite

Chinchillas' ears exposed to extremely cold temperatures will quickly develop frostbite.

Treatment. More severe injuries should be gently cleaned, dried thoroughly and an antibiotic ointment applied. Follow-up cleanings should continue as often as necessary until lesions are completely healed.

Ear haematomas

Ear haematomas are occasionally seen in chinchillas and stem from trauma due to vigorous rubbing of the pinnae. This breaks down the delicate attachment of the skin to the underlying cartilage creating a potential space quickly filled by blood and serum.

Clinical signs. Haematomas usually develop rapidly and are seen as painful swellings of the ear.

Treatment. The haematoma should be lanced at its dependent edge and the contents gently removed to avoid further damage to the ear. To speed healing, the skin over the haematoma must remain in contact with the underlying cartilage and stay immobilised. The ear's rigid anatomy usually holds skin in place, but sutures are sometimes required. Apply antibiotic ointment to open areas to guard against infection.

'Yellow ears'

'Yellow fat' or 'yellow ears' is a common condition seen in chinchillas on diets deficient in choline, methionine or vitamin E. Normally choline and methionine are used by the liver to metabolise ingested plant pigments. When plant pigments are not completely metabolised, they concentrate in the skin and fatty tissues (Kennedy, 1970).

Clinical signs. Initial clinical signs are a slight yellow tinge of the ears that progresses to an orange colour. Advanced stages of the disease reveal discoloration of the genital and perianal areas and the ventral abdomen. In the most severe cases, the entire animal may be discoloured. It is not uncommon for chinchillas with this condition to develop painful, semi-firm swellings on the ventral abdomen of unknown aetiology (Bickel, 1987). Grossly, the liver appears mottled and pale due to fat accumulation.

Treatment. This condition usually responds well to dietary supplementation with choline, methionine and vitamin E.

Vitamin A deficiency

Deficiency due to inadequate dietary vitamin A or the use of rancid cod liver oil produces an ocular condition occasionally reported in chinchilla colonies. Cod liver oil is used as a source of vitamin A in many large chinchilla colonies. It is usually purchased in large quantities and can become rancid when not used by the expiry date. Rancidity destroys vitamins A and D.

Clinical signs. Clinical signs include watery eyes, lens opacity, dull fur, weight loss, weakness, foetal absorptions, abortions, premature births and weakness and blindness in newborn kits.

Treatment. Treatment involves correction of the diet and IM administration of 2,000 IU of vitamin A per day for 7 days, then decreasing to once or twice a week (Kennedy, 1970).

Cataracts and asteroid hyalosis

Cataracts and asteroid hyalosis, which is formation of lipid−calcium complexes within the vitreous humor, are two age-related ocular lesions reported in chinchillas (Kennedy, 1970).

Diseases of the Integument and Musculoskeletal System

Infectious Diseases

Dermatophytosis

Agents. *Trichophyton mentagrophytes* is the most common cause of dermatophytosis in chinchillas, but *Microsporum canis* and *Microsporum gypseum* are occasionally isolated.

Clinical signs. Small alopecic patches are found mainly on the ears, nose and feet (Hoefer, 1994).

Hosts. Outbreaks of fungal infection within a group of chinchillas can often be traced to the addition of a new animal. Fomites contaminated with fungal elements can also serve as a source of transmission (Bleavins, 1984). *T. mentagrophytes* can be transmitted between humans and chinchillas, but this is uncommon (Hagen and Gorham, 1972). Owners should still be cautioned of the zoonotic potential.

Treatment. Griseofulvin and antifungal dips and powders have been used to control dermatophytosis. Oral griseofulvin should be given for 3–4 weeks to control the fungus (Hoefer, 1994). Although not reported in chinchillas, griseofulvin has been associated with teratogenicity when used in pregnant animals of other species (Bleavins, 1984). Lime sulphur dips are a useful adjunct to griseofulvin. Antifungal powders such as Captan (Orthocide) mixed with the dust bath (1 teaspoon to 2 cups of dust mixture) can aid in preventing fungal spread between animals (Hoefer, 1994).

Abscesses

Abscesses in chinchillas occur secondary to bite wounds or other traumatic injuries.

Agents. *Staphylococcus* and *Streptococcus* spp. are most commonly isolated.

Clinical signs. An abscess is often hidden by the chinchilla's thick coat and can progress to the point of rupturing before it is noticed.

Treatment. If the abscess does rupture, the contents should be thoroughly expressed. The area should be liberally flushed with antiseptic solution and coated with an antibiotic ointment. Unruptured abscesses should be surgically removed within their capsule and the animal given parenteral antibiotics based on culture and sensitivity results. Abscesses removed in this manner generally heal better than those that are lanced, drained and flushed (Kennedy, 1970).

Non-Infectious Diseases

Fur-chewing

The phenomenon of fur-chewing may occur in up to 30% of chinchillas (Vanjonack and John-son, 1973). Fur-chewing affects chinchillas in a variety of husbandry conditions and can be a devastating problem. The exact pathogenesis has not been determined but possible causes include boredom (Kennedy, 1970), stress (Jenkins, 1992), unbalanced diet (Kennedy, 1970), hormonal disorders (Hoefer, 1994), adverse environmental conditions (Kennedy, 1970) and inapparent fungal infections. Fur-chewing chinchillas of common ancestry have been reported, suggesting heritability (Zeinert, 1983). Lack of variety in the diet can bore chinchillas and lead to the development of fur-chewing. Chinchillas housed in warm conditions chew hair from their bodies in an attempt to cool themselves. Conversely, draughty conditions that dry the skin and fur can lead to fur-chewing (Kennedy, 1970). Fur-chewing chinchillas consistently have low body temperatures and hyperactive thyroids and adrenal glands. It is not clear if loss of fur insulation is the stimulus for increased endocrine activity or if increased endocrine activity causes the animal to chew its fur (Vanjonack and Johnson, 1973).

Clinical signs. Fur-chewing can range from mild to severe. It is not uncommon for an apparently normal animal to chew as much as half its coat overnight (Zeinert, 1983). The most affected sites include the shoulders, flanks, sides and paws. These areas usually appear darker due to the exposure of darkly coloured underfur. The cropped hair that remains in the chewed areas is easily epilated to expose the flaky, white skin below. Fur-chewing animals frequently have a nervous disposition.

Treatment. Controlling the fur-chewing activity requires a multifaceted approach since the cause of the condition is often unclear. Room humidity and temperature should be lowered. Since hair regrowth will not occur as long as the dense, dark underfur is present, this must be removed from the affected areas. Once the fur is removed, Betadine or Nolvasan should be applied to the skin to disinfect and facilitate scale removal. Within several days, pale, flaky skin will gradually change to pink and later, to blue.

Eventually, the affected skin will appear dark blue or nearly black in colour while unaffected areas will remain lightly coloured (Kennedy, 1970).

'Cotton fur' syndrome

This condition occurs in chinchillas that are fed very high protein rations, for example, substituting turkey or chicken pellets with protein levels of 28% when normal chinchilla diet contains approximately 15%. The hair fibres of affected animals are weakened and wavy, giving the hair coat a cotton-like appearance (Kennedy, 1970).

Fatty acid deficiency

Chinchillas sometimes develop an alopecic skin condition secondary to diets deficient in unsaturated fatty acids (Kennedy, 1970). Diets deficient in linoleic and arachidonic fatty acids are thought to cause reduced hair growth rates and occasional cutaneous ulcers (Hoefer, 1994). This condition is occasionally refered to as 'fungus' or 'fur slip' but this is confusing since the cause is not fungal nor the result of rough handling. Chinchillas are not capable of manufacturing these unsaturated fatty acids to maintain a healthy hair coat, therefore the diet must be supplemented with the proper amounts.

Clinical signs. The fur of affected chinchillas appears dry and epilates easily. The degree of involvement can range from mild skin flakiness to alopecic areas that coalesce and form large denuded areas of pale, flaky skin. In extremely severe cases, the chinchilla becomes debilitated and dies.

Treatment. Treament involves supplementation of the chinchilla's diet with a fresh source of linoleic or undecylenic acid. It is important to store supplements properly and not permit them to become rancid. Often, favourable results are noticed in 4–5 days. When the skin is particularly irritated, an ointment containing linoleic or undecylenic acid can improve systemic absorption and relieve pruritus (Kennedy, 1970).

Pantothenic acid deficiency

If is often difficult to readily distinguish between skin and fur lesions due to unsaturated fatty acid deficiency, pantothenic acid deficiency, or zinc deficiency (Hoefer, 1994; Kennedy, 1970).

Clinical signs. Clinically, chinchillas are hyperactive, anorectic and thin. The fur appears dull grey due to the loss of pigment and is easily epilated, resulting in a patchy alopecia. Affected skin may be thick, roughened and scaly. Pantothenic acid deficiency can also cause stunted growth in young chinchillas.

Treatment. This condition is treated with calcium pantothenate given IM for 2–3 days followed by oral adminstration of propothiouracil.

Calcium : phosphorus imbalance

An imbalance between the ratio of calcium to phosphorus in the diet or a general phosphorus deficiency can often produce a musculoskeletal disorder that is commonly seen in rapidly growing or pregnant chinchillas.

Clinical signs. This dietary insufficiency causes severe cramping of the muscles of the hindlimbs, forelimbs and face. These muscle spasms frequently occur pre-prandially.

Treatment. The muscle spasms are relieved by IM injection of calcium gluconate (Kennedy, 1970). A specific dose for calcium gluconate in chinchillas is not reported but the small animal dose of 94–140 mg/kg IV or IP is suggested (Plumb, 1991). The diet should be balanced and the deficiency corrected.

Systemic Diseases

Infectious Diseases

Systemic infections have been reported frequently in the literature. For these conditions, rapid and aggressive therapy is necessary to save the life of the chinchilla. Most systemic infections are chiefly due to bacteria, but also include fungi and protozoans.

Septicaemia

Agents. Many septicaemic infections begin as one of the bacterial gastroenteritis infections discussed above. If left untreated, the enteritis quickly progresses to septicaemia. Non-enteric bacteria have also been isolated from chinchillas with severe septicaemia, including *Streptococcus* sp., *Enterococcus* sp., *Pasteurella multocida*, *Klebsiella pnuemoniae* and *Actinomyces necrophorum*.

Clinical signs. Clinical signs include rough, dull fur, lethargy, anorexia and severe diarrhoea. Frequently, chinchillas will be found dead with no previous signs. Pathologically, septicaemic organs appear diffusely congested and often contain bacterial emboli.

Diagnosis. Diagnosis is based on culture and isolation of the causative organism from the blood and multiple organs including the gastrointestinal tract, liver and spleen.

Treatment. Treatment consists of antibiotics based on culture and sensitivity and supportive care. Prophylactic antibiotic therapy should be used in severe epizootics. Inoculation with autogenous bacterins also has been effective in decreasing morbidity and mortality (Kennedy, 1970).

Pseudomoniasis

Agent. *Pseudomonas aeruginosa* is considered part of the normal intestinal flora, but it can act as an opportunistic pathogen. Commonly found in drinking water, it causes infections secondary to stress. Routes of transmission include direct contact, aerosol and oral–faecal. In neonatal kits, infection often results from nursing a dam with *Pseudomonas* mastitis.

Clinical signs. Clinical signs vary between adults and young and include anorexia, depression, diarrhoea or constipation, corneal or oral ulcers, intradermal pustules, conjunctivitis, genital swellings, inflamed, blue mammary glands, abortions, infertility and sudden death. Pathological findings include multiple organ abscessation, generalised lymphadenopathy and multi-focal miliary necrosis.

Diagnosis. Definitive diagnosis is based on bacterial culture and isolation.

Treatment. Antibiotic therapy is based on culture and sensitivity. Prophylactic measures against reinfection include acidifying the drinking water to a pH of 2.5–2.8 or hyperchlorinating the water at 12 ppm (Kennedy, 1970; Fox *et al.*, 1984; Lusis and Soltys, 1971; Doerning *et al.*, 1993).

Listeriosis

Chinchillas are highly susceptible to listeriosis.

Agent. Transmission of *Listeria monocytogenes* occurs by the oral–faecal route, usually in conjunction with poor sanitation and contaminated food. Four serotypes of *L. monocytogenes* have been isolated from chinchillas. Type 4 is the most common serotype reported in North America (Cavill, 1967; Finley and Long, 1977).

Hosts. A zoonotic potential exists and is complicated by an asymptomatic carrier state in chinchillas.

Clinical signs. Reports of listeriosis in chinchillas include visceral and encephalitic forms (MacDonald *et al.*, 1972). Clinical signs, if present, typically occur 48–72 h post-infection and include anorexia, depression, weight loss, constipation or diarrhoea and abdominal pain. Central nervous system signs include droopy ears, head tilt, ataxia, circling and convulsions and often precede death. Pathological findings include fibrinous peritonitis, interstitial pneumonia and widespread multifocal miliary necrosis.

Diagnosis. Definitive diagnosis is based on bacterial culture and isolation. A differential diagnosis based on clinical signs and pathological findings includes *Pseudomonas* infection and yersiniosis.

Treatment. Treatment is usually ineffective. Exposed chinchillas not yet exhibiting clinical signs should be inoculated with autogenous bacterins or treated with prophylactic antibiotics, such as chloramphenicol or oxytetracycline (Webb, 1991; Hoefer, 1994; Moreland, 1967; Finley and Long, 1977).

Yersiniosis

Agents. *Yersinia pseudotuberculosis* and *Yersinia enterocolitica* have been isolated from chinchillas.

Hosts. Transmission is via the oral–faecal route and wild rodents, such as *Rattus norvegicus*, serve as reservoir hosts. Transplacental and milk-borne transmission are also reported and an asymptomatic carrier state exists.

Clinical signs. Yersiniosis can cause deadly epizootics in chinchillas. Clinical signs of yersiniosis include sudden death, lethargy, depression, anorexia, weight loss, constipation or diarrhoea and hypersalivation. Pathological findings for each organism are similar with multifocal necrosis, primarily in the liver, spleen and lungs with infection by *Y. pseudotuberculosis*; and in the liver, spleen, intestine, lymph nodes, kidneys and lungs with *Y. enterocolitica* (Hubbert, 1972; Langtoro, 1978).

Diagnosis. Clinically and pathologically, infections with either bacterium are indistinguishable. Definitive differentiation is based on biochemical tests from pure cultures of the organisms. Differential diagnosis includes *Salmonella* sp., *L.*

monocytogenes and *P. aeruginosa* (Hubbert, 1972).

Treatment. Treatment with tetracyclines is not effective for chinchillas with clinical illness, but is effective in preventing further spread within a group (Webb, 1991; Kennedy, 1970).

Toxoplasmosis

Agent. *Toxoplasma gondii*, a protozoan that affects cells of the reticuloendothelial system and gastrointestinal tract, is reported to infect chinchillas.

Hosts. Transmission can be congenital or acquired by ingesting oocysts found within faeces of Felidae or bradyzoites within infected tissue. Members of the Felidae family support sexual production of oocysts in an enteroepithelial cycle.

Clinical signs. Pseudocysts or bradyzoites are seen in the lungs, liver, intestinal tract, pancreas, myocardium and brain. Tachyzoites are seen in the lymph and blood. Clinical signs include lethargy, depression, anorexia, weight loss, dyspnoea, cyanosis, purulent nasal discharge and falling and rolling due to loss of equilibrium.

Diagnosis. Diagnosis is based on the use of such histological stains as Giemsa or periodic acid–Schiff to examine for cysts. Serology based on the Sabin–Feldman dye test also proves useful in diagnosis.

Treatment. Treatment consists of antibiotic therapy with streptomycin or one of the sulphonamides. This treatment is only effective against active infection, not the encysted stage of toxoplasmosis (Kennedy, 1970; Moreland, 1967; Turner, 1978).

Non-Infectious Diseases

Heat prostration

Chinchillas are quite susceptible to heat prostration, particularly when exposed to hot, humid and poorly ventilated environments. Most chinchillas begin to experience heat stress when the ambient temperature reaches 26.7°C. Overweight chinchillas and animals housed in direct sunlight are at a greater risk of overheating.

Clinical signs. Chinchillas will initially appear restless but rapidly become moribund. Untreated, affected animals will become comatose. At post-mortem examination, lungs will be markedly congested and ooze a bloody froth on the cut surface.

Treatment. Excessive handling should be avoided unless absolutely necessary. Animals only mildly affected can be cooled gradually by submersion in lukewarm water and then placed in a cool, dry area. Preventive measures are much more effective than treatment. Close attention to the chinchilla's environment, especially during transport, is required.

References

Balows, A., Hausler, W. J., Herrmann, K. L., Isenberg, H. D. and Shadomy, H. J. (1991) *Manual of Clinical Microbiology*, 5th Ed. American Society for Microbiology, Washington.

Bartoszcze, M., Nowakowska, N., Roszkowski, J., Matras, J., Palec, S. and Wystup, E. (1990) Chinchilla deaths due to *Clostridium perfringens A* enterotoxin. *The Veterinary Record* **126**(14), 341–342.

Bickel, E. (1987) *Chinchilla Handbook*. T. F. H. Publication, Inc., Neptune City.

Bleavins, M. R. (1984) Chinchilla care: Fungus vs. fur-chewing. *Chinchilla World Trade Journal* **6**, 16.

Boettcher, F. A., Bancroft, B. R. and Salv, R. J. (1990) Blood collection from the Transverse Sinus in the Chinchilla. *Laboratory Animal Science* **40**(2), 223–224.

Boisvenue, R. J. and Hendrix, J. C. (1968) Susceptibility of *Chinchilla* sp. to *Hemeonchus contortus*. *The Journal of Parasitology* **54**(1), 183–185.

Brookshyser, K. M., Aulerich, R. J. and Vomachka, A. J. (1977) Adaption of the orbital sinus bleeding technique to the chinchilla (*Chinchilla laniger*). *Laboratory Animal Science* **27**(2), 251–254.

Cartee, R. (1979) Anatomic location and age related changes in the chinchilla thymus. *American Journal of Veterinary Research* **40**(4), 537–540.

Cavill, J. P. (1967) Listeriosis in chinchillas (*Chinchilla laniger*). *The Veterinary Record* **80**(20), 592–594.

Dall, J. A. (1967) Diaphragmatic hernia in a chinchilla. *The Veterinary Record* **81**, 599.

DeVos, A. J. (1970) Studies on the host range of *Eimeria chinchillae*. *Onderstepoort Journal of Veterinary Research* **37**(1), 29–36.

Dieterich, W. H. (1979) Temperature controls for chinchillas. *Chinchilla World Trade Journal* **13**, 24–26.

Doerning, B. J., Brammer, D. W. and Rusa, H. G. (1993) *Pseudomonas aeruginosa*. Infection in a *Chinchilla laniger*. *Laboratory Animals* **27**, 131–133.

Ebino, K. Y. (1993) Studies on coprophagy in experimental animals. *Experimental Animal* **42**(1), 1–9.

Ellett, E. W. and Moellering, A. M. Digestive problems of Chinchilla. *Empress Chinchilla*.

Finley, G. G. and Long J. R. (1977) An epizootic of Listeriosis in chinchillas. *Candian Veterinary Journal* **18**(6), 164–167.

Fox, J. G., Cohen, B. J. and Loew, F. M. (1984) *Laboratory Animal Medicine*. Academic Press, Inc., New York.

Fraser, C. M. and Mays, A. (1986) *The Merck Veterinary Manual*. Merck and Co., Inc., Rahway.

Galton, M. (1968) Chinchilla sex ratio. *Journal of Reproduction and Fertility* **16**, 211–216.

Hagen, K. W. and Gorham, J. R. (1972) Dermatomycoses in fur animals, chinchilla, ferret, mink and rabbit. *Veterinary Medicine, Small Animal Clinician* **67**(1), 43–48.

Heyden, M. J. (1968) Smart chinchillas practice good oral hygiene. *Dental Angles* **9**, 6.

Hoefer, H. L. (1994) Chinchillas. *Veterinary Clinics of North America, Small Animal Practice* **24**(1), 103–111.

Hubbert, W. T. (1972) Yersiniosis in mammals and birds in the United States. *The American Journal of Tropical Medicine and Hygiene* **21**(4), 458–463.

Jarosz, S. (1973) The sexual cycle in chinchilla (*Chinchilla velligera*). *Zoologica Poloniae* **23**(1–2), 120–128.

Jenkins, J. R. (1992) Husbandry and common diseases of the chinchilla (*Chinchilla laniger*). *Journal of Small Animal Exotic Medicine* **2**, 15–17.

Jones, A. K. (1990) Caesarean section in a chinchilla. *The Veterinary Record* **119**(16), 408.

Kennedy, A. H. (1970) *Chinchilla Diseases and Ailments*. Clay Publishing Company, Bewdley.

Kitts, W. D., Krishnamuri, C. R. and Hunson, R. J. (1971) Cellular blood costituents and serum protein fractions of the chinchilla (*Chinchilla lanigera*). *Canadian Journal of Zoology* **49**, 1079–1084.

Kline, A. (1980) The use of solid bottom cages. *Empress Chinchilla Breeder* **35**, *Laboratory Animals* **14**, 331–335.

Kline, A. and Kline, A. (1978) Healthy chinchillas, solving teeth problems. *Empress Chinchilla Breeder* **34**, 7–10.

Langtoro, E. V. (1972) *Pasteurella pseudotuberculosis* infections in Western Canada. *Canadian Veterinary Journal* **13**(4), 85–87.

Lusis, P. I. and Soltys, M. A. *Pseudomonas* infection in man and animals. *Journal of American Veterinary Medical Association* **159**(4), 416.

MacDonald, D. W., Wilton, G. S., Howel, J. and Klavano, G. G. *Listeria monocytogenes* isolations in Alberta (1951–1970). *Canadian Veterinary Journal* **13**, 69–71.

McManus, J. J. Water relation of the chinchilla (*Chinchilla laniger*). *Comparative Biochemical Physiology* **41A**, 445–450.

Moore, R. W. and Greenlee, H. H. (1975) Enterotoxaemia in chinchillas. *Laboratory Animals* **9**(2), 153–154.

Moreland, A. F. (1967) Some common diseases of the chinchilla. *Laboratory Animal Digest* **3**, 8–10.

Mountain, A. (1989) *Salmonella arizona* in a Chinchilla. *Veterinary Record* **125**(1), 25.

Nickelson, D. (1993) Introduction to chinchillas. *Pet-Tec Small Mammal-Reptile Medicine and Surgery for the Practitioner*. Middleton.

Peiffer, R. L. and Johnson, P. T. (1974) Clinical ocular findings in a colony of chinchillas. *Breeder* **30**, 22–23.

Plumb, D. C. (1991) *Veterinary Drug Handbook*. PharmaVet Publishing, White Bear Lake.

Prior, J. E. (1986) Caesarian section in the chinchilla. *Veterinary Record* **119**, 408.

Roberts, C. M. (1971) The early development of some hystricomorph rodents with particular reference to *Chinchilla laniger*. In: *Proceedings of the Society for the Study of Fertility*, Finn, C. A. *et al.* (eds.), pp. 488–489.

Sanford, S. E. (1991) Cerebrospinal nematodiasis caused by *Baylisascaris procyonis* in chinchillas. *Journal Veterinary Diagnostic Investigation* **3**, 77–79.

Strout, H. C. (1976) A restraining device and oral dosing technique for the chinchilla (*Chinchilla laniger*). *Laboratory Animal Science* **26**(4), 610–612.

Strike, W. D. (1970) Hemogram and bone marrow differential of the chinchilla. *Laboratory Animal Care* **20**(1), 33–38.

Tappa, B., Amao, H. and Takahashi, K. W. (1989) A simple method for intravenous injection and blood collection in the chinchilla (*Chinchilla laniger*). *Laboratory Animals* **23**, 73–75.

Thompson, J. B. (1989) Handling your animal properly. *Empress Chinchilla Breeder* **36**, 15–18.

Turner, G. V. S. (1978) Some aspects of the pathogenesis and comparative pathology of toxoplasmosis. *Journal of the South African Veterinary Association* **49**(1), 3–8, 1978.

Vanjonack, W. J. and Johnson, H. D. (1973) Relationship of thyroid and adrenal function to 'fur-chewing' in the chinchilla. *Comparative Biochemical Physiology* **45A**, 115–120.

Volcani, R., Zisling, R., Sklan, D. and Nitzan, Z. (1973) The composition of chinchilla milk. *British Journal of Nutrition* **29**, 121.

Webb, R. A. (1991) Chinchillas. In: *Manual of Exotic Pets*, Benyon, P. H. and J. E. Cooper (eds.). British Small Animal Veterinary Association, pp. 15–22.

Yamini, B. and Raju, N. R. (1986) Gastroenteritis associated with a *Cryptosporidium* sp. in a chinchilla. *Journal of the American Veterinary Medical Association* **189**(9), 1158–1159.

Zeinert, K. (1983) Husbandry of chinchillas. *Veterinary Medicine, Small Animal Clinician* **78**(8), 1292–1294.

(Data Tables follow).

Data Tables

COMMON DISEASES—CHINCHILLAS					
Disease	Aetiology	Diagnosis	Clinical signs	Treatment and control	Zoonotic potential
Respiratory system					
Upper respiratory tract infections	*Streptococcus* spp. *Pseudomonas aeruginosa* *Pasteurella* spp. *Bordetella* spp.	Culture Antibiotic sensitivity	Rhinitis Nasal discharge Conjunctivitis	Antibiotics Supportive care	No
Pneumonia	*Streptococcus* spp. *Pasteurella* spp. *Bordetella* spp.	Culture Antibiotic sensitivity	Dyspnoea Fever	Antibiotics Supportive care	No
Choke	Foreign body	Examination Aspiration	Acute respiratory distress	Sedation and removal Tracheostomy	No
Gastrointestinal system					
Bacterial gastroenteritis	*Escherichia coli, Proteus* sp. *Salmonella* spp.	Culture Antibiotic sensitivity	Diarrhoea Abdominal pain	Roughage, *Lactobacillus* spp. Supportive care	Yes With poor hygiene
Clostridial enterotoxaemia	*Clostridium perfringens* Type D		Weight loss Dehydration	Roughage, *Lactobacillus* spp. Supportive care Toxoid vaccination	No
Corynebacterial enteritis	*Corynebacterium* spp.	Culture Antibiotic sensitivity		Roughage, *Lactobacillus* spp. Supportive care	
Protozoal gastroenteritis	*Giardia* sp. *Trichomonas* sp. *Balantidium* sp. *Cryptosporidium* spp. *Eimeria chinchillae*	Direct faecal examination		Roughage, *Lactobacillus* spp. Supportive care Antiprotozoals	Yes *Giardia* *Crypto-sporidium*
Parasitic gastroenteritis	*Physaloptera* sp. *Hymenolepis* sp. *Haemonchus contortus*	Faecal flotation		Roughage, *Lactobacillus* spp. Supportive care Anthelmintics	Yes
Nutritional gastroenteritis	Change in diet Contaminated feed Vitamin deficiency	History Response to therapy		Roughage, *Lactobacillus* spp. Supportive care	No

Fig. 5.6—continued

COMMON DISEASES—CHINCHILLAS					
Disease	Aetiology	Diagnosis	Clinical signs	Treatment and control	Zoonotic potential
Malocclusion	Inherited condition	Oral examination Radiography	Loss of condition Poor mastication Hypersalivation Oculonasal discharge	Trimming teeth Pumice stone in cage Vitamin and mineral supplementation	No
Gastric tympany	Related to change in diet	Clinical presentation Radiography	Abdominal distension Abdominal pain Respiratory distress	Stomach tube Paracentesis	No
Integument and musculoskeletal system					
Dermatophytosis	*Trichophyton mentagrophytes Microsporum canis Microsporum gypseum*	Skin scraping Fungal culture	Patchy alopecia on ears, nose, feet Crusty dermatitis	Griseofulvin Topical antifungals	Yes *T. mentagrophytes M. canis*
Abscesses	*Streptococcus* sp. *Staphylococcus* sp.	Culture Antibiotic sensitivity	Abscesses	Curettage and drainage Topical antibiotics	No
Fur-chewing	Behavioural, nutritional endocrine, fungal, environment	Clinical examination of fur	Cropped hair exposing darker fur	Lower humidity and temperature Remove exposed underfur Topical antiseptic ointment	No
Fatty acid deficiency	Dietary deficiency of unsaturated fatty acids	Response to therapy	Generalised flaky alopecias	Dietary supplementation with linoleic or undecylenic acids	No
Pantothenic acid deficiency	Dietary deficiency of pantothenic acid	Response to therapy	Patchy alopecia Stunted growth	Calcium pantothenate Propiothiouracil	No
Calcium: phosphorus imbalance	Phosphorus deficiency	Response to therapy	Preprandial muscle spasms	Parenteral calcium gluconate Corrected diet	No
Systemic diseases					
Septicaemias	Enteric bacteria: *Escherichia coli Salmonella typhimurium Salmonella arizona Corynebacterium* sp.	Culture Antibiotic sensitivity	Diarrhoea Paralysis Death	Antibiotics Supportive care	Yes With poor hygiene

Fig. 5.6—continued

COMMON DISEASES—CHINCHILLAS					
Disease	Aetiology	Diagnosis	Clinical signs	Treatment and control	Zoonotic potential
Septicaemias (*Continued*)	Non-enteric bacteria: *Streptococcus* sp. *Enterococcus* sp. *Pasteurella multocida* *Klebsiella pnuemoniae* *Actinomyces necrophorum*		Sudden death		No
Pseudomoniasis	*Pseudomonas aeruginosa*		Diarrhoea Corneal/oral ulcers Mastitis Abortions/ infertility Death		No
Listeriosis	*Listeria monocytogenes*	Culture	Head tilt, ataxia circling Convulsions Death	Chloramphenicol Oxytetracycline Supportive care	No
Yersiniosis	*Yersinia pseudo-tuberculosis* *Yersinia enterocolitica*	Culture Biochemical test	Constipation/ diarrhoea Death	Tetracyclines	No
Toxoplasmosis	*Toxoplasma gondii*	Histology Serology	Lethargy Poor condition Dyspnoea Loss of equilibrium	Antibiotics with active infection	Yes Ingestion of encysted tissue
Genitourinary system					
Abortion	Poor nutrition Trauma Septicaemia Fever	Vaginal examination Radiography	Weight loss Vaginal discharge	Antibiotics Irrigation of uterus	No
Retained foetus	Foetal death late in gestation	Abdominal palpation Radiography	Severe depression Neglects young	Surgery	No
Metritis	Secondary to retained placenta or foetus	Radiography Culture Antibiotic sensitivity	Purulent vaginal discharge Fever	Irrigation of uterus Antibiotics Oxytocin	No
Pyometra	Secondary to retained placenta Sequela to metritis	Radiography Culture Antibiotic sensitivity	Vaginal discharge Weight loss and anorexia	Ovario-hysterectomy Antibiotics	No

Fig. 5.6—continued

COMMON DISEASES—CHINCHILLAS					
Disease	Aetiology	Diagnosis	Clinical signs	Treatment and control	Zoonotic potential
Puerperal septicaemia	Unknown	Examination and history Blood culture Antibiotic sensitivity	Vaginal discharge Fever Agalactia	Antibiotics Irrigation of uterus Supportive care	No
Agalactia	Multiple aetiologies	Examination of dam and kits	Undeveloped mammary glands Weak, thin kits	Oxytocin Hand-rear or cross-foster young	No
Hair rings	Post-copulatory	Examination of penis	Ring of hair around penis	Removal of hair	No
Nervous system					
Thiamine deficiency	Dietary thiamine deficiency	Diet analysis and response to therapy	Trembling Paralysis Circling Convulsions	Parenteral thiamine Dietary thiamine	No
Cerebral nematodiasis	*Baylisascaris procyonis*	Histology	Ataxia Torticollis Paralysis Coma Death	None	Fatal encephalophathy in humans
Lymphocytic choriomeningitis	Arenavirus	Serology	Conjunctivitis Tremors Convulsions	None	Yes Meningitis
Sensory organs					
Otitis media	Miscellaneous bacteria	Otoscopic examination Culture Antibotic sensitivity	Purulent debris Inflammation of ear canal	Flushing ear canal Topical and systemic antibiotics Surgery	No
Otitis interna	Sequela to otitis media	Clinical signs Pathological findings	Torticollis	Systemic antibiotics	No
Ear haematomas	Trauma	Clinical examination	Swelling of the pinna	Lance haematoma Topical antibiotics	No
Yellow ears	Dietary choline, methionine, or vitamin E deficiency	Clinical examination	Yellow discoloration of ears, ventral abdomen, and perineal area	Supplement diet with choline, methionine, and Vitamin E	No

Fig. 5.6—continued

COMMON DISEASES—CHINCHILLAS					
Disease	Aetiology	Diagnosis	Clinical signs	Treatment and control	Zoonotic potential
Conjunctivitis	Foreign body *Staphylococcus* spp. *Pseudomonas aeruginosa*	Clinical signs Culture Antibiotic sensitivity	Conjunctival hyperaemia Palpebral oedema Purulent ocular discharge	Flush eye Topical and systemic antibiotics	No
Vitamin A deficiency	Rancid feed	Diet analysis and response to therapy	Watery eyes Lens opacities Reproductive failure Blind, weak kits	Parenteral vitamin A Dietary supplementation with vitamin A	No

FIG. 5.6 Common diseases — chinchillas.

PHYSIOLOGICAL DATA—CHINCHILLAS	
Body weight of adult female	400–600 g
Body weight of adult male	400–500 g
Life span	Average = 10 years Maximum = 20 years
Rectal temperature	95.8–100.4 °F 35.4–38.0 °C
Heart rate	100 beats per min
Respiratory rate	45–65 per min
Data taken from Jenkins (1992).	

FIG. 5.7 Physiological data — chinchillas.

HAEMATOLOGICAL VALUES—CHINCHILLAS	
	Average (Range)
PCV %	38.0 (25.0–54.0)
Haemoglobin g/dl	11.7 (8.0–15.4)
RBC $\times 10^6$/mm^3	Female = 6.6 Male = 7.3 (5.2–10.3)
Reticulocytes % of RBCs	0.25 (0–2.8)
WBC $\times 10^3$/mm^3	8.7 (4.6–19.5)
Segmented neutrophils %	27.0 (11.0–59.0)
Band cells %	3.8 (0–11.0)
Lymphocytes %	67.0 (35.0–87.0)
Monocytes %	2.8 (0–12.0)
Eosinophils %	0.6 (0–5.0)
Basophils %	0.6 (0–5.0)
Platelets $\times 10^3$/mm^3	276.0 (45.0–740.0)
Blood volume	65 ml/kg
Data taken from Strike (1970) and Kitts *et al.* (1971).	

FIG. 5.8 Haematological values — chinchillas.

CLINICAL CHEMISTRY VALUES—CHINCHILLAS	
	Average (Range)
Sodium mEq/l	153.4 (149–157.8)
Potassium mEq/l	3.8 (3.4–4.2)
Chloride mEq/l	103.1 (98.9–107.3)
Glucose mg/dl	125.7 (106.9–144.5)
LDH mU/ml	521.1 (405.7–636.5)
Total protein g/100 ml	5.5 (5.0–6.0)
Albumin g/100 ml	3.1 (3.0–3.2)
Globulin g/100 ml	2.3 (2.0–2.6)
Albumin/globulin ratio	1.41 (1.28–1.54)
Data taken from Strike (1970) and Kitts *et al.* (1971).	

FIG. 5.9 Clinical chemistry values — chinchillas.

REPRODUCTIVE DATA—CHINCHILLAS	
Puberty	4–12 months
Oestrous season	November–May
Oestrous cycle	40 days (16–69 days)
Duration of oestrous cycle	2 days
Gestation	111 days—*Chinchilla laniger*
	124–128 days—*C. brevicaudata*
Litters per year	2
Litter size	2 kits (1–6 kits)
Birth weight	35 g
Eyes open	At birth
Wean	6–8 weeks
Post-partum oestrus	Onset—12 h post-partum
	Duration—48 h
Number of mammae	4
Data taken from Hoefer (1994), Jenkins (1992), Fox (1984), Kennedy (1970) and Bickel (1987).	

FIG. 5.10 Reproductive data — chinchillas.

6

Rabbits

SUSAN STEIN and SALLY WALSHAW

Introduction

The domestic rabbit, *Oryctolagus cuniculus*, belongs to the class Mammalia, order Lagomorpha (Russell and Schilling, 1973). This rabbit originated from the European wild rabbit. Its ancestors most likely developed on the Iberian Peninsula and spread throughout the Mediterranean area, where Phoenician sailors first observed and described them. The early domestication of the rabbit occurred in Spain during the first century BC. Selective breeding and more skilful domestication were ongoing by the 16th century. Early sailing ships stocked rabbits for meat supplies, inadvertently introducing them throughout the world. Consequently, by the mid-1600s, England and continental Europe were raising these prolific animals to supply meat and fur (Weisbroth *et al.*, 1974).

The mid-1800s saw the initial recorded use of the rabbit in research. An Austrian physician fed deadly nightshade to some randomly selected rabbits. The lack of deleterious effects on these animals led to the discovery of atropinesterase (Russell and Schilling, 1973; Stein, 1980).

There are more than 32 breeds of domestic rabbit, ranging in weight from 1 kg dwarf breeds to 10 kg giants. The larger breeds, such as the New Zealand White and the Californian, are used for commercial meat production. Wool from the Angora rabbit and pelts from the Rex are in demand for the fashion garment industry. The New Zealand White and the Dutch are the most commonly used laboratory rabbits (Cheeke *et al.*, 1987).

Rabbits are growing in popularity as pets, especially in urban areas where space is limited and there are restrictions on keeping dogs and cats as pets. The lively and curious behaviour of rabbits is a source of enjoyment for their owners.

Unique Biology

Rabbits have open-rooted teeth which grow continuously throughout life. The dental formula is $2(I\frac{2}{1}C\frac{0}{0}PM\frac{3}{2}M\frac{2-3}{3})$. The two upper incisors line up one behind the other, with two smaller and more caudal teeth called 'peg' teeth. The upper incisors fit anteriorly to the bottom teeth. Folds of skin between the incisors and premolars limit visibility and access to the rest of the oral cavity.

The digestive system is remarkable for the large caecum, often functionally compared with a rumen. The ileum terminates in a large structure, the sacculus rotundus, frequently called the 'caecal tonsil' (Fig. 6.1). The sacculus rotundus and the terminal portion of the caecum, the caecal appendix, are areas of lymphoid tissue. Two different types of faeces are produced in the colon. The rabbit consumes the soft, clumped, vitamin-rich night faeces directly from the anus (coprophagy). The rabbit leaves the hard droppings.

Normal physiological, haematological and clinical chemistry values are provided in Figs found at the end of the chapter. Rabbit neutrophils, also known as heterophils, may look a lot like eosinophils in other species. True eosinophils in the rabbit usually appear as larger cells with granules that cover the nucleus.

Normal rabbit urine varies in colour and consistency. All of the following are normal: white; turbid; pale yellow; dark yellow; bright orange; brown; bright red. Suspected haematuria must be confirmed by urinalysis. An excess of dietary calcium may be responsible for thick white urine

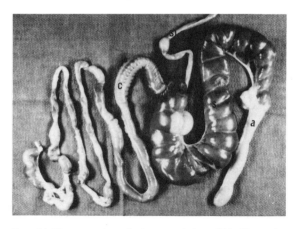

FIG. 6.1 The gastrointestinal tract of the rabbit illustrating the small intestine (si), the sacculus rotundus (s), the caecal appendix (a) and the colon (c).

in the rabbit (Harkness and Wagner, 1989). In a healthy rabbit the urine pH is alkaline, approximately 8.2, but may be as low as 6.0 in an anorectic or fasted rabbit (Burke, 1994). Rabbit urine normally contains albumin, large amounts of calcium carbonate compounds and triple phosphates (Burke, 1994; Mattix, 1993).

Behaviour

Information about rabbit behaviour is largely anecdotal even after 400 years of domestication. Given the opportunity to explore its environment, a rabbit is inquisitive and active. The animal rubs its chin on objects, leaving a scent-mark that is undetected by humans. Wires, wood, paper, upholstery and children's toys become chew toys. Picking up small objects and throwing them is a common behaviour. The rabbit may stretch out quietly for a few minutes and then stand up, shake its head and hop quickly across an open area, twisting its rear quarters in the air. Twitching of the nostrils is normal behaviour in the rabbit but may be absent in rabbits that are resting or sick. Regular exercise for the rabbit will not only help minimise osteoporosis but will also reduce behaviour problems caused by boredom (Morton, 1993; Wemelsfelder, 1994; Harri-

man, 1993). Caged rabbits may be placed in exercise pens, walked on leashes, or given supervised play-time in 'rabbit-proof' areas.

A rabbit (especially if neutered) chooses a single area, in a corner or along a wall, for urination and most of its defaecation (Love and Hammond, 1991; Okerman, 1988). Most rabbits, even adults, will accept a litter pan. During the training phase, it may be helpful to confine the rabbit primarily to its main housing area. A litter pan is placed in the desired location. The food and water bowls are placed in the other corners.

Individual rabbits have clearly discernible 'personalities' ranging from timid to aggressive. The dominant rabbit in a group housed together may be quite fearful of human beings; the opposite can also be true. Rabbits usually learn to trust people who handle them gently and provide food treats, such as small amounts of sweetened breakfast cereal or bits of fresh fruit or vegetables. A caged rabbit will 'beg' for food treats by pressing its nose against the cage or chewing on the cage bars in anticipation. A rabbit out of its cage may beg by circling the owner while making soft humming sounds or by standing on its hind legs near the owner. Many rabbits will lick their owners' hands and arms; this often occurs when the owner has been petting the rabbit.

Thumping with a hind leg is the general alarm call of the rabbit that may last for seconds or an hour or more (Ackerman, 1993a). A timid rabbit may retreat to the back of its cage when approached or thump with a hind foot to signal its alarm at the situation. A severely frightened rabbit may make a terrible scream or, alternatively, may remain immobile. An aggressive rabbit may thump, growl or grunt and attack with teeth and feet when approached. Rabbits act aggressively out of fear, pain, territorial behaviour, or to protect their young or cagemates (Ackerman, 1993b). A rabbit in pain may assume a hunched posture and grind its teeth.

When a female rabbit reaches sexual maturity, she will tend to become aggressive toward humans and other animals. She may bite, dig, chew up such household items as carpeting and engage in nest-building (Shapiro, 1993). She may spray urine and mount or attack other rabbits (even those that have been neutered). If allowed to run in an outdoor garden, the intact female rabbit may dig extensive deep tunnels that necessitate underground peripheral fencing to prevent escape (Okerman, 1988; Love, 1994).

Neutering is recommended for a single pet rabbit as well as for rabbits housed in groups. Between 2 weeks and 2 months after neutering, regardless of age, aggression, territorial behaviour and some other annoying habits should decline (Akerman, 1992).

The rabbit in nature is a social animal (Love, 1994) and it is reasonable to assume that the domestic rabbit needs some opportunities for social behaviour. In addition to interaction with the owner, the rabbit may enjoy some contact with a friendly pet dog, cat or other rabbits. Rabbits may be successfully housed in groups if care is taken to form compatible groups in which ideally all of the rabbits are neutered (Harriman, 1993). Rabbits in groups are less likely to fight if they have hiding places (shelves, barrels or boxes) and materials for chewing (hay, cardboard or paper) (Morton, 1993; Wemelsfelder, 1994; Love and Hammond, 1991; Love, 1994). Rabbits in groups spend considerable time grooming each other and resting next to each other (Love and Hammond, 1991; Love, 1994). Veterinarians have found that a sick rabbit may benefit from a visit from its rabbit companion (Harriman, 1993).

Rabbits are playful, social animals with a varied behavioural repertoire. Patience, gentle handling and neutering will solve most behavioural problems. Selective breeding of rabbits that are sound in temperament, as well as in physical characteristics, should also be valuable in improving the species.

Reproduction

Sexing a young rabbit can be a difficult task. The female vulva appears as a pointed slit (Fig. 6.2) while the male's prepuce assumes a rounded shape (Fig. 6.3). Lateral to the genitalia are the hairless inguinal spaces which may contain white to brown inguinal gland secretions. As adults,

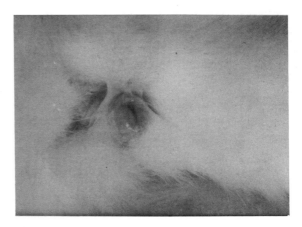

FIG. 6.2 The vulva appears as a pointed slit in a juvenile rabbit. The hairless inguinal spaces are lateral to the vulva.

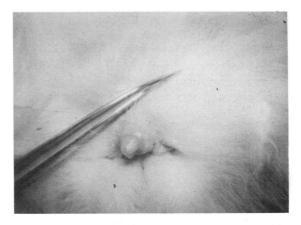

FIG. 6.3 The male rabbit has a rounded prepuce from which the penis can be extruded.

the male has an obvious external scrotum which usually contains the testes, however, the inguinal canal is open and the testes may be retracted into the abdominal cavity.

Mating

Two separate uterine horns and two cervices form the female reproductive tract. Females (does) are induced ovulators with ovulation occurring about 10 h postcoitus. Rabbits become sexually mature at about 4–10 months, the younger end of the range for females and smaller breeds. Rather than exhibiting a regular oe-strous cycle, the female rabbit has a period of receptivity occurring every 5–6 days. There may be no external indication of this receptive state (Walden, 1990). Pseudopregnancies, resulting from sterile matings or mounting by other does, last 15–17 days. Adult female rabbits have a well developed dewlap.

When breeding rabbits, the doe should be taken to the male rabbit's (buck's) cage. This action reduces the territorial aggression exhib-ited by the doe in her home cage. The pair should be observed for up to 10 min (Harkness and Wagner, 1989). If mating does not occur or if fighting ensues, the doe should be removed promptly. Courting behaviour by the buck con-sists of circling the doe followed quickly by mounting and copulation. The buck may hold some skin on the doe's back between his teeth during the mating process. After ejaculation, the buck falls to one side. Breeding behaviour in the sexually mature buck may be directed toward the owner if the rabbit does not have a mate. The buck may hum and circle the owner and try to mount the owner's foot.

Gestation and Birth

Normal gestation averages 32 days. The young are altricial. The doe usually pulls fur from her flanks and belly to form a nest for them. Does will breed immediately post-partum. However, as lactation progresses, receptivity declines until the young are weaned (Walden, 1990). She nurses the young only once or twice daily, leaving them unattended for the majority of the time.

Reproductive information for the rabbit is summarised in Fig. 6.16.

Husbandry

Housing

Rabbits thrive in both indoor and outdoor housing. Outdoor housing should protect rabbits from draughts, predation, wild rabbits, hot summer sun, and, in some environments, mosquitoes and flies. Rabbits gnaw on caging, so caging materials should be non-toxic. Hutches have traditionally been constructed from wood, welded wire and hardware cloth. Large-breed rabbits easily develop hock lesions on the wire surfaces. Wood is difficult to keep clean. Rolled steel bar flooring, despite the high cost, provides the best caging. Rabbit breeders usually house rabbits in cages with flooring which allows faecal material to drop through. The rabbits stay cleaner and it reduces the risk of reinfection with coccidians.

The cage size should be at least 1 m^3 for the average rabbit. Large breeds require more space (Burke, 1994). Group housing of young animals, neutered animals, or adult females previously housed together may work, especially with suf-ficient hiding places (boxes, barrels or tunnels) in the enclosure. Rabbits establish dominance orders and fighting frequently occurs. Grouping sexually intact rabbits together should be avoided. When housing breeding does, place a nest box with hay in the cage one week before 'kindling' or giving birth.

Indoor rabbits frequently adapt to the use of a litter box. Occasionally, rabbits explore and in-gest the bedding in these pans. For that reason corn cob bedding, straw or baled or shredded paper products are better suited than litters with added colour, scents or chemicals. Soft wood shavings, i.e. pine or cedar, may influence liver function and thus are no longer recommended. Rabbits find house plants, electrical cords and detergent boxes tasty fodder. Unsupervised ac-tivity in the house environment should be limited.

Regardless of housing choice, clean the cage or litter pan frequently to prevent the build-up of mould, odour, hair and faeces. Cleaning using commercial kennel preparations or hypochlorite solutions (30 ml/litre water) (Harkness, 1987) assists in removal of microbes. Removal of urine scale and hair may require the use of strong acids or flaming. It is crucial to rinse thoroughly and dry the caging or litter pan adequately be-fore placing the rabbit back into the housing.

Water bottles and automatic watering systems significantly reduce the mess and housekeeping chores associated with heavy water bowls or crocks. Food, hair, or other debris may obstruct sipper tubes. In outdoor housing, water in crocks, sipper tubes and water lines will freeze during cold weather. All water delivery systems must be checked daily.

Traditional housing in the laboratory setting includes the use of commercially produced stainless steel caging. Cage size, environmental temperature, room humidity and frequency of disinfection vary depending on the country and regulatory agencies supervising animals used in research.

Nutrition

A rabbit eats about 5% of its body weight in complete dry diet and drinks approximately 10% of its body weight of water daily (Okerman, 1988). A non-breeding adult rabbit should be maintained on limited feed rather than fed *ad libitum*. The limited quantity of feed should provide enough nutrients to maintain good body condition in the rabbit. This means the fur should be sleek and the vertebrae and ribs detectable on palpation (Cheeke, 1994).

The quantity offered to pregnant does gradually increases until late gestation when *ad libitum* feeding is routinely practised. Lactation peaks at week 3 postpartum. Does may require 2–3 times their nonpregnant intake by that time (Walden, 1990; Okerman, 1988).

Young rabbits show interest in solid food at about 2 weeks of age. Coprophagy starts at around 3 weeks. This facilitates absorption of B vitamins synthesised in the caecum and colon of the rabbit by the resident bacterial population (Cheeke *et al.*, 1987). At 5–6 weeks of age, most rabbits are weaned and provided with commercial diet.

Clean water must be available at all times. Water consumption increases during lactation and hot weather.

Rabbits require a high fibre diet. Commercially available rabbit pelleted diets meet the fibre and other nutritional requirements of the domestic rabbit. Foods used for treats or supplements include hay, cereals, lawn clippings, fruits, vegetables and dead fruit tree prunings. Only feed small quantities of these treats, if at all. Oxalates (in vegetables like spinach), fertilisers, pesticides and cyanide compounds (in most live fruit tree prunings) can cause diarrhoea, illness or even death. Rabbits seem to like grain cereals sold for human consumption as treat foods.

Some individuals maintain that pet rabbits thrive on a mostly hay diet (Burke, 1994). However, nutritional needs of pregnant and lactating rabbits may not be met by such a diet. Deficiencies of vitamin E, in particular, may result in reproductive failure and myopathy (Yamini and Stein, 1989). Vitamin A deficiencies also have an adverse effect on fertility and foetal development and can cause eye lesions involving the cornea and conjunctiva. Hypervitaminosis A results in reproductive problems, high perinatal mortality and various congenital defects (e.g. hydrocephalus) in the rabbit (Mattix, 1993).

Handling, Restraint and Clinical Techniques

Handling and Restraint

It is advisable to observe a rabbit briefly in its cage, pen, or carrier before attempting to handle the animal. Note the rabbit's attitude and whether it is breathing effortlessly at the usual rate of 30–60 breaths/min. Even minimal restraint may cause respiratory arrest in a dyspnoeic rabbit. If the rabbit seems aggressive, additional help and materials may be needed for the clinical assessment and handling.

From a rabbit's point of view, a human being is a large potential predator. A calm, quiet approach is always advisable. The handler should talk quietly to the animal and try to stroke its head, with the hand coming from behind the rabbit's head, before attempting to lift the animal. One does not offer a hand for the rabbit to sniff as with a dog, because a rabbit, with its laterally placed eyes, has relatively poor depth perception and may mistake the person's hand for food. An aggressive rabbit or a nursing doe may quickly inflict painful bites on a hand that is reaching for it.

It is essential to keep the rabbit's back in its normal curved posture during handling and restraint. The rabbit's relatively fragile skeleton and large lumbar muscles render it susceptible to spinal fracture while struggling. Gently lift a rabbit by grasping the skin over the rabbit's

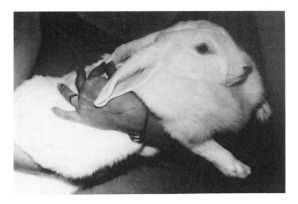

FIG. 6.4 To lift a rabbit, the skin over the dorsal neck should be grasped with one hand while the other hand grasps and supports the heavy hindlimbs.

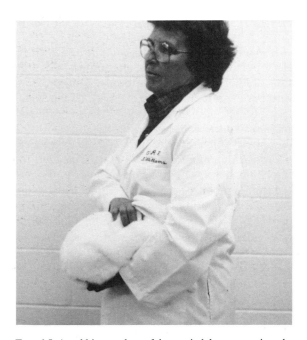

FIG. 6.5 A rabbit can be safely carried by supporting the body with a forearm and stabilising the hindlimbs. Maintain the normal curvature of the back, securing the head between the arm and the body which has a calming effect on the animal.

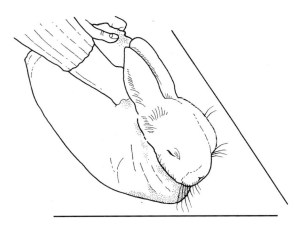

FIG. 6.6 A large towel wrapped securely around the rabbit can be very helpful for restraint.

dorsal neck area with one hand while supporting the rabbit's hind quarters with the other hand (Fig. 6.4). Tuck the rabbit's head and front feet under the upper arm and carry the rabbit a short distance with the rabbit's body supported by the forearm (Fig. 6.5).

A large towel is very useful when restraining a rabbit. The rabbit is placed in the middle of a towel which is then wrapped securely around it, leaving only the head exposed. Cover the rabbit's front feet with the towel to keep the animal from squirming out of the towel (Fig. 6.6). Rabbits seem to tolerate this very well. The rabbit can maintain its normal curved posture. The rabbit's feet and claws are covered, protecting the handler from possible scratches. The towel is warm and comfortable, perhaps explaining why rabbits tend to relax and their ear blood vessels dilate. Do not leave a rabbit, even if wrapped in a towel, unattended on a table. The animal can injure itself if it jumps off the table.

To remove an aggressive rabbit from a cage or carrier, throw a towel over the animal and quickly bundle it up with its head completely covered. It is safer for all involved if the handler then places the 'bundle' of aggressive rabbit on the floor, rather than on a table, for rewrapping in a more efficient manner. In some situations (e.g. when administering oral medication), it may be convenient to kneel on the floor and use the knees and lower legs to hold the rabbit facing outward (Fig. 6.7). Once on the floor, the rabbit cannot

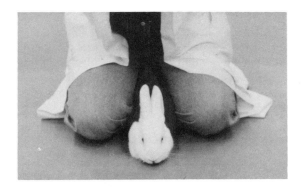

FIG. 6.7 If it is necessary to admininister oral medication, an effective restraint technique involves wrapping the rabbit's body in a towel and holding the animal securely between the knees.

easily scratch the person's face and also may 'freeze' in position in the unfamiliar surroundings. Once out of its cage, the aggressive rabbit may settle down if the handler applies pressure over the rabbit's shoulder area, immobilising the front legs, while also applying pressure over the hip area (Ackerman, 1993b).

Injections

The rabbit does not generally object to a SC injection given in the dorsal neck area. The animal may be left in its cage and just pushed against one side while the SC injection is performed. A small gauge needle (25 or 22 gauge) is suitable.

The preferred location for IM injection in the rabbit is the dorsal lumbar muscle group. This large muscle mass is easily accessible. The quadriceps muscle on the anterior aspect of the femur may also be used. If the quadriceps are used, the injected volume should not exceed approximately 1 ml for a 4 kg rabbit.

Intravenous injections may be made into the marginal ear vein, the cephalic vein, or the saphenous vein. The cephalic and saphenous veins are only practical for use in rabbits that weigh at least 3 kg. Needle size should be 24 gauge or smaller, regardless of the vein used. Rabbit blood clots quickly, especially in metal needles, so IV catheters may be ideal for all IV injection procedures.

For unassisted IM or IV injections restraint with a towel can be useful, with the area to be injected exposed. Covering the rabbit's eyes when approaching it with diagnostic or treatment equipment may help calm the animal.

Specimen Collection

The vessels accessible for blood collection are the central artery of the ear, the marginal ear vein, the jugular vein, the cephalic vein and the lateral saphenous vein. Chemical tranquillisation is a very useful adjunct to the blood collection procedure. Rabbits are timid animals and peripheral vasoconstriction is common in untranquillised rabbits. Towel restraint during blood collection provides warmth and comfort to the rabbit. Using a 24 gauge or smaller IV catheter enables blood collection from the rabbit before the clotting process occurs.

The central artery of the ear is accessible and collection is rapid unless the vessel is constricted in a cold or nervous rabbit. Firm pressure for at least 3 min after blood collection from the central artery is necessary to minimise haematoma formation. When collecting blood from a rabbit's jugular vein, position the rabbit in sternal recumbency with its neck extended and its front legs over a table as for a dog (Hillyer, 1994). Another position for jugular vein blood collection that works well involves placing the towel-wrapped rabbit in dorsal recumbency with its neck extended and body restrained by an assistant (Cranney and Zajac, 1993). The marginal ear vein is a good choice for routine blood collection in any rabbit weighing at least 2 kg. Small amounts (1–3 ml) of blood may be collected from the rabbit's cephalic vein or lateral saphenous vein.

Urine may be collected from the rabbit by cystocentesis or by using non-absorbable veterinary medical litter or aquarium gravel in the rabbit's litter pan.

Oral Medication Administration

Rabbits drink readily from water bottle sipper tubes. They can learn to drink from a small diameter syringe (1–3 ml) if the end of the syringe has been moistened and then dipped into granulated sugar. If the rabbit does not drink readily from the syringe, gently introduce the syringe into the rabbit's mouth behind the incisor teeth and direct the end of the syringe back into the posterior part of the mouth. The dorsal surface of the rabbit's nose should be parallel with the ground to minimise the possibility of aspiration of the liquid into the respiratory tract. It is advisable to administer a small amount of liquid at a time (3 ml in a 4 kg or larger rabbit) and wait until the rabbit swallows before placing any more liquid into the animal's mouth.

If syringe feeding is not successful, an orogastric tube or a naso-oesophageal tube may be placed. A mouth speculum is needed for orogastric tube placement. The speculum can be fashioned from a tongue depressor, wooden dowel or syringe case. It should have a hole drilled in the centre large enough to accommodate a No. 8 French infant feeding tube (Stein, 1980). The passage of the tube and verification of its placement is done as in other species. Instilling a drop of topical ophthalmic anaesthetic at the nostril facilitates passage of a naso-oesophageal tube (Hillyer, 1994).

Diseases—An Introduction

The figure found at the end of the chapter summarises the clincial presentations and suggested treatments for the diseases that are discussed below.

Diseases of the Respiratory System

Bacterial Diseases

Pasteurellosis

Agent. The major respiratory pathogen in the rabbit is *Pasteurella multocida*, a Gram-negative rod. More than 20 serotypes of this bacterium have been described.

Hosts. Other animals that are susceptible to infection with *Pasteurella multocida* include mice, birds, pigs and cattle (Okerman, 1988). *P. multocida* is also a part of the normal nasopharyngeal flora of cats. In general, the serotypes that are found in these other species are different from the serotypes responsible for *Pasteurella*-related disease in the rabbit. Some breeds of rabbits, e.g. Flemish Giants, may be more severely affected by *P. multocida* infections than others, e.g. New Zealand White rabbits (Dillehay *et al.*, 1991).

Clinical signs. *P. multocida* can affect one or more body systems in the rabbit and produce a multitude of clinical signs. The organism can cause nasal discharge, ocular discharge, sneezing, coughing, abscesses under the skin, torticollis, skin ulcers, infertility, lameness, anorexia, dyspnoea and death. Acute and peracute forms of pasteurellosis are manifest as haemorrhagic septicaemia characterised by pericarditis, lung congestion, petechial and ecchymotic haemorrhages and peritonitis (Mattix, 1993). The nasal discharge and sneezing so characteristic of pasteurellosis in the rabbit may reflect sinusitis and even atrophic rhinitis with degeneration of nasal turbinates in some cases (DiGiacomo *et al.*, 1989).

Diagnosis. Diagnosis involves physical examination, including auscultation and percussion of the thorax, radiography and culture of the affected organ system(s). Nasal cultures and ELISA tests are available for diagnosis of respiratory infections caused by *P. multocida*. In cases where death has occurred, a complete necropsy, including microbiological, serological and histopathological determinations, is very useful.

Control / treatment. *P. multocida* is so common in established rabbit colonies that it's eradication is difficult. The organism is transmitted through contact with infected secretions and also by aerosols containing the organism. Reasonable control measures involve attention to environmental factors, e.g. good ventilation, constant temperature and fastidious cage/pen cleaning procedures. Weaning at 4 or 5 weeks of age followed by separation of young rabbits from older, probable carrier rabbits, may be helpful

(Harkness and Wagner, 1989). Symptomatic carrier rabbits should be removed from the breeding colony. Promising new developments include ELISA testing to identify asymptomatic carriers in a colony and vaccines to prevent at least the most virulent forms of pasteurellosis.

Individual animals with respiratory or systemic infection due to bacterial pathogens are best treated with broad-spectrum antibiotics, e.g. tetracyclines, fluoroquinolones. The course of antibiotic therapy may be 1 month or longer. Supportive care includes cleansing the nares, paediatric nasal drops, nasal flushes and nebulisation or vaporiser treatments (Hillyer, 1994). Inflammation and obstruction of the nasolacrimal ducts may commonly occur in rabbits with conjunctivitis. After instilling topical ophthalmic anaesthetic into the conjunctival sac, the duct may be flushed with saline via an 18 or 20 gauge IV catheter inserted into the duct opening at the medial canthus (Hillyer, 1994). If the rabbit is not eating or drinking well, parenteral fluids and force feeding with puréed baby cereal or yogurt are indicated. Dyspnoeic rabbits should receive oxygen therapy and narcotic agents for the anxiety created by the dyspnoea. A chronic carrier state, with or without clinical signs, is very common with *P. multocida* infections even when the rabbit has been treated with appropriate antibiotics for a prolonged period.

Other bacterial respiratory pathogens

Agents. Other infectious agents that may cause respiratory disease in the rabbit include *Staphylococcus aureus* and *Pseudomonas aeruginosa*. *Bordetella bronchiseptica* is considered by a number of authors to be part of the normal flora of rabbits and non-pathogenic in most situations (Harkness and Wagner, 1989; Mattix, 1993; Okerman, 1988).

Viral Diseases

Pleural effusion disease

Agent. A coronavirus causes pleural effusion disease in rabbits. This disease was first reported in 1968, in Scandinavia (Fennestad *et al.*, 1981). The prevalence of this infection worldwide is not known at this time, but the incidence of the disease has remained low.

Clinical signs. Clinical signs of the disease include fever, anorexia, weight loss, hind limb weakness and increased respiratory rate and effort. Mortality is high due to pulmonary oedema, pleural effusion and damage to the heart and liver (Deeb, 1993).

Diseases of the Digestive System

Non-Infectious Diseases

Malocclusion

Malocclusion typically involves the incisors and frequently, the premolars and molars.

Clinical Signs. The affected rabbit may appear anorectic, thin or drooling. Due to the drooling and subsequent dermatitis, the condition is sometimes called 'slobbers'.

Diagnosis. The incisors are easily viewed by retracting the lips. However, observation of the molars requires good restraint or even sedation depending on the temperament of the rabbit. An otoscope, gently placed into the rabbit's mouth, facilitates the examination of the molars, tongue and gums. A radiograph may be required.

Control / treatment. Cutting, followed by filing the overgrown teeth and sharp points, will have to be done periodically throughout the life of the rabbit. Some clinicians prefer to use a dental drill to reshape the affected teeth; others prefer wire cutters, nail trimmers or a jeweller's file used as a small saw. Molar and incisor teeth may have to be extracted if the malocclusion is severe. For a detailed explanation of how to extract incisor teeth, please refer to *Chapter 8*. This condition appears to be inherited, so affected animals should be culled from breeding stock.

Trichobezoars

Also known as hairballs and wool block, this condition is usually seen in mature rabbits. Factors that predispose the rabbit to this condition include an inability to vomit, a small pyloric lumen, excessive fur-chewing, inadequate dietary fibre and deficiencies of copper, protein or magnesium (Walden, 1990). In one of the few controlled studies designed to investigate this syndrome, it was determined that the presence of a latex gastric foreign body, even in the presence of a trichobezoar, did not produce the clinical signs of anorexia and intestinal atony. A necropsy survey also demonstrated that 25% of clinically normal rabbits had one or more trichobezoars present in their stomachs (Leary *et al.*, 1984). Consequently, the pathogenesis of the syndrome remains controversial and a definitive treatment regime has not yet evolved.

Clinical signs. Affected rabbits show gradual onset anorexia, lethargy, weight loss and scant or no faecal production.

Diagnosis. Abdominal palpation, contrast radiography (Fig. 6.8) and possibly exploratory gastrotomy help to confirm the diagnosis. The liver in these animals may have fatty infiltrate and be very friable, so exercise great care on palpation.

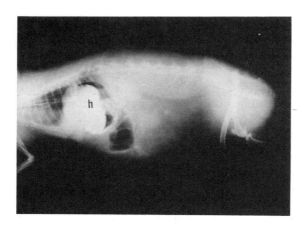

FIG. 6.8 Contrast radiography using air or radiopaque material at 2.5 ml/kg can be used to diagnose the presence of a hairball (h) in the rabbit's stomach.

Control / treatment. The majority of animals respond favourably to medical management, although gastric rupture and peritonitis have been reported (Percy and Barthold, 1993; Bergdall and Dysko, 1994). Survival is dependent upon re-establishing intestinal motility; consequently, it is very important to overcome the anorexia (Gillett *et al.*, 1983). A variety of therapies have been used to treat these animals. These include parenteral fluid support, injectable vitamins and steroids, daily doses of liquid paraffin oil (10–20 ml) followed by gastric massage (Walden, 1990), papaya enzymes or papain tablets, forced feeding with baby food cereals, offering hay, fresh treats and fresh pineapple juice (10 ml) daily for 5 days. Bromelain, an enzyme in the fresh juice, reportedly helps to digest hair. Some authors have recommended using metoclopromide (Hillyer, 1994; Burke, 1994). This should be used cautiously in view of the manufacturer's warning against its use in cases of mechanical obstruction.

Most cases of any duration make poor candidates for surgery (Donnelly, 1990). If surgery is performed to remove the hairball, perioperative supportive therapy must be intense in order to have some assurance of survival.

Infectious Diseases

Bacterial Agents

Enteritis

Many factors may contribute to the clinical presentation of diarrhoea and death in the rabbit. In the newborn or suckling rabbit, for example, hypothermia and maternal neglect may be implicated. Several agents acting in concert may precipitate enteritis.

Bacterial agents in newborn and suckling rabbits. The most commonly identified bacterial agents causing enteritis in newborn and suckling rabbits are *E. coli* and *Staphylococcus*.

Clinical signs. Diarrhoea and death are characteristic in this young age group. Evidence of septicaemia frequently exists in these cases.

Bacterial agents in weanling rabbits. Weanling rabbits most commonly fall victim to enteric diseases. The stress of weaning, changes in diet, insufficient fibre, carbohydrate overload, alteration of gut flora, subsequent intestinal pH changes and crowding all seem to contribute to the enteritis problem. The two main pathogens are *E. coli* and *Clostridium spiroforme*. The *E. coli* involved attaches to the brush border of the intestinal tract, however it does not invade or produce enterotoxins. *C. spiroforme* proliferates and produces enterotoxin in the large bowel under conditions of carbohydrate fermentation, glucose and acid production.

Clinical signs. Weanling rabbits afflicted by this enteritis complex develop diarrhoea, depression and dehydration and usually die rapidly.

Diagnosis. Clearly defining the aetiological agent(s) requires information gleaned from necropsy, histopathology, microbiology and parasitology results.

Control / treatment. Success of treatment for enteritis varies. Therapies include corrective fluid and electrolyte therapy (lactated Ringer's solution either SC or IV), systemic broad spectrum antibiotics, high fibre diets (hay or hay cubes), force feeding cereal baby foods mixed with dextrose, live *Lactobacillus* cultures, high calorie/energy liquids and possibly faeces from a healthy rabbit. Administration of B vitamins and corticosteroids are also indicated. Metoclopromide and commercial anti-diarrhoeals (loperamide or kaolin–pectin combinations) may be helpful.

There may be questions regarding the therapeutic use of *Lactobacillus*. *Lactobacillus* is not a normal inhabitant of the rabbit's gastrointestinal tract, however, anecdotal reports exist of its benefits in many species. If the rabbit will drink voluntarily, certain human oral paediatric electrolytes are very well received and can be added to the water. The average rabbit will tolerate approximately 10–15 ml/kg of orally administered slurries given twice daily (Brown, 1993a). This may prevent the hepatic lipidosis that frequently occurs in these cases. Many of these rabbits appear to be in pain, as evidenced by hunched posture, immobility, resistance to handling and grinding of the teeth. Administration of carefully selected analgesic agents improves the response of these rabbits to therapy (personal observation of the authors). Avoid long-term use of those analgesics associated with gastrointestinal upset (e.g. flunixin); avoid non-steroidal anti-inflammatory agents if the rabbit is being given steroids (Brown, 1993b). If the rabbit tolerates it, consider blood collection to monitor serum chemistry values. Antibiotic therapy should be instituted. Despite intensive efforts, many of these animals die.

Tyzzer's disease

Agent. *Clostridium piliforme*, previously known as *Bacillus piliformis*, is the causative agent of Tyzzer's disease. The Gram-negative organism forms spores which may be infective for long periods. The typical pattern of transmission is via the faecal–oral route, with the possibility of transplacental infection in some host species (Percy and Barthold, 1993).

Hosts. The disease occurs in a variety of hosts, including rabbits, hamsters, gerbils, horses, guinea pigs, cats, dogs and cattle.

Clinical signs. The disease has an acute onset, especially in weanlings and young rabbits. Watery diarrhoea, listless behaviour, anorexia and dehydration usually precede death by a day or so in the majority of cases. Survivors are usually unthrifty animals due to disease-associated changes in the gastrointestinal tract.

Diagnosis. Characteristic changes found at necropsy support the diagnosis of Tyzzer's disease. Such changes include areas of necrosis in the caecum, ileum, colon, liver and myocardium.

Tissue sections stained with the Warthin–Starry silver method or Giemsa demonstrate the typical bundles of filamentous bacilli in affected hepatocytes, enterocytes and myofibres. Complement fixation, indirect immunofluorescent antibody testing and enzyme-linked immunosorbent assays have been used to identify seropositive rabbits.

Control / treatment. Animals have responded poorly to antibiotic treatment and supportive therapy; however, some authors report that tetracycline administration appears to impede the progression of the disease through a colony (Percy and Barthold, 1993; DeLong and Manning, 1994). Minimising stress to the rabbits by the practice of good sanitation, prevention of overcrowding, vermin and dust control should reduce the incidence of disease. Sanitisation using a 0.3% sodium hypochlorite solution has been reported to inactivate the clostridial spores (Ganaway, 1980).

Viral Agents

Rotavirus infection

Agent. Rotaviruses damage villous cells lining the jejunum and ileum with a subsequent onset of diarrhoea in suckling rabbits. Transmission is most likely by the faecal–oral route.

Hosts. Although rotaviruses cause enteric problems in many species, only group A, serotype 3 produces problems in rabbits. Humans and some other animals also may share this serotype (Di-Giacomo and Mare, 1994).

Clinical signs. In those rabbits lacking trans-placentally derived maternal antibody, diarrhoea followed by dehydration and death occurs within one or two days. Those colonies with endemic rotavirus infection have a much reduced incidence of morbidity and mortality. Young rabbits in such colonies may appear clinically normal, while being subclinically infected.

Diagnosis. Diagnosis is confirmed by synthesising the clinical picture, history and necropsy findings with viral identification. Electron microscopy of faecal samples, virus isolation, ELISA tests or a rise in antibody levels all may be used to identify the virus.

Control / treatment. Attempts at treatment are unrewarding. Control measures include closing the colony to new rabbits or stopping breeding for 4–6 weeks to eliminate viral transmission from infected rabbits (DiGiacomo and Mare, 1994). Sterile Caesarean derivation and cross-fostering on to non-shedding does at a different location also may reduce the incidence of rotavirus infection.

Mucoid enteropathy

Mucoid enteropathy also causes enteric disease in rabbits of weaning age and older.

Agents / causes. The exact aetiologic agent remains unknown, however, inadequate dietary fibre and caecal and colonic impactions appear to contribute to the clinical expression of the disease. The use of such antibiotics as clindamycin and lincomycin has also been implicated in causing this complex (Burke, 1994).

Clinical signs. Affected rabbits produce gelatinous or mucoid faeces. If the rabbit is handled, one hears a sound like sloshing water. Clinical signs include mucoid diarrhoea, depression, bloated appearance, grinding teeth, hypothermia and frequently death. Rabbits that survive grow very slowly.

Diagnosis. Diagnosis is based on clinical signs and the post mortem findings of a gas and fluid-filled intestinal tract without evidence of other infectious agents. Marked goblet cell hyperplasia of the large and small intestine is a characteristic histopathological finding and accounts for the clinical presentation.

Control / treatment. Treatment consists of supportive measures but the prognosis in these cases is guarded. Prevention is paramount and involves providing fibre, avoiding sudden dietary changes, using antibiotics judiciously and minimising environmental stress.

Parasitic diseases

Coccidiosis

There are two forms of coccidiosis in the rabbit: the hepatic form and the intestinal form.

Agent. *Eimeria stiedae*, the hepatic form, attacks the bile duct epithelium. The coccidial oocysts emerge from the destroyed lining, enter the bile and exit in the faeces.

Clinical signs. Usually young rabbits show the general unthriftiness, diarrhoea and abdominal distension associated with *E. stiedae* infection.

Agent. Eight species of *Eimeria* cause intestinal coccidiosis, with variable pathogenicity among them.

Clinical signs. All ages of rabbits with intestinal coccidiosis may exhibit the clinical signs of diarrhoea, anorexia, dehydration and death, especially under conditions of stress.

Diagnosis. Faecal examination, oocyst counts, clinical signs and necropsy results (histopathological) assist in differentiating coccidiosis from other enteric diseases.

Control / treatment. Control of the infection requires strict attention to sanitation and husbandry. Avoidance of stress, frequent disinfection of cages, hutches, transport carriers and litter pans with 10% ammonia solutions (Walden, 1990) may reduce or prevent clinical disease.

Treatment programmes include the addition of sulphamerazine or sulphaquinoxaline to the drinking water, robenidine or sulphadimethoxine in the feed (Walden, 1990), lasalocid added to the feed or amprolium added to the feed (Patterson, 1987) or to the water (Hillyer, 1994).

The regulatory agencies in the USA specify a 10 day withdrawal time for sulphaquinoxaline if used in rabbits raised for human consumption. The development of resistance to coccidiostats in the feed has been documented.

Pinworms

Agent. The rabbit pinworm, *Passalurus ambiguus*, has a direct life cycle. Adults live in the colon and caecum, with the eggs being passed in the faeces.

Clinical signs. Infected animals do not usually display clinical signs.

Diagnosis. Faecal flotation for identification of ova or observation of an adult worm passed in the faeces is preferred over the perineal cellophane tape method for diagnosis.

Control / treatment. Treatment is with fenbendazole (Burke, 1994), thiabendazole (Brown, 1993b) or piperazine (Walden, 1990). One author recommends using 2% peracetic acid or formaldehyde vapour to kill pinworm ova in the rabbit housing area (Walden, 1990).

Cysticercosis

Agent. Domestic rabbits are infrequent intermediate hosts for the dog and cat tapeworm, *Taenia pisiformis*.

Clinical signs. This condition is usually an incidental finding at necropsy or slaughter.

Diagnosis. Characteristic lesions at necropsy are vesicles in the liver and mesentery. The organism is evident on histopathological examination.

Control / treatment. Rabbits become infected by consuming food or contacting bedding contaminated with the tapeworm eggs. Eliminating contact between rabbits and cats and dogs breaks the cycle of infection.

Diseases of the Genitourinary System

Bacterial Diseases

Mastitis

Agents. Mastitis in lactating does may be caused by various bacteria including *Staphylococcus*, *Pasteurella* or *Streptococcus*.

Clinical signs. Clinical signs are typical of inflammation with swelling, reddening of the gland, abnormal milk, fever and anorexia. The doe and the young rabbits may die as a result of a severe case of mastitis.

Diagnosis. Diagnosis is based on observation of the clinical signs and bacteriological culture of milk from affected glands.

Control / treatment. Treatment involves the use of antibiotics. Penicillin therapy may be initiated while awaiting the results of bacteriological culture and antibiotic sensitivity testing. Supportive care that must be provided includes parenteral fluids and treatment of infected glands using warm compresses and, if necessary, surgical drainage. Orphaned rabbits can transfer the mastitis organisms to a foster doe, so hand-rearing of orphaned animals is advised in these cases (Mattix, 1993). Prevention includes good housing and hygiene for lactating does and observation of does for several days after the litter is weaned.

Epididymitis, orchitis, metritis, pyometra, ovarian abscesses

Agents. A commonly implicated pathogen in these bacterial infections is *Pasteurella multocida* (Harkness and Wagner, 1989; DeLong and Manning, 1994; Johnson and Wolf, 1993). Metritis in rabbits has also been attributed to Gram-nega-

tive enteric bacteria and to *Treponema cuniculi* (Harkness and Wagner, 1989).

Clinical signs. In both male and female, reduced fertility is characteristic. Male rabbits with orchitis or epididymitis may have obvious signs of inflammation, such as swelling and purulent drainage from abscesses. Clinical signs of metritis, pyometra and ovarian abscesses may include abdominal distension and vaginal discharge.

Diagnosis. Physical examination may be sufficient, although radiographs may provide additional information on does. Orchitis must be differentiated from testicular tumours in bucks.

Treatment. These infections are difficult to treat successfully with antibiotics in any species. Neutering of an affected animal may be a reasonable alternative for a non-breeding rabbit.

Venereal spirochaetosis / rabbit syphilis

Agent. The spirochaete, *T. cuniculi*, causes a rabbit venereal disease known as rabbit syphilis or vent disease. The organism spreads among adult rabbits via breeding and is transmitted to offspring at the time of parturition or lactation.

Clinical signs. The external genitalia, perineal areas, nose, eyelids and lips of affected rabbits develop vesicles and scaliness that progress to ulcers and crusty lesions. Transient infertility may occur in both sexes. Infertility in the female may be attributed to metritis or retained placentas and in the male to preputial inflammation (Harkness and Wagner, 1989).

Diagnosis. Diagnosis may be made by dark field microscopic examination of skin scrapings from lesions and by serological tests.

Control / treatment. Penicillin is effective in treating venereal spirochaetosis in rabbits. Control of the disease in a colony requires either treatment of the entire colony, including neonates, with penicillin or culling of carriers based on serological testing. New animals should be quarantined and tested to prevent introducing this problem into a breeding colony.

Non-Infectious Diseases

Uterine hyperplasia and / or uterine adenocarcinoma

Uterine adenocarcinoma is the most common tumour of the rabbit (Harkness and Wagner, 1989). Female rabbits, if intact after the age of 3 years, may develop uterine hyperplasia or uterine adenocarcinoma, with an incidence reported as high as 80% in does over 5 years of age (Harkness and Wagner, 1989; Percy and Barthold, 1993). There are breed predilections to uterine adenocarcinoma, namely a high incidence in Dutch rabbits and a moderately high incidence in Californian rabbits and New Zealand White rabbits (Mattix, 1993).

Clinical signs. Hyperplasia and adenocarcinoma of the uterus produce similar clinical signs in the rabbit: decreased reproductive performance, bloody vaginal discharge and the development of cystic mammary glands.

Diagnosis. Radiography and biopsy may aid in the diagnosis. Chest radiographs may be used to screen for metastatic lesions.

Treatment. Untreated, adenocarcinoma will lead to death within 24 months (Quesenberry, 1989). Ovariohysterectomy is the treatment of choice for both of these conditions.

Mammary tumours and mammary dysplasia

Mammary dysplasia may occur in association with pituitary adenomas or uterine adenocarcinomas (Lipman et al., 1994; Weisbroth, 1994). Mammary carcinoma has also been associated with uterine adenocarcinoma in the rabbit (Weisbroth, 1994).

Clinical signs. Clinical signs of mammary dysplasia may include enlargement and discoloration of the teats with no evidence of inflammation. Masses or fluid-filled cystic structures may be palpable within the mammary tissue in cases of dysplasia or neoplasia.

Diagnosis. Biopsy is indicated. A positive biopsy for mammary adenocarcinoma should prompt evaluation of the patient for possible uterine adenocarcinoma since these two conditions are known to develop simultaneously.

Treatment. Surgery may be considered for uncomplicated mammary adenocarcinoma, provided thoracic radiographs do not reveal metastatic disease.

Testicular tumours

Interstitial cell tumours occur mainly in 5–7-year-old bucks used for breeding (Mattix, 1993).

Clinical signs. Testicular interstitial cell tumours cause enlargement of the testes with areas of necrosis.

Diagnosis. Clinical signs and age of the buck are indicative. Biopsy would confirm the diagnosis.

Treatment. Castration is indicated.

Ovarian tumours and cysts

Ovarian tumours and cysts have been reported in older female rabbits (Burke, 1994).

Clinical signs. There is a history of decreased reproductive rate or failure to conceive.

Diagnosis. Diagnostic approaches include ultrasonography and laparoscopy.

Treatment. Surgical removal of the ovaries should be curative unless tumour metastasis has already occurred.

Urolithiasis and cystitis

Clinical signs. The clinical signs are similar to those in other species: increased frequency of urination, haematuria, perineal irritation due to urine, straining to urinate. A rabbit with urinary tract obstruction is anorectic and depressed. Straining to urinate may be misinterpreted by owners as an indication of respiratory problems (Okerman, 1988).

Diagnosis. Diagnosis of urolithiasis may be made by physical examination including abdominal palpation, urinalysis and radiography.

Control / treatment. Surgical removal of the urinary calculi is indicated, as well as other treatment based on stone analysis and microbiological culture of the urine (Hillyer, 1994). Fluid therapy is essential since many of these rabbits will be dehydrated at the time of initial examination. Antibiotics are administered if urinary tract infection exists. Urine culture and antibiotic sensitivity testing will determine the best choice of antibiotics for a particular case. Chloramphenicol, tetracycline and trimethoprim/sulpha combinations have been used (Harkness and Wagner, 1989). The rabbit's diet should be assessed to determine if calcium intake is appropriate.

Kidney disease

Kidney disease is fairly common based on necropsy findings in older rabbits, but clinical signs are rare (Okerman, 1988). Kidney damage may have been caused by *Encephalitozoon cuniculi*, *Staphylococcus aureus* and *P. multocida*. Embryonal nephroma is the third most common neoplasm in the rabbit (Mattix, 1993).

Clinical signs. Renal failure is an uncommon problem in rabbits but should be considered if there is a history of polydipsia/polyuria or urine scald in a depressed, thin or aged rabbit.

Diagnosis. Urinalysis and serum chemistry evaluation are essential for making a diagnosis. Abdominal radiographs may be useful.

Treatment. Fluid therapy, a low protein diet and good nursing care to minimise urine scald may help the animal in renal failure feel more comfortable.

Diseases of the Nervous System

Infectious Diseases

Encephalitozoonosis

Agent. The protozoan parasite *E. cuniculi* usually causes latent infection in rabbits. The kidney and brain are the primary target tissues of the parasite.

Clinical signs. Clinically affected animals present with tremors, ataxia, paresis, head tilt and convulsions (Walden, 1990; Okerman, 1988).

Diagnosis. Diagnosis is by serological testing. Necropsy of affected animals and histopathology of the brain and kidney tissues confirm the diagnosis.

Control / treatment. No treatment currently exists. Transmission occurs via urine, although respiratory, faecal and transplacental routes may also play a role. Serological screening, isolation of infected individuals and strict sanitation measures help to eliminate infection from a colony.

Torticollis

Agents. The most common cause of torticollis in the rabbit is infection of the middle or inner ear with *P. multocida*. Head tilt, ataxia and inappetence may also be indicative of infection with *Encephalitozoon*, encephalitis or mechanical trauma due to aberrant parasite migration through the nervous tissue (e.g. *Ascaris* spp.).

Clinical signs. Mild to marked torsion of the neck may be seen as well as inappetence and ataxia.

Diagnosis. Diagnosis and prognosis depend upon the results of serological testing and response to antibiotic and supportive therapy.

Control / treatment. Recommended therapies include the use of enrofloxacin or chloramphenicol, force feeding (Hillyer, 1994) and glucocorticoids. Improvement should be seen in 5–7 days, or the patient should be re-evaluated.

Other Nervous System Problems

Poisoning

Agents poisonous to rabbits with access to home and garden sites include lead (found in certain paints and foil), fertilisers, herbicides and insecticides. In certain cases when rabbits were dipped or sprayed with agents used to control external parasites on cats, rabbits have convulsed and died (Dumonceaux, 1992).

Trauma

Vertebral fracture or dislocation can easily occur in a rabbit that is incorrectly restrained or suddenly kicks out in fear or defence. If the heavy hindlimbs are allowed to thrust unsupported, they can exert significant stress upon the animal's lightweight skeleton which can result in skeletal and spinal cord damage.

Clinical signs. Paralysis of the hind quarters and inability to control defaecation and urination indicate severe spinal cord trauma or transection.

Diagnosis. Radiographs may help to assess the degree of trauma. Fractures most frequently happen at the seventh lumbar vertebra.

Control / treatment. The quality of life for these animals should be taken into account and euthanasia may be the best choice. Animals able to control urination and defaecation may respond to corticosteroid therapy and cage rest.
If spinal cord damage is minimal, surgical treatment (see *Chapter 8*) may be considered. Proper handling and restraint techniques can prevent many of these traumatic episodes.

Epilepsy

Reports indicate that epilepsy occurs in certain breeds of rabbits with white fur and blue eyes (Okerman, 1988).

Diseases of the Special Senses

Ocular Disorders

Buphthalmia / glaucoma

This condition primarily affects New Zealand White rabbits. The inherited autosomal recessive trait compromises drainage of the aqueous humor from the anterior orbital chamber.

Clinical signs. The clinical disease may be bilateral or unilateral with a variable age at onset, perhaps due to the incomplete penetrance of the causative genes. The increased intraocular pressure forces the eye to change in shape and size resulting in megaloglobus and corneal opacity.

Diagnosis. Diagnosis is based on clinical signs. Tonometry may not be diagnostic as it may reveal normal intraocular pressure.

Control / treatment. Treatment is usually not necessary. The rabbit appears to be without pain. Affected individuals should be culled from the breeding programme.

Entropion

Agent / cause. Congenital entropion and entropion resulting from inflammation and infection damage the conjunctiva and cornea (Fox *et al.*, 1979).

Clinical signs. Animals exhibit blepharospasm, conjunctivitis, epiphora and corneal ulceration depending upon the severity of the entropion.

Diagnosis. Bilateral infections, frequently caused by *Pasteurella* or *Staphylococcus* spp., distichiasis, trauma and treponematosis must be ruled out as primary causes of the condition.

Treatment. Surgical correction of the condition involves removing enough tissue to reduce the inward rolling of the lid margin. Secondary bacterial infection and corneal damage must also be resolved by using appropriate ophthalmic preparations and routine monitoring.

Conjunctivitis

Conjunctivitis frequently occurs in the rabbit. The condition may be a primary conjunctivitis or part of an acute or chronic respiratory disease complex.

Agents. *Pasteurella multocida* is most frequently cultured.

Clinical signs. There is a serous or purulent discharge which, if chronic, causes hair loss on the face below the medial canthus. The conjunctival surface appears congested. The eyelids may swell.

Diagnosis. Observation of clinical signs and bacteriological culture of conjunctival swabs assist in diagnosis.

Control / treatment. Using topical ophthalmic preparations containing antibiotics (e.g. chloramphenicol) several times daily is recommended. In more involved cases with persistent conjunctivitis and obstruction of the naso-lacrimal ducts, flushing of the ducts may be attempted. After instilling topical ophthalmic anaesthetic into the conjunctival sac, the duct may be flushed with saline via an 18 or 20 gauge IV catheter inserted into the duct opening at the medial canthus (Hillyer, 1994).

Other eye disorders

Corneal dystrophy, cataracts and intraocular tumours have infrequently been reported in the rabbit (Peiffer *et al.*, 1994). Diagnostics, therapy and prognosis are as for other species.

Otitis Externa

Agent. Otitis externa is usually caused by the mite *Psoroptes cuniculi* (Fig. 6.9).

Clinical signs. Affected rabbits frequently dig at their ears and shake their heads. On inspection, the ear canal and pinna are filled with yellow-grey crusty material. In severe or untreated cases, the infection extends to the base of the ears, along the animal's back and down its legs and feet (Fig. 6.10).

Diagnosis. Microscopic examination of ear debris reveals the presence of the mite.

Control / treatment. The mite requires 21 days to complete its life cycle with females able to survive off the host for several weeks. Although topical treatment with mineral oil and acaricides can be used, this form of therapy can be uncomfortable for the rabbit. Systemic therapy has become more widely used. Ivermectin, administered SC for 3 treatments at 2-week intervals, eradicates the problem. All rabbits in the group must be treated, even if they appear parasite-

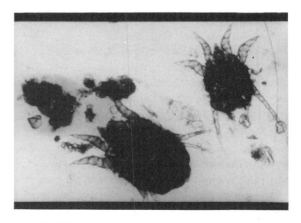

FIG. 6.9 Otitis externa is usually caused by the ear mite, *Psoroptes cuniculi* (magnification ×40).

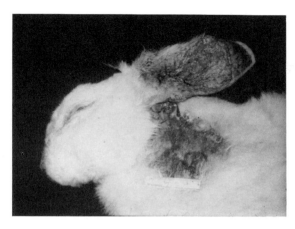

FIG. 6.10 A rabbit suffering from severe infestation by *Psoroptes cuniculi* with spread of the resulting skin lesions from the ear to the shoulder.

free. Possible infection via crusts and debris mandates thorough disinfection of the caging, litter boxes or shared areas.

Otitis Media

Agents. Bacterial agents commonly implicated in otitis media are *Pasteurella multocida*, *Staphylococcus aureus* and *Bordetella bronchiseptica* (DeLong and Manning, 1994).

Clinical signs. Rabbits with otitis media are usually asymptomatic (DeLong and Manning, 1994). In cases where the infection has advanced toward the inner ear, ataxia and torticollis may be evident.

Diagnosis. The diagnosis is presumptive. Other possible causes of these clinical signs are *Encephalitozoon*, encephalitis or mechanical trauma due to aberrant parasite migration through the nervous tissue (e.g. *Ascaris* spp.).

Control / treatment. If bacterial agents are the cause of the clinical signs, improvement may be seen with antibiotic therapy, such as enrofloxacin or chloramphenicol. Bulla osteotomy allows drainage of the tympanic bulla and may be a viable treatment alternative in those animals that are non-responsive to antibiotic therapy.

Diseases of the Integument and Musculoskeletal System

Integumentary System Diseases

Clinical signs of cutaneous problems: General principles

Clinical signs of integumentary diseases include one or more of the following: pruritus, alopecia, reddening, scaliness, purulent material, crusts and swelling. These signs may be a direct consequence of the disease process or caused, totally or in part, by self-trauma. Lacerations and abrasions of the skin may result when a rabbit has a close encounter with sharp objects in the environment, including the teeth and claws of another rabbit.

Painful or pruritic skin problems can change the temperament of a rabbit for the worse. An owner reported that one of her rabbits had inexplicably and suddenly attacked its companion rabbit. Upon examination, she discovered that sharp seeds had become embedded in the animal's perineal skin fold and that the rabbit had fleas. Prompt attention to this problem resulted in a rapid change in the rabbit's attitude toward his companion. As the owner stated, the obvious lesson is to look for physical problems first whenever there is a behaviour change (Harriman, 1992).

Diagnosis of cutaneous problems: General principles

To diagnose integumentary disease, the clinician relies on physical examination, microscopic examination of material from skin scraping or skin vacuuming, aspiration cytology, bacterial and fungal cultures, Wood's lamp examination and skin biopsy. Some of these tests may be repeated to confirm efficacy of treatment.

Ulcerative pododermatitis / 'sore hocks'

Ulcerative pododermatitis or 'sore hocks' is common in rabbits housed on wire mesh or sometimes stainless steel slatted cage floors (Fig. 6.11). The lesions are more dramatic in heavier rabbits (5 kg and larger). Reduced thickness of the foot fur pad, moist cage floors or genetic factors contribute to the development of ulcerative pododermatitis (Harkness and Wagner, 1989).

Clinical signs. Initially there will be alopecia and reddening on the plantar surfaces of the hind feet and the palmar surfaces of the front feet. These lesions may be replaced by thick scar tissue or may ulcerate. Secondary bacterial infection of the ulcers occurs.

Control / treatment. Treatment of severe lesions can be lengthy and may involve bandaging (and rebandaging) for weeks. Some rabbits will not tolerate bandages. All cases of pododermatitis show improvement if the rabbit is housed on solid flooring. Providing rabbits with adequate solid floor resting areas may prevent and control this problem.

Cutaneous abscesses

Agents. Microbiological culture of an abscess in a rabbit usually yields *S. aureus* or *P. multocida* (Okerman, 1988).

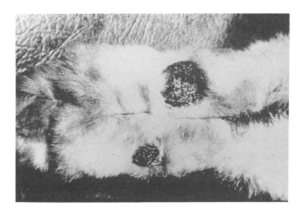

FIG. 6.11 Ulcerative pododermatitis or 'sore hocks' is frequently seen in obese animals housed on wire mesh floors.

Treatment. Treatment consists of draining the abscess and flushing the cavity daily for several days with a dilute antiseptic solution. Systemic antibiotics may prevent haematogenous spread of the organism to other tissues.

Blue fur disease

Agent. *Pseudomonas aeruginosa* is the offending organism in a moist dermatitis called blue fur disease in the rabbit.

Clinical signs. This condition affects skin folds in areas that may be constantly wet, such as the dewlap.

Control / treatment. Blue fur disease is controlled by eliminating the organism from the water crocks or the sipper tubes of water bottles and by treating the rabbit with topical or injectable gentamicin (Okerman, 1988). It is also important to check the husbandry routine to ensure that the rabbit's environment remains dry.

Ectoparasites

Ectoparasites are a common cause of skin problems in the rabbit. *Psoroptes cuniculi* is an ear mite. The rabbit fur mites are *Cheyletiella parasitovorax* and *Listrophorus gibbus*. *Notoedres*, *Dermanyssus gallinae* (red fowl mite) and *Sarcoptes* spp. may all infect rabbits.

Cheyletiella

Agent. *Cheyletiella parasitovorax* is the most common fur mite in the rabbit. It may be a vector for myxomatosis.

Hosts. This mite is found on many mammalian hosts, including dogs, cats and rabbits. It may cause dermatitis in humans.

Clinical signs. The mite causes minor hair loss, scaling and some itching in the rabbit.

Diagnosis. Skin scraping and examination of hairs from the lesion sites are traditional diagnostic techniques for recovering skin mites from animals. Additionally, gently vacuuming the animal with a pipette attached to a suction unit or small commercial vacuum works very well. A small piece of milk filter paper placed in the line traps debris which can be examined microscopically. Pruritic animals especially seem to enjoy the motion of the pipette and the technique is atraumatic and efficient for recovering ectoparasites.

Control / treatment. An effective treatment for *Cheyletiella* infestation is ivermectin. Cat flea powders and aerosol preparations have also been used. Control measures include disinfection of the premises. The bedding should also be changed or dusted with the same powders used on the animals.

Lice and fleas

Lice and fleas occasionally occur on pet rabbits.

Hosts. Domestic rabbits housed outdoors can acquire the rabbit flea, a vector for myxomatosis, by contact with wild rabbits. Pet rabbits occasionally acquire fleas, such as the cat flea, from other domestic animals (Okerman, 1988).

Clinical signs. Rabbits infested with the louse *Haemeodipsus ventricosis* may be anaemic, pruritic and in generally poor condition (Harkness and Wagner, 1989).

Diagnosis. Careful physical examination may reveal louse nits and evidence of fleas from their excrement. The skin vacuuming procedure described for *Cheyletiella* in this chapter may also be used to recover the organisms.

Control / treatment. Treatment and environmental control of lice and fleas are the same as for the cat.

Cuterebra

Cuterebra larvae may pupate in the subcutaneous tissues of rabbits that spend time out of doors.

Clinical signs. The larva frequently appears to be moving back and forth inside a swollen tunnel on the rabbit's neck or throat area.

Treatment. Treatment requires removing the larva by gentle extraction through the enlarged airhole or attempting to kill the larva by applying ether to the site before removal. Special handling and storage are necessary when using ether, an explosive, flammable agent.

Myiasis / fly strike

Fly strike or maggot infestation also occurs in rabbits, especially obese or debilitated animals.

Control / treatment. Affected animals should be sedated before the fur is clipped, the maggots removed and the damaged tissues gently irrigated. Treatment should include systemic fluid therapy, antibiotics and gentle cleaning of the wound sites as required. Ivermectin given as two doses 2 weeks apart has been recommended (Hillyer, 1994). Prevention involves using fly control, screening outdoor pens and frequent examination of rabbits spending time outside.

Aged or overweight pet rabbits may have difficulty grooming the perineal area. Faeces and urine accumulate in this 'pouch' of flabby skin, a prime site for fly strike (maggot infestation). A surgical corrective procedure called perineal skin fold reduction has improved the activity level of a number of aged rabbits (Waidhofer, 1989).

Psoroptes cuniculi

P. cuniculi causes ear mange, also referred to as ear canker.

Dermatophytosis

Agent. The most common dermatophyte in the rabbit is *Trichophyton mentagrophytes*.

Hosts. Many mammalian domestic animals are susceptible to *Trichophyton* infection. This is a zoonotic disease, with some humans easily infected.

Clinical signs. Some rabbits are carriers with no clinical signs although they can transmit the organism to people and to other animals. Ringworm, especially in young rabbits, may cause hair loss and crusty lesions on the face, front legs and ears (Harkness and Wagner, 1989).

Control / treatment. Treatment for dermatophytosis may require only topical antifungal agents daily for 2–4 weeks or, in severe cases, oral griseofulvin for several weeks. Two other treatment regimens described for *Trichophyton* are: (1) a topically applied two-component commerical cold disinfectant (MECA: metastabilised chlorous acid/chlorine dioxide; USA trade name Alcide®) diluted 1 part base compound to 1 part activator compound to 10 parts tap water, massaged into the rabbit's fur; (2) a 1% copper sulphate dip (Franklin *et al.*, 1991).

Viral Cutaneous Diseases

There are viral diseases that cause neoplasia in the rabbit: the Shope fibroma virus and the myxoma virus. Fibromatosis is generally a benign disease in wild rabbits. The Shope fibroma virus is utilised in the manufacture of vaccines for myxomatosis and can cause severe illness if administered to domestic rabbits younger than 3 weeks of age (Okerman, 1988). The Shope papilloma virus of wild rabbits occasionally causes skin warts in domestic rabbits. These warts are usually on the eyelids and ears of the rabbit and may eventually become carcinomas (Burke, 1994). These viral diseases are spread by arthropod vectors from wild to domestic rabbits. Control can be achieved by thoroughly screening outdoor rabbit pens.

Skin tumours

Other skin neoplasias in the rabbit include lipoma, squamous cell carcinoma, trichoepithe-lioma and basal cell tumour (Hillyer, 1994; Mattix, 1993; Weisbroth, 1994). Surgical excision is the recommended treatment. Most are slow to metastasise.

Musculoskeletal System Diseases

Fractures

Vertebral fracture results in neurological signs. A young rabbit can fracture a leg if running in a cage with wire flooring that has holes large enough to trap its foot. Such injuries are assessed and managed as for leg fractures in dogs and cats.

Osteomyelitis and osteosarcoma

The mandible of the rabbit is the primary site for osteomyelitis and osteosarcoma. Radiographs and biopsy will differentiate these two problems. Osteomyelitis is very difficult to treat successfully even with aggressive surgical debridement and antibiotic therapy. Euthanasia is a humane course of action with a rabbit with osteosarcoma.

Splay leg

Animals with this condition keep one or more legs spread and appear unable to adduct the affected limbs. The condition becomes noticeable when the young leave the nest box. There seems to be a heritable basis for this defect. No effective treatment exists.

Systemic Diseases

Bacterial Diseases

Staphylococcosis

Agent. *Staphylococcus* spp. may cause disease in multiple systems.

Hosts. *Staphylococcus* in the rabbit may be of human or rabbit origin.

Clinical signs. The clinical problems precipitated by this agent include bacterial dermatitis, conjunctivitis, rhinitis, mastitis with subsequent septicaemia and associated death in does and their offspring, pneumonia, subcutaneous abscesses and renal infarction.

Diagnosis. Culture and sensitivity will determine the presence of the organism. Strains of rabbit origin cause more virulent disease problems, therefore biotyping of the isolated strain should be performed.

Control / treatment. Antibiotic therapy minimises clinical expression of the disease but does not eliminate the problem. Rabbits can harbour the organism in their nasal passages, providing a source for reinfection. Eradication of the problem requires elimination of all current stock and thorough disinfection of the premises.

Salmonellosis

Agent. *Salmonella typhimurium* or *Salmonella enteritidis* are the serovars most commonly isolated in disease outbreaks in the rabbit.

Hosts. *Salmonella* spp. are common in all vertebrate animals.

Clinical signs. Rabbits infrequently develop salmonellosis. Clinical signs of this primarily septicaemic disease range from depression, fever, abortion and diarrhoea to sudden death.

Diagnosis. Culturing tissues or faeces from suspect carriers most frequently yields the agent. The viscera of affected rabbits appear congested, haemorrhagic and necrotic. In acute infections, splenomegaly may be the outstanding gross finding.

Control / treatment. Reported cases seem to occur under conditions of poor hygiene, stress or contaminated feed. Factors contributing to the disease must be identified and eliminated. Treated animals may become inapparent carriers. If possible, the recommendation is to euthanase the remaining colony and thoroughly disinfect the premises.

Pet owners and rabbit breeders need to be reminded of the potential for human infection, interspecies transmission and carrier status. Faecal culture may be used to identify human carriers.

Parasitic Diseases

Toxoplasmosis

Agent. *Toxoplasma gondii* is a protozoan.

Hosts. Definitive hosts are members of the cat family. *T. gondii* infection occurs when rabbits ingest feed contaminated with cat faeces containing the oocyst stage of the parasite. The parasite proliferates with cyst formation in the rabbit's tissues.

Clinical signs. Usually, the chronic infection remains inapparent. However, in the more acute form, clinical signs include anorexia, listlessness, fever, tremors, muscle weakness and paralysis (Okerman, 1988).

Diagnosis. Rabbits dying from the acute form have congested tissues and marked splenomegaly.

Control / treatment. To remove rabbits from the *Toxoplasma* reservoir loop, avoid potentially contaminated feed. There is a report in the literature of a suspected transmission of toxoplasmosis from a pet rabbit to its owner (Ishikawa *et al.*, 1991).

Viral Diseases

Myxomatosis

Agent. The agent is a poxvirus. Exposure occurs via direct contact, indirect contact or parasite vector, i.e. mosquitoes and fleas.

Clinical signs. Oedema of the face, ears and genitalia, nasal and ocular discharge, followed by diffuse cutaneous lumps used to be thought pathognomonic for the disease. However, a variant strain of the virus only affects the respiratory system, sometimes resulting in pneumonia (Okerman, 1988). Domestic rabbits infected with this pox-virus almost always die.

Diagnosis. The diagnosis is confirmed by histopathological examination of the typical gross lesions.

Control / treatment. Symptomatic treatment is usually unrewarding and these animals may be a source of infection for others. Prevention methods centre around vector control. Control includes reducing contact with wild rabbits and hares, which harbour the virus with far less clinical involvement. The availability of vaccines varies from country to country. Infected rabbitries should not rely on cold, dry conditions to eliminate the virus, but rather use chemical disinfectants.

Viral haemorrhagic disease

Agent. At present, the agent is considered to be a calicivirus (Percy and Barthold, 1993; DiGiacomo and Mare, 1994).

Hosts. Both domestic and wild rabbits are susceptible to the disease. Infected rabbits and contaminated fomites serve as sources of infection.

Clinical signs. The disease usually follows an acute course with high morbidity and mortality. Clinical signs, if seen, include depression, anorexia, fever, inco-ordination, progressing to death.

Diagnosis. Pathology produced by the causative calicivirus includes hepatic necrosis and haemorrhages in the lungs, kidneys and other tissues. These findings, together with serological tests, confirm the diagnosis.

Control / treatment. Vaccines against the virus are currently available in Europe and China (Hillyer, 1994; Fuller et al., 1993). Vaccinated rabbits can still acquire subclinical infections (DiGiacomo and Maré, 1994). In endemic areas or after an outbreak, strict quarantine measures and fastidious disinfection of premises are essential. The virus can be inactivated with 0.5% sodium hypochlorite (DiGiacomo and Maré, 1994). Treatment for clinically ill rabbits is empirical, with parenteral fluids and other supportive measures, as for any severe systemic disease.

Diseases of the Haematopoietic and Cardiovascular Systems

Rabbit (Viral) Haemorrhagic Disease, a fatal disease, has been reported in Europe, China and Mexico.

Lymphosarcoma

Lymphosarcoma is the second most common tumour of rabbits. Genetic predisposition may play a role in the occurrence of lymphosarcoma.

Clinical signs. Clinical signs of lymphosarcoma in the rabbit may include lethargy, anorexia, weight loss and pale mucous membranes (Toth et al., 1990).

Diagnosis. Lymphosarcoma occurs mainly in young adult or even juvenile rabbits (Harkness and Wagner, 1989). The most common form of lymphosarcoma is the visceral form, involving the liver, spleen, kidney, mesenteric lymph nodes, stomach, adrenal glands, lungs and bone marrow. Haematology and biopsy of bone marrow and lymph nodes should aid in diagnosis.

Control / treatment. Veterinary oncologists could suggest chemotherapeutic combinations to try in the rabbit since well defined protocols are available for the treatment of lymphosarcoma in the dog and cat.

Cardiomyopathy

Agent. Rabbit coronavirus has been implicated as a possible cause of rabbit cardiomyopathy. This develops in conjunction with pleural effusion disease.

Clinical signs. Clinical signs are those associated with congestive heart failure, such as increased respiratory rate and effort and generalised muscle weakness (DiGiacomo and Maré, 1994).

Diagnosis. Thoracic radiographs and echo-cardiography reveal pleural effusion, a dilated right ventricle and pulmonary oedema.

Control / treatment. Treatment has not been defined in the rabbit but palliative treatment could be based on similar conditions in the dog or cat.

Arteriosclerosis

Arteriosclerosis in the rabbit is a well recognised problem in many breeds.

Clinical signs. Clinical signs may include anorexia, dehydration and weight loss (Mattix, 1993). In one case report, seizures were the presenting sign in a rabbit whose necropsy later revealed arteriosclerosis (Shell and Saunders, 1989).

Diagnosis. The most common sites for mineralisation are the aortic arch and the thoracic aorta. Thoracic radiographs and necropsy results confirm the diagnosis.

Control / treatment. The cause of arteriosclerosis in the rabbit is believed by some to be hypervitaminosis D in the diet (Mattix, 1993). There is no effective treatment.

Atherosclerosis

Hypercholesterolaemia is a hereditary defect in Watanabe rabbits. These animals develop severe atherosclerosis and are used as a research model for the human disease. Experimental gene therapy has corrected this defect in research rabbits.

Metabolic Diseases

Pregnancy Toxaemia

Pregnancy toxaemia affects obese rabbits (even males and non-pregnant does). If the obese animal becomes inappetent, its fat stores will be mobilised. The rabbit's liver is not well suited to handle a large fat load and liver necrosis ensues.

Clinical signs. The animal will show signs of depression and anorexia, may abort or even convulse and die. The urine from an affected animal will be clear with evidence of protein and ketones on analysis.

Diagnosis. At postmortem examination an empty stomach, obesity, a pale yellow liver and kidneys and possible dead foetuses and uterine haemorrhage are found.

Treatment. Treatment is often unrewarding (Walden, 1990). Treatment must include parenteral fluids containing glucose. It is important to encourage the rabbit to resume eating. The rabbit may accept such treat foods as fresh clover or vegetables, hay and breakfast cereal. Force feeding the rabbit puréed baby rice cereal with fruit or suspensions of softened rabbit feed or yogurt may be necessary. Propylene glycol and corticosteroids may be administered.

Diabetes mellitus

Diabetes mellitus has been reported in New Zealand White rabbits. The disease resembles maturity-onset diabetes in people (Mattix, 1993). Insulin injections are probably not necessary provided the diet is closely monitored and obesity is prevented.

Antibiotic Toxicity in the Rabbit

The normal gastrointestinal flora in the rabbit consists of at least 16 predominantly Gram-positive bacteria (Deeb, 1991). Certain antibiotic agents alter the bacterial population resulting in the overgrowth of enterotoxic *Clostridium*. This is not to be confused with spontaneous bacterial enteritis.

Agents. The following antibiotics have been reported to cause this indirect toxicity: lincomycin, ampicillin, amoxicillin, procaine penicillin, cephalexin, erythromycin, clindamycin, tylosin and metronidazole. The toxic effect is not uniform and varies from animal to animal.

Clinical signs. Within 2 weeks of antibiotic treatment, a rabbit that is sensitive to a particular antibiotic will become anorectic, develop diarrhoea and may die.

Diagnosis. Diagnosis is presumptive and requires careful attention to the history. Inflammation and haemorrhage in the caecum coupled with the history are diagnostic (Okerman, 1988).

Control / treatment. Judicious selection of antibiotics is critical in the rabbit. However, in some situations, culture/sensitivity test results or the presence of resistant strains of a bacterial pathogen may necessitate the use of the afore-mentioned antibiotics. Hospitalisation to enable careful patient monitoring and feeding of a high fibre diet may permit prompt response to an antibiotic toxicity problem if it occurs (Mitchell, 1992; Harkness, 1990). Use of cholestyramine resin has been suggested as being effective in preventing experimentally induced antibiotic enterotoxaemia (Lipman *et al.*, 1992).

Antimicrobials frequently used in the rabbit are trimethaprim–sulphur combinations, chloramphenicol, polymixin, neomycin, tetracycline and streptomycin at lower doses and fluorinated quinolones. Use of chloramphenicol and sulphonamides should be avoided in meat rabbits as they may be hazardous or allergenic to humans.

This chapter is dedicated to some of the rabbits we have known: Cotton, Peter, Sunny, Bartles and James, Bonnie and Clyde, Larry and Daryl, Mr Bugs, Snowshoes, Fancy Sweets, Domino, Thumper, Max, Monroe, Butterscotch and Tulip.

References

Ackerman, S. (1992) Sexual behaviour after neutering. *Rabbit Health News* **6**, 1.

Ackerman, S. (1993a) Why does my rabbit...? *Rabbit Health News* **9**, 5–6.

Ackerman, S. (1993b) Aggressive rabbits. *Rabbit Health News* **8**, 4–5.

Bergdall, V. K. and Dysko, R. C. (1994) Metabolic, traumatic, mycotic and miscellaneous diseases. In: *The Biology of the Laboratory Rabbit*, 2nd edn, Manning, P. J., Ringler, D. H. and Newcomer, C. H. (eds.). Academic Press, San Diego, p. 339.

Brown, S. (1993a) Anorectic rabbit protocol. *Rabbit Health News* **9**, 3–4.

Brown, S. (1993b) Rabbit drug dosages. *Rabbit Health News* **10**, 6–7.

Burke, J. (1994) Clinical care and medicine of pet rabbits. In: *Proceedings of the Michigan Veterinary Conference*, pp. 49–77.

Cheeke, P. R. (1994) Nutrition and nutritional diseases. In: *The Biology of the Laboratory Rabbit*, 2nd edn, Manning, P. J., Ringler, D. H. and Newcomer, C. H. (eds.). Academic Press, San Diego, pp. 323–325.

Cheeke, P. R., Patton, N. M., Lukefahr, S. D. and McNitt, J. I. (1987) *Rabbit Production*. Interstate Printers & Publishers Inc, Danville.

Cranney, J. and Zajac, A. (1993) A method for jugular blood collection in rabbits. *Contemporary Topics /AALAS* **32**(6), 6.

Cruise, L. J. and Brewer, N. R. (1994) Anatomy. In: *The Biology of the Laboratory Rabbit*, 2nd edn, Manning, P. J., Ringler, D.H. and Newcomer, C. H. (eds.). Academic Press, San Diego, pp. 52–53.

Deeb, B. (1991) Digestive physiology — key in rabbit antibiotic therapy. *Rabbit Health News* **4**,2.

Deeb, B. (1993) Viral infections of domestic rabbits. *Rabbit Health News* **10**, 4–5.

DeLong, D. and Manning, P. J. (1994) Bacterial diseases. In: *The Biology of the Laboratory Rabbit*, 2nd edn, Manning, P. J., Ringler, D. H. and Newcomer, C. H. (eds.). Academic Press, San Diego, pp. 134–136, 144, 146.

DiGiacomo, R. F. and Maré, C. J. (1994) Viral diseases. In: *The Biology of the Laboratory Rabbit*, 2nd edn, Manning, P. J., Ringler, D. H. and Newcomer, C. H. (eds.). Academic Press, San Diego, pp. 188, 190, 195.

DiGiacomo, R. F., Deeb, B. J., Giddens, W. E., Bernard, B. L. and Chengappa, M. M. (1989) Atrophic rhinitis in New Zealand rabbits infected with *Pasteurella multocida*. *American Journal of Veterinary Research* **50**, 1460–1465.

Dillehay, D. L., Paul, K. S., DiGiacomo, R. F. and Chengappa, M. M. (1991) Pathogenicity of *Pasteurella multocida* A:3 in Flemish Giant and New Zealand White rabbits. *Laboratory Animals* **25**, 337–341.

Donnelly, T. (1990) Rabbits and rodents as pets – special considerations. In: *Proceedings 142. Rabbits and Rodents Laboratory Animal Science.* Post Graduate Committee in Veterinary Science, University of Sydney, Sydney.

Dumonceaux, G. A. (1992) Household toxicosis in exotic animals and pet birds. In: *Current Veterinary Therapy XI*, Kirk, R. W. and Bonagura, J. D. (eds.). W.B. Saunders, Philadelphia, pp. 178–182.

Fennestad, K. L., Mansa, B. and Larsen, S. (1981) Pleural effusion disease in rabbits. *Archives of Virology* **70**, 11–19.

Fox, J. G., Shalev, M., Beaucage, C. M. and Smith, M. (1979) Congenital entropion in a litter of rabbits. *Laboratory Animal Science* **29**(4), 509–511.

Franklin, C. L., Gibson, S. V., Caffrey, C. J., Wagner, J. E. and Steffen, E. K. (1991) Treatment of *Trichophyton mentagrophytes* infection in rabbits. *Journal of the American Veterinary Association* **198**(9), 1625–1630.

Fuller, H. E., Chasey, D., Lucas, M. H. and Gibbens, J. C. (1993) Rabbit haemeorrhagic disease in the United Kingdom. *Veterinary Record* **133**, 611–613.

Ganaway, J. R. (1980) Effect of heat and selected chemical disinfectants upon infectivity of spores of *Bacillus piliformis* (Tyzzer's disease). *Laboratory Animal Science* **30**, 192–196.

Gillett, N. A., Brooks, D. L. and Tillman, P. C. (1983) Medical and surgical management of gastric obstruction from a hairball in the rabbit. *Journal of American Veterinary Medical Association* **183**(11), 1176–1178.

Harkness, J. E. (1987) Rabbit husbandry and medicine. *The Veterinary Clinics of North America, Small Animal Practice* **17**(5), 1019–1044.

Harkness, J. E. and Wagner, J. E. (1989) *The Biology and Medicine of Rabbits and Rodents*, 3rd edn. Lea and Febiger, Philadelphia.

Harkness, J. R. (1990) Diseases of rabbits: gastrointestinal. In: *Proceedings 142. Rabbits and Rodents Laboratory Animal Science.* Post Graduate Committee in Veterinary Science, University of Sydney, Sydney.

Harriman, M. (1992) The violent itch. *House Rabbit Journal* **2**(10), 8–9.

Harriman, M. (1993) Rabbit lifestyles that promote longevity. *Rabbit Health News* **8**, 1–3.

Hillyer, E. V. (1994) Pet rabbits. *The Veterinary Clinics of North America, Small Animal Practice* **24**(1), 25–65.

Ishikawa, T., Nishino, H., Ohara, M., Shimosato, T. and Nanba, K. (1991) The identification of a rabbit-transmitted cervical toxoplasmosis mimicking malignant lymphoma. *American Journal of Clinical Pathology* **94**(1), 107–111.

Jain, N. C. (1986) *Schalm's Veterinary Hematology*, 4th edn. Lea and Febiger, Philadelphia, pp. 277–279.

Johnson, J. H. and Wolf, A. M. (1993) Ovarian abscesses and pyometra in a domestic rabbit. *Journal of the American Veterinary Medical Association* **203**(5), 667–669.

Leary, S. L., Manning, P. J. and Anderson, L. C. (1984) Experimental and naturally-occurring gastric foreign bodies in laboratory rabbits. *Laboratory Animal Science* **34**(1), 58–61.

Lipman, N. S., Connors, M. J., Olsen, D. A. and Taylor, N. S. (1992) Utilisation of cholestyramine resin as a preventive treatment for antibiotic (clindamycin) induced enterotoxaemia in the rabbit. *Lab Animal* **26**, 1–8

Lipman, N. S., Zhi-Bo, Z., Andrutis, K. A., Hurley, R. J., Fox, J. G. and White, H. J. (1994) Prolactin-secreting pituitary adenomas with mammary dysplasia in New Zealand White rabbits. *Laboratory Animal Science* **44**(2), 114–120.

Love, A. and Hammond, K. (1991) Group-housing rabbits. *Lab Animal* **20**(8), 37–43.

Love, J. A. (1994) Group housing: meeting the physical and social needs of the laboratory rabbit. *Laboratory Animal Science* **44**(1), 5–11.

Mattix, M. E. (1993) Diseases of rabbits. Presented at Pathology of Laboratory Animals. Washington, DC, Armed Forces Institute of Pathology.

McLaughlin, R. M. and Fish, R. E. (1994) Clinical biochemistry and hematology. In: *The Biology of the Laboratory Rabbit*, 2nd edn, Manning, P. J., Ringler, D. H. and Newcomer, C. H. (eds.). Academic Press, San Diego, pp. 118, 124.

Mitchell, D. (1992) Injectable antibiotics versus oral antibiotics. *Rabbit Health News* **6**, 1.

Mitruka, B. M. and Rawnsley, H. M. (1977) *Clinical Biochemical and Hematological Reference Values in Normal Experimental Animals.* Masson Publishing USA, Inc., pp. 83, 134–135.

Morton, D. (1993) Enrichment techniques for rodents and rabbits. In: *SCAW (Scientists Center for Ani-*

mal Welfare) Newsletter **15**(2), 6.

Okerman, L. (1988, 1994 2nd edn) *Diseases of Domestic Rabbits*. Blackwell Scientific Publications, Oxford.

Patterson, L. T. (1987) Rabbit coccidiosis. *Veterinary Human Toxicology* **29**(Supplement 1), 73–79.

Patton, N. M. (1994) Colony husbandry. In: *The Biology of the Laboratory Rabbit*, 2nd edn, Manning, P. J., Ringler, D. H. and Newcomer, C. H. (eds.). Academic Press, San Diego, p. 34.

Peiffer, R., Pohm-Thorsen, L. and Corcoran, K. (1994) Models in ophthalmology and vision research. In: *The Biology of the Laboratory Rabbit*, 2nd edn, Manning, P. J., Ringler, D. H. and Newcomer, C. H. (eds.). Academic Press, San Diego, pp. 418–419.

Percy, D. H. and Barthold, S. W. (1993) *Pathology of Laboratory Rodents and Rabbits*. Iowa State University Press, Ames.

Quesenberry, K. (1989) Potpourri of rabbit medical entities. *Proceedings of the Second Annual Conference: Ferret-Rabbit Medicine and Surgery for the Practitioner*, Madison.

Russell, J. R. and Schilling, P. W. (1973) *The Rabbit. Aeromedical Review, Selected Topics in Laboratory Animal Medicine XXI*, pp. 1–24.

Shapiro A. (1993) Tools of the trade. *House Rabbit Journal* **2**(12), 4–7.

Shell, L. G. and Saunders, G. (1989) Arteriosclerosis in a rabbit. *Journal of the American Veterinary Association* **194**(5), 679–680.

Stein, S. (1980) A rabbit in the clinic. *The Animal Health Technician* **1**(5), 214–219.

Toth, L. A., Olson, G. A., Wilson, E., Rehg, J. E. and Claasen, E. (1990) Lymphocytic leukemia and lymphosarcoma in a rabbit. *Journal of the American Veterinary Association* **197**(5), 627–629.

Waidhofer, K. (1989) Perineal skin fold reduction. *House Rabbit Journal* **1**(10), 9.

Walden, N. B. (1990) *Rabbits: A Compendium* (The T G Hungerford VADE MECUM series for Domestic Animals: Series C.13). Post Graduate Foundation in Veterinary Science, University of Sydney, Sydney.

Weisbroth, S. H., (1994) Neoplastic diseases. In: *The Biology of the Laboratory Rabbit*, 2nd edn, Manning, P. J., Ringler, D. H. and Newcomer, C. H. (eds.). Academic Press, San Diego, pp. 262–266.

Weisbroth, S. H., Flatt, R. E. and Kraus, A. L. (eds.) (1974) *The Biology of the Laboratory Rabbit*. Academic Press, New York.

Wemelsfelder, F. (1994) Animal boredom. *Wards* **5**(2), 1–4.

Yamini, B. and Stein, S. (1989) Abortion, stillbirth, neonatal death and nutritional myodegeneration in a rabbit breeding colony. *Journal of American Veterinary Association* **194**(4), 561–562.

Further Reading

Bell, J. C. (1988) *The Zoonoses*. Edward Arnold, London.

Bowman, D. D., Fogelson, M. L. and Carbone, L. G. (1992) Effect of ivermectin on the control of ear mites (*Psoroptes cuniculi*) in naturally infested rabbits. *American Journal of Veterinary Research* **53**(1), 105–109.

Brooks, D. L. (1983) Rabbit gastrointestinal disorders. In: *Current Veterinary Therapy VIII*, Kirk, R. W. (ed.). W.B. Saunders Company, Philadelphia, pp. 654–656.

Broome, R. L. and Brooks, D. L. (1991) Efficacy of enrofloxacin in the treatment of respiratory pasteurellosis in rabbits. *Laboratory Animal Science* **41**(6), 572–576.

Broome, R. L., Brooks, D. L., Babish, J. G., Copeland, D. D. and Conzelman, G. M. (1991) Pharmacokinetic properties of enrofloxacin in rabbits. *American Journal of Veterinary Research* **52**(11), 1835–1841.

Burke, T. J. (1992) Skin disorders of rodents, rabbits and ferrets. In: *Current Veterinary Therapy XI, Small Animal Practice*, Kirk, R. W. and Bonagura, J. D. (eds.). W.B. Saunders Company, Philadelphia, pp. 1170–1175.

BVAAWF/FRAME/RSPCA/UFAW Joint Working Group on Refinement (1993) Refinements in rabbit husbandry. *Laboratory Animals* **27**, 301–329.

Colby, E. D. (1986) The rabbit. In: *Current Therapy in Theriogenology 2*, Morrow, D. A. (ed.). W. B. Saunders Company, Philadelphia, pp. 1005–1008.

Deeb, B. J., DiGiacomo, R. F., Evermann, J. F. and Thouless, M. E. (1993) Prevalence of coronavirus antibodies in rabbits. *Laboratory Animal Science* **43**(5), 431–433.

Dille, S. E., Wall, H. G. and Latendresse, J. R. (1991) Red, enlarged and bulbous nose on a rabbit. *Lab Animal* **20**(9), 16–19.

Eisele, P. H. (1986) Dental problems in rabbits and rodents. In: *Current Veterinary Therapy IX*, Kirk, R. W. (ed.). W.B. Saunders Company, Philadelphia, pp. 759–762.

Fish, R. E. and Besch-Williford, C. (1992) Reproductive disorders in the rabbit and guinea pig. In: *Current Veterinary Therapy XI, Small Animal Practice*, Kirk, R. W. and Bonagura, J. D. (eds.). W.B. Saunders Company, Philadelphia, pp. 1175–1178.

Hamlen, H. J. and MacInnes, S. (1992) A randomised trial using oral and parenteral enrofloxacin and parental ceftiofur to treat lapine pasteurellosis in a biomedical research facility. *AALAS Contemporary Topics* **31**(4), 24.

Okerman, L., DeVriese, L. A., Gevaert, D., Uyttebroek, E. and Haesebrouck, F. (1990) *In vivo* activity of orally administered antibiotics and chemotherapeutics against acute septicaemic pasteurellosis in rabbits. *Lab Animal* **24**, 341–344.

Popilskis, S. J., Oz, M. C., Bass, L. S. and Popp, H. (1991) Abdominal pregnancy in rabbits. *Lab Animal* **20**(5), 14–18.

Shapiro, A. (1992) Honorary rabbit. *House Rabbit Journal* **2**(8), 4–5.

Smith, J. (1993) Thumper and me. *House Rabbit Journal* **2**(12), 1–2, 6–7.

Williams, C. S. F. (1976) *Practical Guide to Laboratory Animals*, C.V. Mosby Company, St. Louis, pp. 148–171.

(Data Tables follow).

Data Tables

COMMON DISEASES—RABBITS				
Disease	Aetiology	Clinical signs	Treatment and control	Zoonotic potential
Respiratory system				
Pasteurellosis	*Pasteurella multocida*	Nasal/ocular discharge Sneezing Coughing Skin ulcers Torticollis Lameness Anorexia Dyspnoea Infertility Metritis Pyometra Ovarian abscesses Orchitis Epididymitis Death	Broad spectrum antibiotics Nasal drops Nasal flushes Nebulisation Supportive therapy Castration	± Bite wound
Pleural effusion disease	Coronavirus	Fever Anorexia Weight loss Hind limb weakness Dyspnoea Death	Supportive therapy	No
Gastrointestinal system				
Malocclusion	Genetic factors	Drooling Anorexia	Trimming and reshaping teeth	No
Trichobezoars	Fur-chewing Diet	Anorexia Lethargy Weight loss Decreased faeces	Supportive therapy Surgery as required	No
Bacterial enteritis	*Escherichia coli* *Staphylococcus* *Clostridium spiroforme* *Clostridium piliforme* Rotavirus	Diarrhoea Depression Hypothermia Abdominal distension Death	Supportive therapy	No

Mucoid enteropathy	Unknown but dietary
	  changes contributory
		Mucoid diarrhoea
		Bloating
		Depression
		Hypothermia
		Death
			Supportive measures,
			  guarded prognosis
			Prevent by providing
			  fibre and avoiding
			  sudden diet changes
				No

Fig. 6.12—continued

COMMON DISEASES—RABBITS				
Disease	Aetiology	Clinical signs	Treatment and control	Zoonotic potential
Coccidiosis	*Eimeria* spp.	Unthriftiness Diarrhoea Anorexia Dehydration Death	Disinfection Anticoccidial agents	No
Pinworms	*Passalurus ambiguus*	Usually none	Anthelmintics	No
Cysticercosis	*Taenia pisiformis*	None	Eliminate contact between rabbits and cats and dogs	No
Genitourinary system				
Uterine adenocarcinoma	Age and breed related	Decreased reproductive performance Vaginal discharge Cystic mammary glands	Ovariohysterectomy	No
Mastitis	*Staphylococcus* *Pasteurella* *Streptococcus*	Inflamed glands Fever Abnormal milk Anorexia	Antibiotics Supportive care Improved sanitation	No
Epididymitis Orchitis Metritis Pyometra	*Pasteurella multocida* *Treponema cuniculi*	Reduced fertility Inflammation	Antibiotics Neutering	No
Venereal spirochaetosis/ Rabbit syphilis	*Treponema cuniculi*	Infertility, Genital lesions	Penicillin	No
Urolithiasis Cystitis	Bacteria Diet	Increased frequency of urination, straining to urinate, haematuria, perineal irritation	Surgical removal of calculi Antibiotics Supportive therapy	No
Nervous system				
Encephalito- zoonosis	*Encephalitozoon* *cuniculi*	Latent, may cause tremors, ataxia, paresis, head tilt, convulsions	None	No
Vertebral fracture	Trauma	Paralysis of hind quarters, inability to control urination and defaecation	Corticosteroids Cage rest depending on severity of signs	No

Fig. 6.12—continued

COMMON DISEASES—RABBITS				
Disease	Aetiology	Clinical signs	Treatment and control	Zoonotic potential
Torticollis/Wry neck	*Pasteurella multocida* Middle/inner ear infection	Head tilt, ataxia Inappetance	Supportive therapy Antibiotics	No
Sensory organs				
Buphthalmia/ Glaucoma	Genetic factors	Megaloglobus, Corneal opacity	Usually none	No
Entropion	Infection Congenital	Blepharospasm, epiphora, conjunctivitis corneal ulcer	Surgery Topical ophthalmic antibiotics	No
Conjunctivitis	*Pasteurella multocida* Other bacteria	Ocular discharge	Topical ophthalmic antibiotics Flushing of nasolacrimal ducts	No
Otitis externa	*Psoroptes cuniculi*	Head shaking, digging at ears, crusts in ear canals	Ivermectin	No
Otitis media	*Pasteurella multocida* *Staphylococcus aureus* *Bordetella bronchiseptica*	None, ataxia, head tilt	Antibiotics	No
Integument and musculoskeletal system				
Ulcerative Pododermatitis 'Sore Hocks'	Thin foot fur pads, moist cage floor, mesh or slatted floor, genetic factors	Alopecia, ulcerative lesions on plantar/palmar surfaces of feet	Place on solid floor, Bandage severe lesions	No
Abscesses	*Pasteurella multocida* *Staphylococcus aureus*	Fluctuant or firm cutaneous mass ± Draining tracks	Drain and flush Antibiotics	No
Blue fur disease	*Pseudomonas aeruginosa*	Blue discoloration of fur in areas of moist skin (dewlap)	Eliminate organism from water crocks and sipper tubes Gentamicin	No
Fur mites	*Cheyletiella parasitovorax* *Listrophorus gibbus*	Alopecia, scaling, itching	Ivermectin, disinfect housing, flea powders	Yes

Fig. 6.12—continued

COMMON DISEASES—RABBITS				
Disease	Aetiology	Clinical signs	Treatment and control	Zoonotic potential
Fleas, Lice	*Ctenocephalides felis* (cat flea) *Haemodipsus ventricosis* (louse)	Poor condition of rabbit	Insecticides as for cats	Yes (fleas)
Fly strike/Myiasis		Maggot infestation	Removal of maggots Supportive therapy Antibiotics	No
"Ringworm" Dermatophytosis	*Trichophyton mentagrophytes*	Hair loss, Crusty lesions	Topical antifungal agents Oral griseofulvin, Alcide®	Yes
Shope papilloma infection	Shope papilloma virus	Skin warts (eyelids, ears)	Control by screening outdoor rabbit pens to prevent transmission by arthopods from wild to domestic rabbits	No
Osteomyelitis	Bacteria	Mandible most commonly involved	Surgical debridement and antibiotics can be tried—poor prognosis	No
Systemic diseases				
Staphylococcosis	*Staphylococcus* spp.	Dermatitis Conjunctivitis Rhinitis Mastitis Septicaemia Pneumonia Abscessation Renal infarct	Therapy to minimise condition (not eradicate) Antibiotics	No
Salmonellosis	*Salmonella typhimurium* *Salmonella enteritidis*	Depression Abortion Fever Diarrhoea Death	Culture to confirm then euthanasia	Yes
Toxoplasmosis	*Toxoplasma gondii*	Inapparent—death in acute form	Prevent by avoiding faecal contaminated feed	Yes Consuming undercooked infected rabbit meat

Fig. 6.12—continued

COMMON DISEASES—RABBITS				
Disease	Aetiology	Clinical signs	Treatment and control	Zoonotic potential
Myxomatosis	Myxoma virus	Oedema of face, ears, genitalia, nasal/ocular discharge, cutaneous lumps, possible respiratory problems	Supportive therapy, usually unsuccessful Preventive vaccination in UK and Europe	No
Viral haemorrhagic disease	Calicivirus	Depression Fever Ataxia—peracute form Sudden death	Preventive vaccination	No
Haematopoietic and cardiovascular systems				
Lymphosarcoma	Genetic factors	Lethargy Anorexia Weight loss Pale mucous membranes	Undocumented	No
Cardiomyopathy	Coronavirus	Increased respiratory rate and effort Muscle weakness	Undocumented	No
Arteriosclerosis	Hypervitaminosis D	Anorexia Dehydration Weight loss Seizures	Reduce vitamin D content in feed	No
Other systems				
Hypovitaminosis E	Dietary deficiency	Skeletal and cardiac muscle necrosis Impaired reproductive performance	Increase vitamin E content in feed	No
Hypervitaminosis A	Dietary excess	Congenital defects Impaired reproductive performance	Reduce vitamin A content in feed	No
Pregnancy toxaemia	Obesity and inappetance	Depression Anorexia Abortion Seizures Death	Supportive therapy, fluids containing glucose Poor prognosis	No
Antibiotic toxicity				
Enterotoxaemia/ Gastrointestinal bacterial overgrowth	*Clostridium* overgrowth due to antibiotic administration	Anorexia Diarrhoea Death	Supportive care; prevent by careful selection of antibiotic therapy and monitoring of any rabbit receiving antibiotic	No

FIG. 6.12 Common diseases — rabbits.

PHYSIOLOGICAL DATA—RABBITS	
Life span	5–8 years
H_2O consumption	10 ml/100 g b.w.
Temperature	38–39.6 °C
Food consumption	100–150 g
Heart rate	120–325/min
Respiratory rate	30–60/min
Urine volume	20–350 ml/24 h
Urine pH	7.6–8.8

Data taken from Burke (1994), Harkness (1987), Hillyer (1994), McLaughlin and Fish (1994) and Walden (1990).

FIG. 6.13 Physiological data — rabbits.

HAEMATOLOGICAL VALUES—RABBITS	
RBC $\times 10^6/mm^3$	3.8–7.9
PCV %	30–50
Haemoglobin g/dl	9.4–17.4
WBC $\times 10^3/mm^3$	2.6–12.5
Neutrophils %	12–55
Eosinophils %	0–3.4
Basophils %	0–6
Lymphocytes %	28–85
Monocytes %	0–13
Platelets $\times 10^3/mm^3$	270–480
Blood volume ml/kg	54 ± 5

Data taken from Jain (1986), Mitruka and Rawnsley (1977) and Walden (1990).

FIG. 6.14 Haematological values — rabbits.

CLINICAL CHEMISTRY VALUES—RABBITS	
Calcium mg/dl	5.5–12.5
Phosphorus mg/dl	4.0–6.9
Sodium mEq/l	130–155
Chloride mEq/l	92–120
Potassium mEq/l	3.7–10
Glucose mg/dl	78–155
BUN mg/dl	13–30
Creatinine mg/dl	0.5–2.6
Total bilirubin mg/dl	0–0.75
Total protein g/dl	5.4–8.3
Albumin g/dl	2.4–4.6
Cholesterol mg/dl	10–80
Alk phos IU/l	4–16
SGOT IU/l	35–100
SGPT IU/l	48–80
LDH IU/l	34–129

Data taken from Burke (1994), Hillyer (1994), Mitruka and Rawnsley (1977), Okerman (1988) and Walden (1990).

FIG. 6.15 Clinical chemistry values — rabbits.

REPRODUCTIVE DATA—RABBITS	
Breeding age	5–9 months
Gestation	28–35 days
Average litter size	6–7
Birth weight	40–100 g
Eyes open	7 days
Wean	4–6 weeks
Postpartum receptivity	yes
Number of mammae	8
Breeding duration	1–6 years

Data taken from Harkness (1987), Patton (1994) and Walden (1990).

FIG. 6.16 Reproductive data — rabbits.

7

Anaesthesia and analgesia for rodents and rabbits

PAUL FLECKNELL

Pre-anaesthetic Preparations

Small rodents and rabbits can be anaesthetised safely and reliably, provided special attention is given at all stages of anaesthesia and the anaesthetic regimen is chosen with care. When selecting the method of anaesthesia, remember that one major cause of peri-operative morbidity and mortality in rodents and small rabbits is hypothermia. This can result in a prolonged recovery period, which seems to predispose some species such as the guinea pig and chinchilla to the development of post-operative inappetence. A second major factor that will influence the outcome of anaesthesia is the initial health of the animal. Sub-clinical respiratory infections are common in small rodents and rabbits. Pre-operative clinical assessment of the animal should be undertaken, giving particular attention to the respiratory system. Auscultation and percussion of the chest may enable detection of more severe respiratory disease, but even in larger species such as rabbits, they are of limited value because of the relatively restricted lung fields. It is advisable to assume that all of these patients have some degree of pre-existing pulmonary damage. Since all anaesthetic regimens cause some degree of respiratory depression, it follows that these animals may be at greater risk of respiratory failure. To minimise this risk, oxygen should always be administered during anaesthesia, respiratory stimulants should be available and when practicable, some method of monitoring respiratory function should be used.

These considerations apply to all small mammals presented for anaesthesia, including apparently healthy patients requiring elective surgery such as castration. The risks of anaesthetic death are much greater with animals in obviously poor clinical condition. For example, animals requiring dental procedures may have become almost completely inappetent and be significantly dehydrated. Although the incisor teeth can be clipped without anaesthetic, attention to the molars and premolars may require anaesthesia. Before undertaking this, it is advisable to administer fluid therapy. The IV route is usually considered impracticable in small rodents and even in rabbits venepuncture can be difficult if peripheral circulatory shut-down has occurred. Although it is possible to place a small 'over-the-needle' catheter into the lateral tail vein in the rat, this technique is difficult and IV injection, even in clinically healthy mice and gerbils is even more technically demanding. In the guinea pig, the lateral or medial saphenous veins situated on either side of the foot can be cannulated with practice. In all of these smaller species, placement of a tourniquet to dilate the vessel will increase the likelihood of successful cannulation. An elastic band wrapped around the limb or tail is suitable for most animals. In rabbits, a 'butterfly' type infusion set or over the needle catheter can be inserted into the marginal ear vein (Fig. 7.1). Over-the-needle catheters are preferable, since there is then no risk of a needle becoming displaced should the rabbit move or be repositioned during fluid infusions. To anchor a winged catheter firmly, the technique illustrated in Fig. 7.1 should be followed. Following completion of the fluid infusion, the catheter can be filled with heparin/saline (100

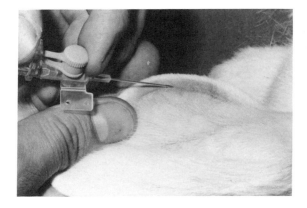

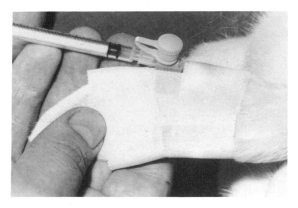

FIG. 7.1 Insertion of a 22 gauge over-the-needle catheter into the marginal ear vein of the rabbit. One wing of the catheter is removed, the hair overlying the vessel shaved using a scalpel blade, and the catheter introduced. The appearance of blood usually indicates successful placement, and the stylet is then withdrawn and the catheter advanced into the vessel. A strip of adhesive tape is then placed along the length of the ear covering the remaining wing of the catheter. Two further strips of tape are then applied around the ear above and below the point of insertion, anchoring the catheter firmly to the ear.

IU/ml heparin in 0.9% NaCl) and bandaged in place, enabling further infusions over a 24–36 h period.

A more rapid technique in small rodents is to administer fluids by the IP or SC routes. Suitable volumes are listed in Fig. 7.2. Standard considerations as to choice of fluid apply. For a predominant water deficit 0.18% NaCl:4% dextrose should be used whereas mixed water and electrolyte deficits should be corrected using lactated Ringer's solution (Hartmanns solution) or nor-

mal saline. All fluids used should be warmed to 38°C before use. Fluid administered by the SC route will be absorbed over 6–12 h, but if marked dehydration is present, as indicated by loss of skin tone and tenting of the skin, then absorption may be too slow to be of benefit. IP administration may be a less familiar technique, but fluid administered by this route is absorbed more rapidly than following SC injection.

Prior to anaesthesia, it is not necessary to withhold food from rodents or rabbits as these species do not vomit. In some circumstances withholding food can be detrimental, since prolonged periods of fasting can cause significant hypoglycaemia. Atropine (0.05 mg/kg SC or IM) is not usually necessary as a pre-medication in small rodents, but can be useful for reducing respiratory secretions in animals with obvious respiratory disease. A high proportion of rabbits have high levels of atropinase, and atropine is short acting in these animals, so glycopyrrolate (0.1 mg/kg SC) should be used in this species.

All equipment which may be required during anaesthesia should be checked and prepared before use. It is particularly important to set up a suitable post-operative recovery area and to stabilise the environmental temperature in this facility. Ensure that any emergency drugs which may be required are available and if necessary, with high-risk patients, ensure that an appropriate small quantity of drug has been diluted ready for administration.

Anaesthetic Selection

A major concern during anaesthesia of small mammals is respiratory depression and hypothermia, so anaesthetic regimens that result in rapid recovery and easy adjustment of the depth of anaesthesia are preferable. In larger species, this is easy to achieve using either short-acting, non-cumulative IV agents such as propofol, or by use of inhalation agents. In small rodents, IV administration of injectable anaesthetics is rarely considered practical, so these agents are given by the IP, IM or SC routes. In larger animals, anaesthetics are usually administered IV and the

APPROXIMATE VOLUMES FOR FLUID REPLACEMENT THERAPY		
	Subcutaneous (ml)	Intraperitoneal (ml)
Chinchilla (500 g)	10	10
Gerbil (60 g)	1–2	2–3
Guinea pig (1 kg)	10–20	20
Hamster (100 g)	3	3
Mouse (30 g)	1–2	2
Rabbit (3 kg)	30–50	50
Rat (200 g)	5	5

FIG. 7.2 Approximate volumes for fluid replacement therapy IP and SC administration.

estimated dose of drug can be given gradually and adjusted to match the response of the individual animal. This adjustment of the estimated dose is not usually possible in small mammals, since a single injection of drug is given by the IP, SC, or IM routes. It has been shown that variations in drug response occur between different strains of laboratory rodents and it is likely that similar variations occur in pet animals. In addition, the safety margin of some anaesthetics is low with the anaesthetic dose being very close to the lethal dose in many individuals. These factors combine to make some injectable anaesthetic regimens particularly hazardous in small rodents, especially when dealing with the individual pet animal, rather than a group of laboratory animals.

Given these considerations, in most circumstances it is preferable to use an inhalational anaesthetic such as halothane, isoflurane or methoxyflurane. If injectable anaesthetics are used, then those with a wide safety margin are preferred, particularly those agents which can be reversed by means of specific antagonists.

Inhalational Agents

All of the commonly used inhalational agents can be used safely in small rodents provided appropriate apparatus is available. Halothane, isoflurane and methoxyflurane provide good skeletal muscle relaxation and cause only mild to moderate depression of the cardiovascular and respiratory systems. As with larger domestic species, recovery is rapid, particularly with isoflurane.

Older anaesthetic agents such as ether should not be used, since they are irritating to the respiratory tract and unpleasant for the animals to inhale. Ether also represents a significant safety hazard because it forms explosive mixtures with air or oxygen.

Anaesthetic Induction Chambers

Induction of anaesthesia is most easily carried out using an anaesthetic induction chamber. These can be purchased commercially, or can be constructed from readily available materials, such as a clear plastic food container. A chamber size of 30 cm × 30 cm × 20 cm is suitable for small rodents and guinea pigs. The anaesthetic agent should be supplied from a calibrated vaporiser and surplus anaesthetic gas should be ducted away from the chamber using a suitable gas-scavenging system. The animal should be placed in the chamber and an appropriate induction concentration of the anaesthetic (Fig. 7.3) delivered in 100% oxygen. There is little advantage in using nitrous oxide, since the concentration required to make a significant contribution to anaesthesia is high in these species. Anaesthesia is induced within a few minutes of exposure to halothane or isoflurane, since the high respiratory rates of these small animals result in rapid uptake and equilibration of anaesthetic. Induction with methoxyflurane is slightly slower and takes about 5–6 min. After the animal has lost its righting reflex, it can be removed from the chamber and anaesthetic delivered via a face-mask to maintain anaesthesia. Alternatively, if a rapid procedure is to be undertaken, the animal can be removed from the chamber and the procedure carried out immediately. Recovery will occur within 30–120 s depending upon the agent used. If the animal recovers too rapidly, it can be replaced in the chamber until anaesthesia deepens again. Alternatively, the anaesthetic concentration can be reduced to the maintenance concentration and the animal allowed to remain in the chamber for about 5 min. When removed, recovery will take slightly longer, allowing a little more time for minor procedures such as blood sampling or teeth clipping.

A range of alternative induction systems have been described, for example using a large glass jar, with liquid anaesthetic placed on cotton wool in its base. This crude technique has little to recommend it apart from its low cost. If it is used, then it is essential that the liquid anaesthetic cannot come into direct contact with the animal. In addition, only methoxyflurane should be used, since halothane and isoflurane produce dangerously high concentrations of anaesthetic vapour when used in this way.

Although a larger size of chamber can be used to induce anaesthesia in rabbits, problems can arise because of the physical characteristics of the anaesthetic vapour, coupled with the be-haviour of many rabbits. The vapour of volatile anaesthetics is significantly denser than air and most anaesthetic chambers fill gradually from the base. A small chamber, with a volume of 10–12 litres, with anaesthetic delivered at a fresh gas flow of 4 litres/min will fill within approximately 3 min. Large chambers suitable for rabbits may have a volume of approximately 40 litres and even at a flow rate of 8 litres/min, filling will occur only after 5 or 6 min. With small rodents this is relatively unimportant, since isoflurane, halothane and methoxyflurane do not appear unpleasant to inhale and the animals frequently remain in the base of the chamber and become anaesthetised rapidly. In contrast, many rabbits try to avoid inhaling halothane or isoflurane and sit with their noses pressed into the top part of the chamber. They eventually breathe high concentrations of vapour and also show periods of breath-holding during this period.

Induction Using a Face-Mask

An alternative to using an anaesthetic chamber is to administer the anaesthetic via a face-mask while physically restraining the animal. Induction of anaesthesia of rodents is easier and smoother if a sedative or tranquiliser is administered about 45–60 min before induction (Fig. 7.4). If rabbits are anaesthetised in this way, many animals show marked breath-holding behaviour and develop hypoxia, hypercapnia and

RECOMMENDED CONCENTRATIONS OF INHALATIONAL ANAESTHETICS		
Anaesthetic	Induction concentration %	Maintenance concentration %
Enflurane	3–5	1–3
Ether	10–20	4–5
Halothane	3–4	1–2
Isoflurane	3–4	1.5–3
Methoxyflurane	3–3.5	0.4–1

FIG. 7.3 Recommended concentrations of inhalational anaesthetics for induction and maintenance of anaesthesia. The concentrations required can be reduced by administration of pre-anaesthetic medication or concurrent use of injectable anaesthetics.

SEDATIVE AND TRANQUILLISER DOSE RATES					
Species	Acepromazine	Diazepam	Medetomidine	Midazolam	Xylazine
Chinchilla	0.5 mg/kg IM	5 mg/kg IP	—	—	—
Gerbil	3 mg/kg IM	5 mg/kg IP	—	5 mg/kg IP	2 mg/kg IP
Guinea pig	5 mg/kg IM	5 mg/kg IM	—	5 mg/kg IM	—
Hamster	5 mg/kg IP	5 mg/kg IP	100 μg/kg SC	5 mg/kg IP	5 mg/kg IP
Mouse	5 mg/kg IP	5 mg/kg IP	30–100 μg/kg SC	5 mg/kg IP	10 mg/kg IP
Rabbit	1–2 mg/kg IM	2 mg/kg IM	500 μg/kg SC	2 mg/kg IM	2.5 mg/kg IM
Rat	2.5 mg/kg IP	2.5 mg/kg IP	30–100 μg/kg SC	2.5 mg/kg IP	10 mg/kg IP

Fig. 7.4 Sedative and tranquilliser dose rates for small animals. Considerable variation in effect occurs between different strains.

a bradycardia (Flecknell *et al.*, 1995). This behaviour may account for some of the cases of sudden death during induction of anaesthesia. Pre-anaesthetic medication may not prevent this behaviour, even when very heavy sedation has been produced.

It is recommended that whenever possible, rabbits receive pre-anaesthetic medication and that inhalational agents are administered via a face-mask. Before delivery of any anaesthetic, allow the animal to inhale 100% oxygen for 1–2 min. Observe the animal closely as the anaesthetic is introduced and only increase the inhaled concentration when the rabbit is breathing.

Anaesthetic Maintenance: Masks and Circuits

Whichever induction technique is used, the animal will require maintenance using an appropriate anaesthetic circuit. Although the same considerations apply as with larger species, two practical points simplify the choice of circuit in rodents. The small size of the animal, coupled with the anatomy of the oropharynx, make endotracheal intubation difficult. The animal will therefore almost always be connected to the anaesthetic circuit using a face-mask. Since these species are small (30–1000 g), the fresh gas flow rates needed to prevent rebreathing using a simple open circuit are of the order of 200–2500 ml. In most circumstances a face-mask is all that is needed. It is only when anaesthetising larger guinea pigs that it might be appropriate to use a T-piece or Bain's circuit. When using a face-mask, scavenging of waste anaesthetic gases can be difficult and it is worth considering use of the commercially available concentric mask system (Fig. 7.5).

Rabbits can range in body-weight from 500 g to over 8–10 kg, so most individuals can be maintained successfully using an unmodified Bain's circuit or a T-piece. In smaller rabbits, low-dead space T-pieces designed for human paediatric use are particularly suitable. Endotracheal intubation can be achieved either using an appropriate laryngoscope blade (Wisconsin size 1 (2–6 kg) or 0) or otoscope in smaller rabbits (500 g to 2 kg) (Fig. 7.6) or a blind intubation technique can be used. Before attempting intubation, the rabbit should be allowed to inhale 100% oxygen for 3 or 4 min.

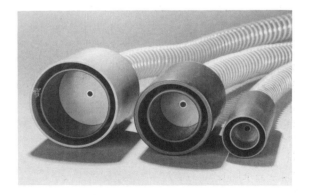

Fig. 7.5 Concentric face mask system to allow effective removal of waste anaesthetic gases. An extraction fan is attached to the outer tube and mask; the inner tube and mask deliver fresh gas from the anaesthetic machine.

When using a laryngoscope or otoscope, the anaesthetised rabbit is positioned on its back and the larynx visualised and sprayed with local anaesthetic to minimise the risk of laryngospasm. If using an otoscope, a smooth, blunt-ended introducer should be inserted through the otoscope, into the larynx and passed down the trachea. The otoscope is then carefully withdrawn and the endotracheal tube (2–4 mm outside diameter) can then be threaded over the introducer and passed into the trachea. The introducer is then withdrawn, leaving the tube in place. When using a laryngoscope the introducer is placed through the endotracheal tube and used to guide it into the larynx. The introducer is then withdrawn.

To intubate using the blind technique, the anaesthetised rabbit is held in sternal recumbency, with its head and neck extended. The endotracheal tube is passed over the tongue and advanced until exhalation can be detected either by auscultation at the tip of the tube, or by the presence of condensation at each breath if a clear plastic endotracheal tube is used. The endotracheal tube is then advanced gently as the rabbit inhales. If timed correctly, the tube will slide easily into the trachea. Often the rabbit will cough at this point. Correct positioning is confirmed either by the appearance of condensation of water vapour in the tube lumen, or by

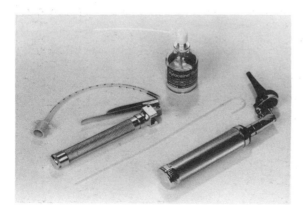

FIG. 7.6 Apparatus for intubation of the rabbit under direct vision. Laryngoscope with Wisconsin size 1 blade. Otoscope, local anaesthetic spray, endotracheal tube (3.5 mm), blunt tipped introducer.

chest movements in response to assisted ventilation. If the tube is not correctly positioned then the procedure can be repeated. With all of these intubation techniques, it is important not to attempt to force the tube into the airway. If more than slight resistance is felt, then the tube should be withdrawn slightly and then advanced again. The larynx is a delicate structure which can easily be traumatised during intubation, resulting in haemorrhage or oedema and consequent respiratory obstruction post-operatively.

Injectable Anaesthetics

Whatever injectable anaesthetics are used, always weigh the animal accurately as it is not easy to guess the weight of a 35 g mouse, especially if the anaesthetist is more familiar with larger species. The appropriate dose of anaesthetic can then be calculated. If necessary the commercial preparation should first be diluted 1:10 or 1:5 to enable accurate measurement of the required volume. Suitable volumes for IP injection will be of the order of 0.2–0.3 ml for a 30 g mouse, 0.5–1.0 ml for larger species. Use of an insulin syringe will enable more accurate dosing. Irrespective of the choice of injectable anaesthetic, oxygen should be administered by face mask throughout the period of anaesthesia. When anaesthetising small rodents, the anaesthetic will usually be administered by IP injection, so it is not possible to adjust the dose to match the individual animal's requirements. After administration of the anaesthetic, observe the animal carefully during the induction period. If the animal fails to become anaesthetised to the required depth, it is possible to deepen anaesthesia by injecting an additional dose of anaesthetic. In general, additional doses of 20–25% of the initial dose are required. This is a somewhat hazardous procedure and it is much safer to deepen anaesthesia using a low concentration of volatile anaesthetic. Dose rates for injectable anaesthetics are given in Fig. 7.7.

INJECTABLE ANAESTHETIC DOSE RATES				
Drug	Dose rate (mg/kg)	Effect	Duration of anaesthesia (min)	Sleep-time (min)
Chinchilla				
Ketamine/acepromazine	40 mg/kg+0.5 mg/kg IM	Surgical anaesthesia	30–40	120–180
Ketamine/diazepam	20 mg/kg+5 mg/kg IP	Light anaesthesia	20–30	60–120
Pentobarbital	40 mg/kg IP	Light anaesthesia	?	?
Tiletamine/zolezepam	22–44 mg/kg IM	Immobilisation/light anaesthesia	20–40	180–420
Gerbil				
Alphaxalone/alphadolone	80–120 mg/kg IP	Immobilisation	—	60–90
Fentanyl/fluanisone	0.5–1.0 ml/kg IM	Immobilisation/analgesia	20	60–90
Fentanyl/fluanisone/ midazolam	8.0 ml/kg IP*	Surgical anaesthesia	20	60–90
Ketamine/acepromazine	75 mg/kg+3 mg/kg IP	Immobilisation	—	60–90
Ketamine/diazepam	50 mg/kg+5 mg/kg IP	Immobilisation	—	30–60
Ketamine/xylazine	50 mg/kg+2 mg/kg IP	Immobilisation	—	20–60
Pentobarbital	60–80 mg/kg IP	Immobilisation/anaesthesia	20	60–90
Guinea pig				
Alphaxalone/alphadolone	40 mg/kg IP	Immobilisation	—	90–120
Fentanyl/fluanisone	1.0 ml/kg IM	Immobilisation/analgesia	60 (analgesia only)	120–180
Fentanyl/fluanisone/ midazolam	8.0 ml/kg IP*	Surgical anaesthesia	45–60	120–180
Fentanyl/droperidol	0.44–8 ml/kg IM		60–120 (analgesia only)	180
Ketamine/acepromazine	125 mg/kg+5 mg/kg IM	Immobilisation/anaesthesia	45–120	90–180
Ketamine/diazepam	100 mg/kg+5 mg/kg IM	Immobilisation/anaesthesia	30–45	90–120
Ketamine/medetomidine	40 mg/kg+0.5 mg/kg IP	Immobilisation	—	90–120
Ketamine/xylazine	50 mg/kg+2 mg/kg IP	Immobilisation/anaesthesia	30	90–120
Methohexital	31 mg/kg IP	Immobilisation	—	20
Pentobarbital	37 mg/kg IP	Immobilisation/anaesthesia	60–90	240–300
Tiletamine/zolezepam	40–60 mg/kg IM	Immobilisation	—	70–160
Urethane	1500 mg/kg IV, IP	Surgical anaesthesia	360–480	non-recovery only
Hamster				
Alphaxalone/alphadolone	150 mg/kg IP	Immobilisation/anaesthesia	20–60	120–150
Fentanyl/fluanisone	0.5 ml/kg IP	Immobilisation/analgesia	20–30	60–120
Fentanyl/fluanisone/ midazolam	4.0 ml/kg IP*	Surgical anaesthesia	40–50	60–90
Fentanyl/droperidol	0.9 ml/kg IM	Analgesia, unpredictable degree of sedation	—	90

Fig. 7.7—continued

INJECTABLE ANAESTHETIC DOSE RATES				
Drug	Dose rate (mg/kg)	Effect	Duration of anaesthesia (min)	Sleep-time (min)
Ketamine/acepromazine	150 mg/kg + 5 mg/kg IP	Immobilisation/anaesthesia	45–120	75–180
Ketamine/diazepam	70 mg/kg + 2 mg/kg IP	Immobilisation/anaesthesia	30–45	90–120
Ketamine/medetomidine	100 mg/kg + 250 μg/kg IP	Surgical anaesthesia	30–60	60–120
Ketamine/xylazine	200 mg/kg + 10 mg/kg IP	Surgical anaesthesia	30–60	90–150
Pentobarbital	50–90 mg/kg IP	Immobilisation/anaesthesia	30–60	120–180
Tiletamine/zolezepam	50–80 mg/kg IP	Immobilisation/anaesthesia	20–30	30–60
Tiletamine/zolezepam/ xylazine	30 mg/kg + 10 mg/kg IP	Immobilisation/anaesthesia	30	40–60
Urethane	1000–2000 mg/kg	Surgical anaesthesia	360–480	non-recovery only
Mouse				
Alphaxalone/alphadolone	10–15 mg/kg IV	Surgical anaesthesia	5	10
Fentanyl/fluanisone	0.4 ml/kg IM	Immobilisation/analgesia	20	60
Fentanyl/fluanisone/ midazolam	10.0 ml/kg IP*	Surgical anaesthesia	45–60	120–240
Fentanyl/droperidol	0.5 ml/kg IM	Immobilisation/analgesia	20–30	60–120
Ketamine/acepromazine	100 mg/kg + 5 mg/kg IP	Immobilisation/anaesthesia	20–30	40–120
Ketamine/diazepam	100 mg/kg + 5 mg/kg IP	Immobilisation/anaesthesia	20–30	60–120
Ketamine/medetomidine	75 mg/kg + 1.0 mg/kg IP	Immobilisation/anaesthesia	20–30	60–100
Ketamine/xylazine	100 mg/kg + 10 mg/kg IP	Immobilisation/anaesthesia	20–30	60–120
Methohexital	10 mg/kg IV	Surgical anaesthesia	5	10
Pentobarbital	40–50 mg/kg IP	Immobilisation/anaesthesia	20–40	120–180
Propofol	26 mg/kg IV	Surgical anaesthesia	5–10	10–15
Thiopental	30–40 mg/kg IV	Surgical anaesthesia	5–10	10–15
Tiletamine/zolezepam	80 mg/kg IP	Immobilisation	—	60–120
Tribromoethanol	240 mg/kg IP	Surgical anaesthesia	15–45	60–120
Rabbit				
Alphaxalone/alphadolone	6–9 mg/kg IV	Light anaesthesia	5–10	10–20
Fentanyl/fluanisone	0.5 ml/kg IM	Immobilisation/analgesia	20–30 (analgesia only)	—
Fentanyl/fluanisone and midazolam	0.3 ml/kg IM + 2 mg/kg IV or IP	Surgical anaesthesia	30–60	60–120
Fentanyl/droperidol	0.22 ml/kg IM	Immobilisation/analgesia	40–60	40–60
Ketamine/acepromazine	50 mg/kg + 1 mg/kg IM	Surgical anaesthesia	20–30	60–90
Ketamine/diazepam	25 mg/kg + 5 mg/kg IM	Surgical anaesthesia	20–30	60–90
Ketamine/medetomidine	25 mg/kg + 0.5 mg/kg IM	Surgical anaesthesia	60–90	120–240
Ketamine/xylazine	35 mg/kg + 5 mg/kg IM	Surgical anaesthesia	40–60	60–120
Ketamine/xylazine/ butorphanol	35 mg/kg + 5 mg/kg IM + 0.1 mg/kg IM	Surgical anaesthesia	60–90	120–180

Fig. 7.7—continued

INJECTABLE ANAESTHETIC DOSE RATES				
Drug	Dose rate (mg/kg)	Effect	Duration of anaesthesia (min)	Sleep-time (min)
Methohexital	10 mg/kg IV	Surgical anaesthesia	4–5	5–10
Pentobarbital	45 mg/kg IV	Immobilisation/anaesthesia	20–30	60–120
Propofol	10 mg/kg IV	Light anaesthesia	5–10	10–15
Thiopental	30 mg/kg IV	Surgical anaesthesia	5–10	10–15
Urethane	1000 mg/kg IV	Surgical anaesthesia	360–480	non-recovery only
Rat				
Alphaxalone/alphadolone	10–12 mg/kg IV	Surgical anaesthesia	5	10
Fentanyl/fluanisone	0.4 ml/kg IM	Immobilisation/analgesia	20	60
Fentanyl/fluanisone midazolam	2.7 ml/kg IP*	Surgical anaesthesia	45–60	120–240
Fentanyl/droperidol	0.5 ml/kg IM	Immobilisation/analgesia	20–30	60–120
Ketamine/acepromazine	75 mg/kg + 2.5 mg/kg IP	Light anaesthesia	20–30	120
Ketamine/diazepam	75 mg/kg + 8 mg/kg IP	Light anaesthesia	20–30	120
Ketamine/medetomidine	75 mg/kg + 0.5 mg/kg IP	Surgical anaesthesia	20–30	120–240
Ketamine/xylazine	75–100 mg/kg +10 mg/kg IP	Surgical anaesthesia	20–30	120–240
Methohexital	7–10 mg/kg IV	Surgical anaesthesia	5	10
Pentobarbital	40–50 mg/kg IP	Light anaesthesia	15–60	120–240
Propofol	10 mg/kg IV	Surgical anaesthesia	5	10
Thiopental	30 mg/kg IV	Surgical anaesthesia	10	15
Tiletamine/zolezepam	40 mg/kg IP	Light anaesthesia	15–25	60–120
Chloralose	55–65 mg/kg IP	Light anaesthesia	480–600	non-recovery only
Inactin	80 mg/kg IP	Surgical anaesthesia	60–240	120–300
Urethane	1000 mg/kg IP	Surgical anaesthesia	360–480	non-recovery only

*Dose in ml/kg of a mixture of 1 part fentanyl/fluanisone plus 2 parts water for injection and 1 part midazolam (5 mg/ml initial concentration).

FIG. 7.7 Injectable anaesthetic dose rates. Duration of anaesthesia and sleep times are provided as a guide only since considerable variation between animals occurs.

Ketamine and Ketamine / Sedative Combinations

Ketamine is a dissociative anaesthetic, a term used to describe a functional dissociation between the cortex and lower brain systems. In some larger animal species and in man, ketamine can produce good analgesia and immobilise the patient for minor surgery. In small rodents, when administered as the sole anaesthetic agent, ketamine fails to produce immobility until excessively high doses have been used. Even at high dose rates, the degree of analgesia produced is inadequate even for minor surgical procedures. Suturing of skin wounds may be possible, but some animals will require additional analgesia, for example infiltration of the skin with local anaesthetics (e.g. lidocaine). In rabbits, ketamine produces sedation and loss of the righting reflex, but insufficient analgesia even for minor surgery. However, when administered with a sedative or tranquiliser, light or moderate surgical anaesthesia is produced, with good muscle relaxation.

Ketamine / Xylazine and Ketamine / Medetomidine

Ketamine in combination with either xylazine or medetomidine usually provides more effective surgical anaesthesia than other ketamine mixtures. Both xylazine and medetomidine have analgesic as well as sedative properties and have the added advantage that they can be reversed by administration of specific antagonists. Older antagonists such as yohimbine (0.2 mg/kg IV, 0.5 mg/kg IM) can be effective, but they may have other, non-specific side-effects. The more recently introduced antagonist, atipamezole, is highly specific and devoid of undesirable side-effects (1 mg/kg IM, IP, SC or IV). The combination of ketamine/xylazine or ketamine/medetomidine produces medium planes of surgical anaesthesia in most animals. A significant number of small rodents will fail to lose their withdrawal reflex and may be responsive to surgical stimuli. Rather than inject additional anaesthetic, it is preferable to administer a low concentration of volatile anaesthetic, or to infiltrate the surgical field with local anaesthetic.

The use of these ketamine combinations causes a moderate depression in respiration and it is advisable to administer oxygen by face-mask to prevent hypoxia. It is important to note that xylazine and medetomidine cause significant cardiovascular system depression. Although ketamine used alone causes a rise in blood pressure, when this drug is administered in combination with xylazine or medetomidine, or with other sedatives, hypotension occurs. A further non-specific effect of xylazine and medetomidine is the production of a diuresis and glycosuria. All of these effects are rapidly

and completely reversed by the specific antagonist atipamezole.

Ketamine and either xylazine or medetomidine can be mixed together and given as a single injection. In rodents this is best administered by the IP route, since IM injection of ketamine can result in muscle damage in these small animals (Smiler *et al.*, 1990). In rabbits, IM injection into the quadriceps is preferable. Onset of anaesthesia occurs in approximately 5 min, but full surgical anaesthesia may not develop until 10–15 min after injection. Recovery period can be prolonged (Fig. 7.7), but can be dramatically reduced by administration of atipamezole (1 mg/kg IM, IP, SC or IV).

In rabbits, additional analgesia which may be required for major surgery can be provided by the inclusion of butorphanol in the regimen (Marini *et al.*, 1992). The addition of butorphanol has the additional advantage of providing some post-operative analgesia.

Other Ketamine Combinations

Ketamine in combination with either acepromazine, promazine, midazolam or diazepam has been suggested as an anaesthetic mixture for small rodents. These sedatives and tranquilisers have no analgesic action and the depth of anaesthesia produced is usually insufficient for major surgery in small rodents. In some strains of rodent, surgical anaesthesia can be produced and it may be worthwhile assessing these combinations in certain circumstances. In small animal practice, when only individual animals are dealt with, it is preferable to select ketamine/xylazine or ketamine/medetomidine for rodents.

In rabbits, ketamine together with acepromazine, midazolam or diazepam provides light to moderate surgical anaesthesia and is more effective in this species than in small rodents. However, even in rabbits, the degree of analgesia is neither as good nor as consistent as that produced by ketamine in combination with medetomidine or xylazine.

Tiletamine/Zolezepam

Tiletamine is a dissociative anaesthetic which resembles ketamine in its activity. It is marketed in North America and Europe as a mixture of tiletamine and zolezepam, a benzodiazepine. This tiletamine/zolezepam mixture can be used to provide light anaesthesia in rodents and rabbits. In rabbits, there have been reports of renal damage associated with use of high dose rates of this compound (32–64 mg/kg) (Brammer *et al.*, 1991) and it is suggested that tiletamine/zolezepam should only be used in low doses, in combination with other anaesthetic agents, in this species.

Fentanyl/Droperidol

The neuroleptanalgesic mixture of fentanyl and droperidol can be used to sedate and immobilise rodents and rabbits. This anaesthetic mixture produces good analgesia, but very poor muscle relaxation. It also causes marked respiratory depression, particularly at higher dose rates. It is best used only for providing restraint for minor surgical procedures.

Fentanyl/Fluanisone

When used as the sole anaesthetic regimen fentanyl/fluanisone resembles fentanyl/droperidol in its actions. It produces marked depression of respiration and good analgesia but poor muscle relaxation. When combined with either midazolam or diazepam, surgical anaesthesia with good muscle relaxation and only mild or moderate respiratory depression is produced. Unfortunately, mixtures of fentanyl/droperidol and benzodiazepines do not appear to produce such successful results. An added advantage of using fentanyl/fluanisone or fentanyl/fluanisone and midazolam is that the fentanyl component can be reversed using opioid antagonists such as naloxone. Since use of pure μ antagonists such as naloxone removes all analgesic effects, it is preferable to use mixed antagonist/agonist opioids such as buprenorphine, butorphanol or nalbuphine. These analgesics reverse the respiratory depressant effects of fentanyl, reduce the degree of sedation, but provide an analgesic effect (Flecknell *et al.*, 1989).

Barbiturates

Pentobarbital

Pentobarbital, a barbiturate with a medium duration of action (30–240 min) has poor analgesic properties and a narrow margin of safety in rodents and rabbits. Inadvertent over- or under-dosage is common and it is preferable to use alternative anaesthetics whenever possible. If pentobarbital is used, then low dose rates should be administered to provide loss of consciousness, with inhalational agents used to deepen anaesthesia.

Thiopental, thiamylal and methohexital

Thiopental, methohexital and thiamylal have short durations of action (5–15 min) and when administered IV can provide short periods of anaesthesia in rodents and rabbits. In these small animals, thiopental should be reconstituted at a concentration of 1.25% or less, to allow a more controllable volume for injection.

Propofol

Propofol is a compound which is unrelated to the barbiturates, steroids or other anaesthetic agents. It is an alkyl phenol and to overcome problems associated with its poor water-solubility, it is formulated as an emulsion with soya-bean oil and glycerol. When administered IV propofol produces surgical anaesthesia in rodents. In the rabbit, surgical anaesthesia is only produced after administration of high dose rates which result in apnoea. No data on the effects of propofol in the chinchilla appear to be available. Unlike the short-acting barbiturates, propofol is relatively non-cumulative and so has been used in a variety of species for long-term anaesthesia, administered by continuous IV infusion. Infusion rates for rats are approximately 0.6 mg/kg/min and 2.2 mg/kg/min for mice.

Local Anaesthetic Techniques

The use of local anaesthesia is frequently overlooked as an option when anaesthetising rodents and rabbits. The lack of cooperation on the part of the patient limits the use of local anaesthesia as the sole anaesthetic, but low dose rates of other injectable or inhalational agents can be used in combination with infiltration of the surgical field with local anaesthetic. This technique can reduce the risks associated with producing deep planes of general anaesthesia in high risk patients.

In addition to local infiltration, techniques of epidural and spinal anaesthesia have been described in rabbits and guinea pigs and these methods may be of use in certain special situations (Hughes *et al.*, 1993).

Topical Anaesthesia

Local anaesthetic gel and sprays can be used to produce anaesthesia of mucous membranes in small mammals, in the same manner as in larger species. Ophthalmic preparations containing local anaesthetic can be used to anaesthetise the surface of the eye. A local anaesthetic cream, consisting of a mixture of lignocaine and prilocaine, can be used to produce full skin-thickness anaesthesia in animals and man. In the rabbit, this cream is particularly useful for providing local anaesthesia prior to passing an over-the-needle catheter into an ear vein (Flecknell *et al.*, 1990). The cream is applied to the ear, covered by an occlusive dressing and left in contact with the skin for approximately 45 min.

Intra-Operative Care

Irrespective of the method of anaesthesia, successful recovery depends critically on the provision of high standards of intra-operative care. Although this applies to all patients, it is especially important in small rodents because of their susceptibility to hypothermia. As mentioned earlier, a final point to consider is that many small mammals which are kept as pets will often be in a poor state of health when presented for anaesthesia. They may be dehydrated, be in poor body condition and frequently have subclinical infections, such as bronchopneumonia. Aside from general debility, the main areas of concern are maintenance of body temperature, prevention of hypoxia and hypercapnia, and avoidance of hypotension. In all instances, prevention of these problems is preferable to attempting to correct them after they have occurred. It is therefore worth adopting a set of routine practices which will tend to minimise the incidence of hypothermia, hypoxia and hypotension and use simple monitoring procedures to try to ensure the continued well being of these small patients.

Hypothermia

Small mammals have a relatively large body surface area relative to their body weight and so lose heat rapidly. Anaesthetics depress homeostatic mechanisms and suppress the normal responses which would correct hypothermia. Anaesthetics may also cause peripheral vasodilation, which leads to an increase in heat loss. The use of cold fluids and exposure of the viscera during surgery will also increase heat loss. In small animals, the cooling effect of cold anaesthetic gases from an anaesthetic machine can also represent a significant source of cooling.

If small rodents are simply allowed to remain at room temperature when anaesthetised, they cool rapidly, the degree of cooling being markedly influenced by the environmental temperature. The fall in body temperature reduces metabolic rate and slows recovery from anaesthesia. Prolongation of recovery leads to further falls in temperature and the end result may be that the animal fails to recover. As a general guide, once the body temperature has fallen below 25°C, circulatory failure occurs and the animal will die.

To prevent hypothermia, animals should be insulated and supplemental heating provided. A range of different materials are suitable for insulating animals. Cotton wool, aluminium cooking foil, 'bubble pack' and more sophisticated purpose-made materials can be used. The animal should be wrapped immediately after induction of anaesthesia, although some compromises will need to be made to allow access to a surgical field. Although less effective, the advantage of using inexpensive material such as bubble-packing is that these materials can be cut to provide access to the surgical field and disposed of after use. As an alternative, supplemental heating can be used, provided by heating pads or lamps. If heating lamps are used, they should be placed in the required position in advance and the temperature produced monitored to prevent over-heating and injury to the animal. Heating pads are generally preferable and most will provide a stable temperature with little risk of injury to the patient. Many heat blankets require a short period to reach their operating temperature and although this delay would be insignificant in a large animal with a slow rate of cooling, in small mammals it can result in a marked temperature drop. To avoid this problem, blankets should be activated about 30 min before they are required. Over-heating is rarely a problem, but it is advisable to monitor the surface temperature of the pad, to check it remains below 40°C.

Whatever the method of heating used, the animal's body temperature should be monitored to ensure that the methods used are adequate. Inexpensive electronic thermometers can be obtained which combine measurement of temperature with provision of high and low temperature alarms. A probe diameter of 2–2.5 mm is suitable for rats and larger species and instruments of this size are readily available. Smaller probe sizes (1 mm), which are suitable for mice, are relatively expensive and more difficult to obtain. Mercury clinical thermometers and some electronic clinical thermometers are unsuitable for use in small patients, since the lowest temperature they are capable of recording is 35°C. In some instances the animal's rectal temperatures will have already fallen below this level during induction and pre-operative preparations.

When preparing an animal for surgery, the degree of heat loss can be reduced by removing only sufficient hair to allow aseptic surgery to be undertaken and by keeping the use of skin disinfection to a minimum. Whenever possible, any fluids used should be warmed to body temperature before administration and this can often be achieved quickly and easily by use of a microwave oven.

Respiratory Function

Virtually all of the anaesthetics used will depress respiration and this will produce hypoxia, hypercapnia and acidosis. If the degree of depression is severe, then cardiovascular failure may result. Animals with pre-existing respiratory diseases are obviously at greater risk, but even apparently healthy animals may become cyanosed and develop respiratory failure when anaesthetised.

A number of different techniques are available to monitor the respiratory system. The simplest method is to observe the pattern and depth of respiration and to note the colour of the mucous membranes. In albino rodents and rabbits the colour of the muzzle and ears will indicate the development of cyanosis. Obvious colour change will only occur after the development of severe hypoxia and when noted will require immediate corrective action. Since in many instances the duties of anaesthetist and surgeon are combined, it is often more convenient to use electronic monitoring devices to record respiratory rate and pattern. Relatively inexpensive respiratory monitors often use a thermistor, placed close to the animal's nose, to detect respiration. Temperature changes caused by exhaled gases are detected by the thermistor and trigger the monitor. These simple devices will usually function reliably in animals weighing more than 200 g, but it is advisable to check the sensitivity of any monitor before purchase. A fall in respiratory rate of more than 50% is usually an indication of the onset of significant respiratory depression, which should be corrected. Since most rodents and rabbits are tachypnoeic before induction, because of fear or apprehension, this general guide may be difficult to interpret. If a normal resting respiratory rate cannot be obtained, then published data on predicted normal rates must be used.

Measurement of respiratory rate is a fairly crude index of respiratory depression and a much better assessment of respiratory function can be obtained by using a pulse oximeter. These instruments are extremely useful, but two problems arise when monitoring small mammals. Some instruments do not detect the small signals from these species, or discard the signal as an artifact because of its low amplitude and rapid frequency. The rapid heart rates also result in instruments failing to display a correct rate, since the upper rate which can be recognised may be only 250 beats per min. Although this prevents the use of the upper heart rate alarm in some patients, most instruments will still display a correct value of oxygen saturation. Instruments specifically designed for veterinary use are now becoming available and these can accurately measure a wider range of heart rates. When breathing air and using injectable anaesthetic regimens, saturations of 85–90% are usual. A fall in saturation below 75% requires corrective action.

Respiratory Arrest

Although respiratory depression results in both hypercapnia and hypoxia, administration of oxygen by face-mask will prevent hypoxia and this appears to reduce the overall detrimental effects of respiratory depression. If significant respiratory depression or respiratory arrest occurs, quickly check that the animal's airway is unobstructed. If an endotracheal tube has been used, check that it is still correctly positioned and is not kinked. If the animal has not been intubated, extend its head and neck and pull its tongue forwards. If oxygen is being delivered from an anaesthetic machine, check that the supply has not been exhausted. If oxygen was not being administered, supply 100% oxygen immediately via a face-mask. Assist ventilation, either by appropriate use of the anaesthetic circuit, or by manual compression of the thorax. Even in small rodents, compression of the chest using the thumb and forefinger can provide effective ventilation. Compress the chest at a rate of around 60 compressions per min. Once respiratory function has improved, continue to observe the animal closely for a few minutes to ensure that the depth and rate of respiration stabilise.

Respiration can also be stimulated centrally by administration of doxapram (10 mg/kg, IV, IP or sublingual), which will increase the rate and depth of respiration in all small mammals. If surgery has been completed, then it may be possible to reverse anaesthesia using a specific antagonist.

Cardiovascular Function

Both hypothermia and respiratory depression can lead to cardiovascular failure, but the most common cause of failure in small mammals is hypovolaemia caused either by pre-existing fluid deficit, or by haemorrhage during surgery. Although it is self-evident that small animals have correspondingly small circulatory volumes, the relative importance of haemorrhage is often underestimated. It is important to minimise blood loss by careful surgical technique and meticulous attention to haemostasis. Blood loss can be corrected by administration of whole blood, colloids or crystalloids, as in other species. The small size of the animals may make IV administration impracticable, but IP administration of crystalloids is an easy technique, which is effective in correcting pre-operative deficits, or providing post-operative circulatory support. The relatively slow rate of absorption makes this route unsuitable for treating acute blood loss.

A second common cause of cardiovascular and respiratory failure is overdose of anaesthetic. The risk of overdose of an individual animal can be minimised by carefully weighing the animal to calculate the dose of injectable anaesthetic required. If inadvertent overdose of anaesthetic is suspected, then a specific antagonist drug, or non-specific respiratory stimulant (e.g. doxapram, 10 mg/kg, IV, IP or sublingual) should be administered.

Cardiac Arrest

If complete cardiac arrest has occurred, it is helpful to assess the likely cause. However irrespective of the underlying problem, an immediate priority is to ensure that the airway is unobstructed and 100% oxygen is being supplied. If respiration has ceased it should be assisted as described above. In addition, external cardiac massage by intermittent compression of the chest wall should be commenced. The chest should be held between the anaesthetist's thumb and forefinger and the area over the heart compressed regularly and rapidly, about 90 times/min. This technique enables some circulatory support to be maintained while other corrective measures are instigated. Combining assisted ventilation and external cardiac massage requires practice and it is usually easier to compress all areas of the thorax simultaneously.

In larger species, in addition to correction of hypovolaemia, it is usual to administer drugs to help restore normal cardiac function, but to do this effectively usually requires monitoring of arterial pressure and the electrocardiogram. In small mammals, measurement of the ECG is hampered by the low-amplitude signal and rapid heart rate found in these species. It is possible, however, using specifically designed monitors. If asystole is diagnosed, adrenaline (0.1 ml/kg of 1:10,000) should be given, or if ventricular fibrillation has occurred, lidocaine (lignocaine) should be administered (1–2 mg/kg). Tachy-arrhythmias may respond to propranolol (0.1 mg/kg), although atropine may also be required to counteract any bradycardia caused by the propranolol. Complete heart block or low cardiac output can be treated by administration of isoprenaline (0.1–1 mg/kg/min). IV administration of these agents is possible in the rabbit, but in small rodents the intracardiac route may be necessary. If intracardiac injection is carried out, a 25 gauge needle should be used, to minimise the risk of myocardial injury.

Other factors that can cause either respiratory or cardiovascular depression can arise from a failure to appreciate fully some of the consequences of the small body-weight of these animals. Placement of surgical instruments across the thorax, or resting the operator's hands on the patient's body are tolerated by dogs and cats, but the weight of a retractor or clamp can easily interfere with normal thoracic movements in small rodents.

Post-Operative Care

As discussed earlier, a special recovery area should have been prepared prior to induction of anaesthesia. This can consist of a specially designed incubator or may simply be a cage equipped with a heating pad. Preparation of this facility well in advance will allow heating pads or blankets to stabilise at a suitable temperature. Initially, small rodents require a temperature of 35–37°C and rabbits 30–35°C, but this can be reduced to 25–30°C once the animal is recovering and has regained its righting reflex. After full recovery, it is advisable to provide a warm environment (20–25°C) as activity is often markedly reduced in the first 24 h following surgery. As a routine, dextrose–saline (0.18% saline, 4% dextrose) should be administered by SC or IP injection. Most small rodents will have a reduced fluid intake during the first 24 h following surgery and administration of fluid at the end of surgery will help maintain normal fluid balance. If oral administration is not well tolerated, then SC administration should be repeated every 6–12 h. Many small mammals can be hand-fed fluids relatively easily however and may also benefit from being fed cereal-based semi-liquid human infant foods. Rabbits and guinea pigs may find liquefied vegetables particularly palatable.

Small rodents and rabbits should not be allowed to recover on sawdust or wood-shavings as these can clog the eyes, nose and mouth. More suitable materials such as synthetic sheepskin, or towelling should be used. Tissue paper is relatively ineffective as it is easily pushed aside and the animal then lies on the cage base and often becomes covered in urine and faeces. Urine soiling can occur even when using suitable bedding, so the animal should be dried at appropriate intervals to minimise the risk of hypothermia and irritation of the skin. The response to human contact varies considerably amongst different individuals, but in general these smaller animals are less responsive to nursing care than are dogs and cats. Frequent handling, stroking and other disturbances can be counterproductive and cause unnecessary stress to the animal. It is therefore necessary to judge carefully the degree of disturbance that is appropriate in the immediate post-operative period.

If the animal is still showing signs of respiratory depression, then it is advisable to continue administering oxygen until normal respiratory function has resumed. It is relatively simple to make an oxygen chamber for small animals, e.g. by using a clear plastic or polyethylene container as a recovery cage.

Analgesia and Pain Assessment

Post-operative pain can slow recovery and may have other undesirable consequences. Despite the growing body of evidence that animals experience pain (Popilskis *et al.*, 1993; Nolan and Reid, 1993) and that analgesic therapy in the post-operative period can be beneficial (Liles and Flecknell, 1993, 1994), few animals receive pain-relieving drugs following surgery. This is particularly ironic in the case of small rodents, since the initial studies of the pharmacology and modes of action of many analgesics have been undertaken in these species. Because of their

widespread use in research laboratories, basic data on safety and efficacy of many analgesics are readily available. These data enable suitable dose rates to be suggested (Fig. 7.8).

As with other animals, a number of concerns may arise when analgesic use is contemplated. Since pain has a protective function, it has been suggested that analgesics should be withheld because an animal that is pain-free following surgery may injure the operative site. This concern is unwarranted and in the author's experience, routine use of analgesics has presented no difficulties in this respect. In any event, producing immobility by allowing the animal to experience unrelieved pain is ethically unacceptable, since alternative methods of protecting surgically repaired tissues are available. For example, following orthopaedic procedures, the affected limb can be splinted or bandaged and the animal confined in a small cage to restrict its movements.

A second concern is that the undesirable side-effects of some analgesics could be detrimental to the animal. The most significant of these side-effects in man is respiratory depression following opioid administration. In animals, respiratory depression is much less severe and is very rarely seen when mixed agonist/antagonist opioids such as buprenor-

ANALGESIC DOSE RATES			
	Buprenorphine	Butorphanol	Carprofen
Guinea pig	0.05 mg/kg SC q 8 h	?	?
Mouse	0.05–0.1 mg/kg SC, q 12 h	1–5 mg/kg SC q 3–4 h	?
Rabbit	0.01–0.05 mg/kg IV, SC q 8–12 h	0.1–0.5 mg/kg IV, SC q 4 h	?
Rat	0.01–0.05 mg/kg SC q 8–12 h	2.0 mg/kg SC q 3–4 h	5 mg/kg SC? q 8–12 h
	Flunixin	Morphine	Nalbuphine
Guinea pig	?	2–5 mg/kg SC, IM q 4 h	?
Mouse	2.3 mg/kg SC	2–5 mg/kg SC q 4 h	4–8 mg/kg SC
Rabbit	1.1 mg/kg SC, IM ? q 8 h	2–5 mg/kg q 4 h	1–2 mg/kg IV, SC q 4 h
Rat	2.5–5.0 mg/kg SC	2–5 mg/kg SC q 4 h	1–2 mg/kg SC q 3 h

FIG. 7.8 Analgesic dose rates. Dose rates based on clinical experience and published data on analgesiometry and pharmacokinetics (Flecknell, 1984; Flecknell and Liles, 1990, 1992; Liles and Flecknell, 1992). Frequency of administration should be based on clinical assessment of the individual animal, but where reasonable estimates of average duration or drug action are available, these are provided. No data are available for analgesic dose rates in chinchillas, hamsters or gerbils.

phine or butorphanol are administered (Pircio *et al.*, 1976; Flecknell and Liles, 1990). The only occasion in which respiratory depression is likely to be seen is administration of pure μ agonists such as morphine after use of similar analgesics during anaesthesia. If butorphanol, buprenorphine or nalbuphine are used instead, then any residual respiratory depression caused by the anaesthetic regimen is reversed and analgesia is maintained by the second opioid.

A commonly held misconception is that opioids should not be given to animals with head injuries. In man, opioids are withheld under these circumstances because of the effects on consciousness, which makes neurological assessment difficult and because respiratory depression may cause an increase in cerebral blood flow and raised intracranial pressure. As mentioned earlier, opioids rarely produce clinically significant respiratory depression in animals and neurological assessment of the type undertaken in human patients is rarely, if ever, undertaken in veterinary patients. There is therefore no reason not to alleviate the pain associated with cranial injury or trauma.

A final point to consider is the view that because of their hypotensive effects, opioids should be withheld from animals which may have hypovolaemia. Once again, this advice is based upon out-dated observations. Although rapid IV injection of morphine can cause hypotension in some species, the mixed agonist/antagonist opioids do not have this effect (Cowan *et al.*, 1977; O'Hair *et al.*, 1988) and can be given safely to animals which are hypovolaemic.

Recognition of Pain in Rodents and Rabbits

One of the main reasons why analgesics are used relatively infrequently in animals is that we are unable to assess accurately the degree of pain experienced by our patients. In many instances, we may even be unable to recognise that the animal is in pain. To overcome this problem, it is necessary to become familiar with the normal behaviour and appearance of small mammals and to appreciate that easily recognised signs of pain are rarely present. One problem is that some species, for example rats, are more active at night and observing them during the day may give a poor indication of their normal behaviour. A second difficulty is that unlike cats and dogs, small mammals may not respond positively to human contact and may remain immobile when examined. This behaviour can severely limit attempts to use behaviour and posture to detect pain.

Despite these difficulties, it may be possible to recognise some clinical signs which may be associated with pain. The posture of the animal may be abnormal and it may appear hunched and remain immobile. When encouraged to move, the animal may have an abnormal gait or posture, may be reluctant to continue moving and may show uncharacteristic signs of aggression when approached or handled. The animal may also vocalise when approached or handled. Rabbits may position themselves in the back of their cage or pen, facing away from any observers. The external appearance of the animal may be altered, notably because of lack of grooming behaviour. The coat may appear unkempt and ruffled. In rats, a blackish discharge may be present around the eyes and nose. This discharge is secretion from the Harderian gland and when removed with damp cotton wool, it has a red colour. It is not certain whether stress increases the quantity secreted, or whether the build-up is due primarily to reduced grooming. Food and water intake and consequently body-weight, are reduced and these latter indices can provide a simple and relatively objective means of monitoring an animal's progress.

The clinical signs outlined above are relatively non-specific and can occur because of non-painful conditions such as infectious disease. When attempting to assess pain, the clinical appearance of the animal should be considered in conjunction with the nature of the surgical interference. In the author's experience, most surgical procedures in rodents and rabbits cause very few signs of pain that are detectable during a brief clinical inspection. Detailed longer term monitoring of behaviour and assessment of variables such as body-weight do, however, provide a clear indication of changes in response to surgery and positive responses to the administration of analgesics can be demonstrated (Liles and Flecknell, 1993, 1994).

Choice of Analgesic Therapy

The main problems associated with the use of opioids arise from their relatively short duration of action. The exception is buprenorphine, which although not always as effective an analgesic as morphine, does have a much greater duration of action. Repeated dosing at 8–12 h intervals appears effective in controlling most post-surgical pain.

Most rodents and rabbits seem to benefit from administration of a single dose of buprenorphine either intra-operatively or immediately post-operatively (Flecknell, 1991; Flecknell and Liles, 1992). If the animal appears to be in pain when reassessed 8 h later, then a second dose can be administered. This appears to be sufficient for all but the most severe surgical procedures.

An alternative to the use of opioids is to administer non-steroidal anti-inflammatory drugs (NSAIDs) or local anaesthetics. Once again, considerable basic data are available concerning likely effective dose rates of these agents (Liles and Flecknell, 1992). When attempting to control post-operative pain, the more potent NSAIDs such as carprofen and flunixin should be selected, rather than weak NSAIDs such as aspirin. The duration of action of these more potent NSAIDs in rodents is uncertain, but clinical experience suggests that a single dose may provide up to 24 h analgesia.

Long-acting local anaesthetics such as bupivacaine can be used to infiltrate a surgical field, but the results produced are very variable. This may be because the duration of action of bupivacaine appears to be shorter in rats than in larger species such as dogs, farm animals and human patients

Chronic Pain

Aside from the requirement to control acute post-operative pain, animals may suffer from a range of conditions which may cause significant chronic pain. For example, arthritis is common in old (> 2 years old) rats, all species may develop neoplasia and localised infection and associated inflammation may cause pain. In these circumstances, NSAIDs are most suitable and suggested dose rates are listed in Fig. 7.8.

Conclusions and Recommendations

Provided that sound clinical principles are adopted, anaesthesia of small rodents should present no greater risk than that associated with similar procedures in larger species. Critical points to consider are the need for pre-operative evaluation of the animal and the provision of high standards of intra-operative care, especially the prevention of hypothermia and administration of oxygen to provide some respiratory support. Inhalational anaesthetics are strongly recommended for use in these species since the onset and recovery from anaesthesia is rapid and the depth of anaesthesia can be rapidly adjusted to that required for a particular procedure. If injectable anaesthetics are used, then ketamine in combination with medetomidine or xylazine, or fentanyl/fluanisone/midazolam, are recommended. Whenever possible these combinations should be partly reversed by administration of specific antagonists. Finally, high standards of post-operative care, including administration of fluid therapy, provision of analgesia and a warm and comfortable environment must be considered essential.

References

Brammer, D., Doerning, B. J., Chrisp, C. E. and Rush, H. G. (1991) Anaesthetic and nephrotoxic effects of tiletamine/zolezepam in New Zealand White rabbits. *Laboratory Animal Science* **41**, 432–435.

Cowan, A., Doxey, J. C. and Harry, E. J. R. (1977) The animal pharmacology of buprenorphine, an oripavine analgesic agent. *British Journal of Pharmacology* **60**, 547–554.

Flecknell, P. A. (1984) Relief of pain in laboratory animals. *Laboratory Animals* **18**, 147–160.

Flecknell, P. A. (1991) Postoperative analgesia in rabbits and rodents. *Lab. Animal* **20**, 34–37.

Flecknell, P. A. and Liles, J. H. (1990) Assessment of the analgesic action of opioid agonist-antagonists in the rabbit. *Journal of the Association of Veterinary Anaesthetists* **17**, 24–29.

Flecknell, P. A. and Liles, J. H. (1992) Evaluation of locomotor activity and food and water consumption as a method of assessing postoperative pain in rodents. In: *Animal Pain*, Short, C. E. and Van Poznak, A. (eds.). Churchill Livingstone, pp. 482–488.

Flecknell, P. A., Liles, J. H. and Williamson, H. A. (1990) The use of lignocaine–prilocaine local anaesthetic cream for pain-free venepuncture in laboratory animals. *Laboratory Animals* **24**, 142–146.

Flecknell, P. A., Liles, J. H. and Wootton, R. (1989) Reversal of fentanyl/fluanisone neuroleptanalgesia in the rabbit using mixed agonist/antagonist opioids. *Laboratory Animals* **23**, 147–155.

Hughes, P. J., Doherty, M. M. and Charman, W. N. (1993) A rabbit model for the evaluation of epidurally administered local anaesthetic agents. *Anaesthesia and Intensive Care* **21**, 298–303.

Liles, J. H. and Flecknell, P. A. (1992) The use of non-steroidal anti-inflammatory drugs for the relief of pain in laboratory rodents and rabbits. *Laboratory Animals* **26**, 241–255.

Liles, J. H. and Flecknell, P. A. (1993) The effects of surgical stimulus on the rat and the influence of analgesic treatment. *British Veterinary Journal* **149**, 515–525.

Liles, J. H. and Flecknell, P. A. (1994) A comparison of the effects of buprenorphine, carprofen and flunixin following laparotomy in rats. *Journal of Veterinary Pharmacology and Therapeutics* **17**, 284–290.

Marini, R., Avison, D. L., Corning, B. F. and Lipman, N. S. (1992) Ketamine/xylazine/butorphanol: a new anaesthetic combination for rabbits. *Laboratory Animal Science* **42**, 57–62.

Nolan, A. and Reid, J. (1993) Comparison of the post-operative analgesic and sedative effects of carprofen and papaveretum in the dog. *The Veterinary Record* **133**, 240–242.

O'Hair, K. C., Dodd, K. T., Phillips, Y. Y. and Beattie, R. J. (1988) Cardiopulmonary effects of nalbuphine hydrochloride and butorphanol tartrate in sheep. *Laboratory Animal Science* **38**, 58–61.

Pircio, A. W., Gylys, J. A., Cavanagh, R. L., Buyniski, J. P. and Bierwagen, M. E. (1976) The pharmacology of butorphanol a 3,14-dihydroxymorphinan narcotic antagonist analgesic. *Archives Internationales de Pharmacodynamie et de Therapie* **220**, 231–257.

Popilskis, S., Kohn, D. F., Laurent, L. and Danilo, P. (1993) Efficacy of epidural morphine versus IV morphine for post-thoracotomy pain in dogs. *Journal of Veterinary Anaesthesia* **20**, 21–28.

Smiler, K., Stein, S., Hrapkiewicz, K. L. and Hiben, J. R. (1990) Tissue response to IM and IP injections of ketamine and xylazine in rats. *Laboratory Animal Science* **40**, 60–64.

8

Common surgical procedures in rodents and rabbits

M. MICHAEL SWINDLE and PAUL M. SHEALY

Veterinarians are increasingly called upon to perform surgery on pet rabbits and rodents. Most practitioners are generally unfamiliar with anaesthesia and surgery in these species. The purpose of this chapter is to provide a general overview of surgical principles and perioperative care for rabbits and rodents. Some of the more common surgical techniques are discussed in detail. More detailed information on the diseases discussed in this chapter may be found in the various species chapters. The chapter on anaesthesia and analgesia should be used to supplement the general information provided in this chapter.

General Surgical Principles

The most common indications for surgery encountered in private practice include: traumatic wounds, fractures, tumours, dystocia, gastro-intestinal foreign bodies, malocclusion and sterilization. General surgical principles apply to all species and surgical techniques performed on larger animals may be transposed to rodents and rabbits, with careful attention given to anatomical differences. It is important to adhere to Halsted's principles of asepsis, haemostasis, gentle handling of tissues, careful approximation of the wound, avoiding tension, closing dead space and minimising foreign material such as sutures. These species cannot tolerate major losses of blood and are prone to fatal shock with traumatic experiences. The caecum is large and friable and care should be taken to avoid injuring it with surgical instruments when performing abdominal procedures. The use of electrocoagu-

lation on low settings or hand-held battery-powered disposable cauteries minimises blood loss. Careful approximation of the wound eliminates dead space without the overuse of sutures. Inflammation due to a foreign body reaction to sutures or placing sutures too tightly will rapidly lead to self-inflicted trauma and dehiscence of the wound. Rodents and rabbits are susceptible to subclinical and clinical infections of surgical wounds without appropriate aseptic technique. Standard surgeon and surgical site preparation, caps, masks, gown, gloves, draping and sterilised instruments are recommended (Swindle, 1993; Gentry and French, 1994).

Suture selection is important to minimise inflammation. Highly reactive suture materials such as plain or chromic gut and silk should be avoided. Synthetic absorbable suture material is less likely to produce reactions. The thin muscle layers in these species generally allow the peritoneum and abdominal muscles to be closed in a single layer. Subcuticular suture patterns are recommended for skin closure, but are difficult to perform in animals with minimal skin and subcutaneous tissue thickness. Stainless steel suture or staple closure of surgical incisions can lead to wound infection from the accumulation on the wound of foreign material such as bedding and hair. This is not such a problem if the surgical wound is on the dorsum of the body. These species are capable of chewing out sutures or staples regardless of the strength of the material. If subcuticular suture patterns are not used, 3/0–4/0 synthetic monofilament suture in a simple interrupted or mattress pattern is recommended, taking care to avoid excess tension.

Tissue glues can also be used for skin closure, however, their efficacy has not been evaluated in a controlled study in these species.

Supportive care must be provided to avoid hypothermia and to maintain homeostasis. Intravenous (IV) fluid administration can be difficult in rodents due to minimal venous access, however, they tolerate intraosseous (IO), subcutaneous (SC) or intraperitoneal (IP) injections of warmed solutions. Fluids can easily be administered via the ear vein in rabbits. Circulating water blankets are recommended to maintain body temperature during surgery. If they are not available, a table pad or drapes should be used between the animal and the surgery table. Heat lamps or electrical heating pads are also used, but it is very easy to induce fatal hyperthermia in these species or to dry and damage tissue by using these techniques.

Anaesthetic depth should be monitored using corneal, pinnae, pedal or tail twitch reflexes. Pulse oximetry can be performed by attaching a standard finger probe of appropriate size to the ear, tail or tongue. Care must be taken to observe the respiratory rate and pattern continuously. A femoral pulse can generally be palpated in all of these species provided there is access to the limb during surgery. Alternatively, observing the lingual pulse and monitoring capillary refill time and mucous membrane colour is useful. Small animals can be resuscitated by chest compression in the early stages of cardiopulmonary arrest. More detailed information is available in *Chapter 7*.

Intubation of most of these species is difficult at best and impractical in smaller rodents such as rats and mice. Intubation can be accomplished in larger species such as rabbits, guinea pigs and hamsters, using commercially available tubes and laryngoscopes, but requires experience and practice for routine use. The use of small curved blades on paediatric laryngoscopes allows optimum visualisation of the larynx. Small tubes or modified IV tubing are used to maintain the airway. However, it is more important to minimise anaesthetic time than to repeat unsuccessful attempts at intubation.

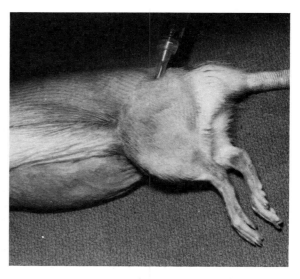

Fig. 8.1 Intraosseus injection into the aseptically prepared femoral trochanter of a rat.

Fluid replacement and nutritional support after surgery may be provided by SC or IP administration of small volumes (5–25 ml) of warmed lactated Ringer's solution or other parenteral fluids to rodents. Femoral IO injection using a hypodermic needle can be substituted for IV administration (Fig. 8.1). Generally, the precautions for asepsis and perioperative considerations for fluid administration that are followed for dogs and cats are applicable to these animals. Oral supplementation with commercial nutritional substitutes or peanut butter on fruit may also be given to rodents to provide for their high caloric requirements during the postoperative period. Rabbits are easier to manage after surgery and techniques applicable for supporting cats are appropriate including IV fluids, nutritional supplements and warmth. Rabbits will frequently eat hay or shredded wheat biscuits and fresh fruits and vegetables when they are anorectic.

Antibiotic, anaesthetic and analgesic dosages are given in mg/kg but actual body weights of rodents are in grams. The following typical adult body weights of these species may be useful in calculating drug dosages:

mouse 25 g
rat 300–400 g
gerbil 80–100 g
hamster 100–120 g
guinea pig 500–600 g.

For the purpose of calculating dosages, an adult mouse weight of 0.025 kg would be used. Because calculations of injectables result in such small volumes, the use of microlitre syringes is recommended. However, tuberculin syringes are adequate for most injections as the injectate can be added to saline for volume. IM injections are administered in the rear legs, SC injections in the scruff or flanks and IP injections in the lower left quadrant of the abdomen while the animals are held in a head down position. IV injections are routinely administered in the ear veins of rabbits and often in the tail vein or saphenous vein of some rodents. The technique of metabolic scaling for calculating drug dosage and administration frequency is described elsewhere (Sedgwick and Martin, 1994). Although probably more accurate than more common interpolation methods, calculations are difficult to perform and blood levels of administered pharmaceuticals have rarely been validated with this technique.

Surgical Techniques

Specific surgical techniques that may be commonly performed in pet rodents and rabbits are discussed in this section. The discussion in the previous section on general principles should be read to complement the surgical description.

Orchidectomy (Castration)

Neutering of rodents and rabbits is performed to prevent reproduction and to reduce fighting, especially between males. Castration may also be indicated following traumatic injury.

Both rodents and rabbits have open inguinal canals from birth. If testicles are not palpable at the time of surgery, a gentle caudal pushing motion on the abdomen will force them into the scrotum. Care must be taken, especially in the rabbit, to avoid traumatising the skin and scrotum during clipping and surgical preparation.

Techniques

The surgical approach may be scrotal, prescrotal or midline intra-abdominal. A direct single midline scrotal incision or a bilateral scrotal incision is most commonly performed. Prescrotal incisions may be on the midline or over the inguinal ring if closure of the ring is desired. The intra-abdominal approach also allows the surgeon to close the inguinal rings. The non-scrotal approaches or combined scrotal and non-scrotal approaches may be indicated in cases of trauma or in any case where hernia and evisceration is considered likely.

Orchidectomy may be performed with either an open or a closed tunica albuginea (Figs 8.2–8.7). The simplest method, the open technique, is to incise the tunic, exposing the testicle and the structures of the spermatic cord. The vas deferens is clamped and ligated with the spermatic vessels. The ligament of the testicle and epididymis is ligated in the same manner. There is anecdotal evidence that preservation of the epididymal fat pad may reduce the incidence of herniation. The tunic is closed with simple interrupted or continuous sutures followed by skin closure.

The closed technique is performed by placing circumferential or transfixion ligatures around the spermatic cord and ligament of the

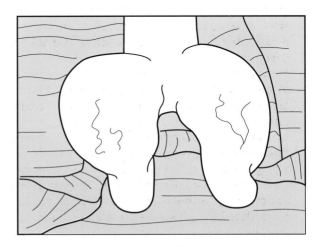

FIG. 8.2 Rabbit testicles are positioned for a scrotal castration approach.

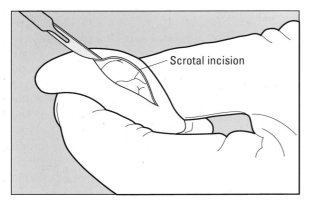

FIG. 8.3 The skin incision is made after tensing the the skin.

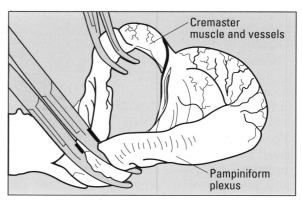

FIG. 8.6 When using an open technique, the tunic is incised and the vessels of the spermatic cord are ligated separately from the vas deferens.

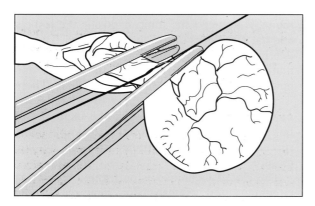

FIG. 8.4 When using the closed technique, the tunic is not incised prior to ligation of the spermatic cord.

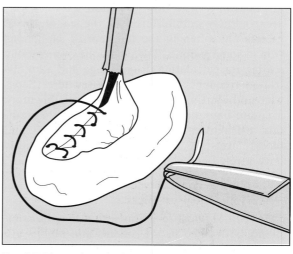

FIG. 8.7 The tunic and subcutaneous tissues are closed with a continuous suture pattern.

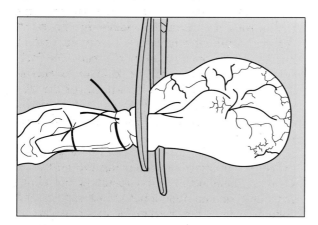

FIG. 8.5 After double ligation, the testicle and epididymis are excised.

epididymis without incising the tunic. The tunic may also be twisted and ligated when performing this technique.

Closure of the inguinal canal usually requires only a few non-absorbable sutures. No definitive studies have been performed to determine whether any of these techniques are superior in these species. From experience, any of these methods are effective and complications are minimal if care is taken to avoid tissue trauma. If irritation is present, these animals will frequently eviscerate themselves.

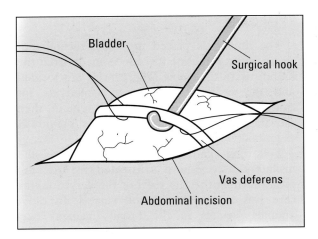

FIG. 8.8 The vas deferens of a rat has been exteriorised with a surgical hook.

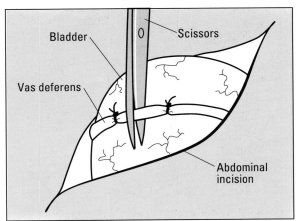

FIG. 8.9 The vas deferens is transected after double ligation.

Vasectomy

If sterility is the only goal, a vasectomy may be performed.

Technique

A vasectomy may be performed open through a scrotal or prescrotal approach by ligating and transecting the vas deferens. Care should be taken to avoid incising the testes with the scalpel if they are to be preserved.

A more common approach in rodents is a midline caudal abdominal incision (Figs 8.8 and 8.9). Upon entering the abdomen, the turgid, white ductus deferens can be identified in the region of the neck of the bladder. Usually a fat pad near the bladder must be retracted caudally to visualise the structures. Double ligation of each ductus deferens is performed with non-absorbable sutures. The ductus deferens is transected with scissors between the ligatures. It is unnecessary to remove a section of the ductus deferens.

The midline coeliotomy incision is closed in one layer with continuous or simple interrupted sutures, followed by closure of the skin.

Ovariectomy / Fallopian Tube Ligation

Surgical neutering of females may be performed by either ovariectomy or Fallopian tube ligation. The decision is based upon the presence or absence of pathological conditions such as cystic ovaries or tumours, and the behaviour of the pet during oestrus.

Technique

Although the ovary may be approached through a midline coeliotomy incision, it may be preferable in obese animals to make paired dorsoventral flank incisions with the animal in sternal recumbency. The ovaries are approached through the flank with a midline dorsal skin incision followed by blunt dissection of the muscle layers on either side of the vertebral wings (Fig. 8.10). Usually the kidneys are palpable and the ovaries are located caudally in the same surgical plane. Alternatively, a routine ventral midline coeliotomy can be performed. The incision is made caudal to the kidneys extending approximately one-half to two-thirds of the distance between the xiphoid process and the pelvis on the dorsal flank or the ventral midline, respectively.

Care should be taken to avoid damaging the ovary or only partially removing the structure. Ovarian remnants will re-implant in the abdomen and remain functional. Most rabbits and rodents have a periovarian fat pad that can be manipulated with forceps to avoid this complication.

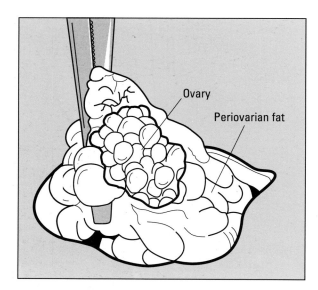

FIG. 8.10 Exteriorisation of the left ovary of a rat using a dorsal midline incision and blunt dissection through the muscle layers.

With ovariectomy, the ovarian vessels and Fallopian tube are ligated individually and the ovary and periovarian fat are removed.

The same approach is performed in Fallopian tube ligation. The Fallopian tubes are double ligated and divided. In larger rodents and in rabbits, haemostatic vascular clips can be substituted for suture ligation of tubules.

The midline incision of the dorsal flank muscle is closed routinely with simple interrupted or continuous sutures. Skin closure is routine. The dorsal approach is a common research technique and the skin incision is closed with wound clips. With experience, this technique has relatively few complications.

Ovariohysterectomy / Hysterectomy

The uterus, ovaries or both may be removed when performing routine neutering, or following a C-section for dystocia or pregnancy toxaemia. Other indications include neoplasia. In older animals, there is usually substantial adipose tissue associated with the uterine horns which can make dissection of the reproductive tract difficult (Sedgwick, 1982).

Technique

The animal is placed in dorsal recumbency and a ventral midline incision is made from the umbilicus to the pubis. The ovaries are located and the ovarian vessels are ligated as for ovariectomy. If the ovaries are to remain, then the Fallopian tubes are ligated as previously described (Fig. 8.11).

Following ligation of the ovarian vessels, the ipsilateral uterine horn is dissected free from the broad ligament to the level of the cervix, taking care not to tear any blood vessels. In older animals, vessels in the broad ligament may require ligation. Uterine vessels should be ligated separately in the larger species such as the rabbit. A single ligature around the vessels and the vagina caudal to the cervix may be all that is necessary in small rodents (Fig. 8.12). With a gravid or large uterus, the uterine stump may require closure using an inverting suture pattern or transfixion sutures.

The abdominal incision and skin are closed routinely.

Caesarian Section

Dystocia is an acute emergency situation in rodents and rabbits. An endotoxic shock syndrome can occur following the death of a foetus *in utero*. In guinea pigs, a pregnancy toxaemia syndrome may occur secondary to uteroplacental ischaemia. C-section may be necessary as part of the emergency treatment.

Technique

The animal is placed in dorsal recumbency and a ventral midline incision is made from the pubis to the umbilicus. The body of the uterus in rodents and rabbits is generally too small to remove all foetuses from a single incision. Consequently, an incision is made centrally in each horn. The incision should be made in an avascular area on the antimesometrial surface of the uterus.

Each foetus is removed individually while an assistant removes the membranes and ligates the

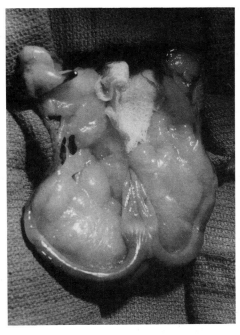

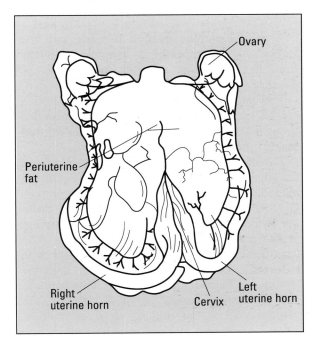

FIG. 8.11 The ovaries and uterus of a rabbit after exteriorisation. The right ovarian pedicle has been clamped.

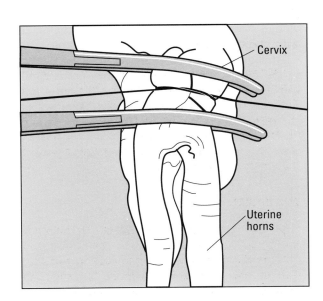

FIG. 8.12 A transfixion suture has been placed in the vagina prior to excision of the uterus.

placental vessels. The newborn should be stimulated by rubbing and clearing the oronasal passages and kept warm.

After careful palpation, each uterine horn may be closed with a single layer inverting suture pattern. However, it is advisable to perform a hysterectomy or ovariohysterectomy to prevent further pregnancies.

The same procedure described above for ovariohysterectomy should be followed. The midline incision is closed routinely.

Cystotomy

Guinea pigs and rabbits commonly develop uroliths (or cystic calculi). Generally uroliths are small and sand-like, passing without complication in the urine during voiding. However, large uroliths associated with cystitis commonly affect aged guinea pigs. Complications in rabbits are most frequently associated with larger numbers of the small uroliths which accumulate over time, although large uroliths may occasionally be seen. Urolithiasis is generally asymptomatic in the other species discussed in this text.

Technique

A ventral midline incision is made with the animal in dorsal recumbency extending cranially from the pubis approximately one-fourth the distance to the xiphoid cartilage.

The bladder is exteriorised so that an incision can be made in an avascular plane. Moistened sponges are used to pack off the bladder prior to making the incision.

The incision is made in the avascular area of the dorsal, ventral or apical surface of the bladder, taking care to avoid injury to the ureters. Uroliths can be removed manually and by flushing with saline. Proper technique will prevent urine and urolith contamination of the peritoneal cavity. The bladder is closed with absorbable suture material using an inverting continuous Lembert pattern or a simple continuous pattern. Generally in these animals, the bladder wall is too thin to close in multiple layers. Additional sutures may be required to obtain a watertight seal. After replacing the bladder into the abdomen, a two-layer closure of the abdomen is routine.

Gastrotomy/Enterotomy/Miscellaneous GI Techniques

Foreign bodies including indigestible materials, such as plastic, are encountered in these species because of their chewing behaviour. Gastroenteritis, enterocolitis or obstruction may occur secondarily. Trichobezoar development in rabbits is a complex syndrome and is discussed in *Chapter 6*. Trichobezoar removal may be necessary as part of the medical management of the syndrome (Leary *et al.*, 1984; Gillett *et al.*, 1983). If it is performed, then the perioperative care must be intense and directed towards overcoming anorexia and reestablishing intestinal motility.

Technique

With the animal placed in dorsal recumbency, a ventral midline coeliotomy is performed extending from the xiphoid process to the umbilicus. For gastrotomy, the stomach is exteriorised and packed off with moistened sponges. A gas-

trotomy incision of adequate length is made in the avascular area of the body of the stomach (Fig. 8.13). Foreign material is removed and the gastric lumen is flushed and suctioned to assess gastric mucosal integrity. The gastrotomy incision is closed with either a single or two-layer inverting suture pattern, depending on the size of the stomach. A continuous Cushing pattern oversewn with a continuous Lembert pattern, using absorbable suture, is the preferred method of closure. The Lembert suture is the preferred method if only a single layer closure is used. Gauze sponges used to pack off the stomach are removed and the abdomen is copiously flushed with warm sterile saline and suctioned.

If an enterotomy is performed, the same precautions to prevent septic contamination should be followed. A linear enterotomy incision should be made proximal to the foreign body in the avascular area of the antimesenteric border of the intestine. The enterotomy incision should be closed in a simple interrupted pattern using absorbable suture. Inverting or multiple layers of sutures are contraindicated because of less wound strength and the loss of lumen diameter with potential to create stricture formation.

Appendicitis can be experimentally produced in the rabbit and consequently may occur clinically (Swindle and Adams, 1988), although it has not been conclusively documented. Removal of the vermiform appendix may be performed using

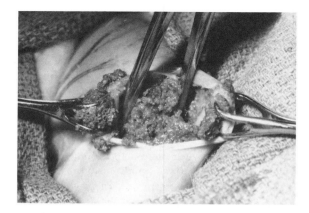

FIG. 8.13 An incision has been made in the avascular plane of the greater curvature of the stomach of the rabbit. A trichobezoar is present in the lumen.

these techniques. However, extreme caution should be used in handling the thin walled caecum to avoid traumatic rupture.

After replacing the intestines into the abdominal cavity, the laparotomy incision is closed routinely. Postoperative considerations for gastrotomies or enterotomies include the administration of fluids and soft foods aforementioned in the general principles of surgery.

Oncological Surgery (Tumour Removal)

The veterinarian is commonly presented with animals which have superficial masses such as mammary gland tumours. Visceral neoplasia is more life threatening and disease is generally advanced at diagnosis. If visceral neoplasia is diagnosed, it should be approached in the same manner as in dogs and cats.

When considering the surgical treatment of tumours in these species, it is important to remember that some laboratory species are bred for susceptibility to tumours. For example, C3H mice have a 100% incidence of mammary tumour by one year of age. Additionally, many tumours are also caused by viruses. Consequently, tumour recurrence is high after surgery. Surgical neutering may slow the growth or prevent recurrence of tumours under hormonal influence. Histopathological examination of all tumours is recommended in order to provide an accurate diagnosis and prognosis.

Techniques

The general principles of oncological surgery apply to the removal of tumours in rodents and rabbits. Principles which apply specifically to tumour removal in these species will be discussed.

Haemostasis is extremely important in these cases. Many superficial tumours, such as mammary tumours, are highly vascular. Minimising surgical time is important in order to maintain homeostasis and prevent hypothermia. Consequently, the use of electrosurgical or cautery techniques is recommended. Regardless of technique, it is important to identify and ligate, coagulate, or cauterise blood vessels in advance of severing them during surgery.

It is also important to leave enough skin to close the incision properly in order for first intention healing to occur. Careful dissection beyond the edges of the tumour into normal tissues is important. Conversely, if the surgeon is unsure that all of the edges of the tumour can be removed with such an incision, use of skin flaps may be indicated. Second intention healing may lead to self-mutilation in these species. Closure of dead space is essential to prevent haematomas and seromas. Tension on the suture line should be avoided because of the potential for self-mutilation.

Most tumours that are encountered will be either mammary gland, adnexal or sebaceous gland in origin. Most are fast-growing and can rapidly become clinically significant. A presumptive diagnosis can be made on the basis of location, size and the information presented in the species chapters in this text. Surgical treatment should be based on a balance of this information in conjunction with the owner's desires.

Trauma Surgery / Fractures / Amputations

Trauma due to fighting among cagemates or secondary to inappropriate handling will be commonly encountered by the clinician (Goring, 1994). Lacerations, abscesses, fractures and internal injuries are the most common presentations. The general principles of trauma surgery, as practised for dogs and cats, apply to rabbits and rodents.

Technique

Fighting among cagemates commonly leads to lacerations, abscesses or traumatic castration. Trauma in these species should be treated as an emergency and the animal stabilised to prevent shock and maintain homeostasis.

Standard techniques for wound cleansing and debridement are appropriate in these situations.

It is important to be gentle in tissue handling and to avoid irritating solutions in order to prevent self-mutilation. Wounds are best flushed with warmed sterile saline, utilising a 35 ml syringe and 18 gauge needle. Wound closure may be performed using standard techniques. Topical antibacterials have been associated with clostridial enterotoxaemia because animals ingest them during grooming. Caution must be used in rabbits, guinea pigs and hamsters to avoid antibacterial agents associated with this complication of enterocolitis.

Fractures of the axial skeleton are most often encountered in long bones. Fracture healing is rapid in small mammals and callous formation is commonly noted after 7–10 days. Most fractures in rodents can be treated by external coaptation (Figs 8.14–8.17). Splints and slings can be fashioned from tongue depressors and tape. Plastic syringe barrels, small metal rods (coat hangers) or lightweight polymer casting material can also be used to fashion splints in larger animals. If external coaptation devices are used, chewing can be discouraged by hardening of tape using glue, by application of noxious substances, such as hot sauce, or by use of Elizabethan collars.

Internal fixation may be indicated for certain fractures. Kirschner wires or hypodermic needles without the hub are used. It is best to use the closed pinning techniques to avoid complications of post surgical self-inflicted trauma. Larger

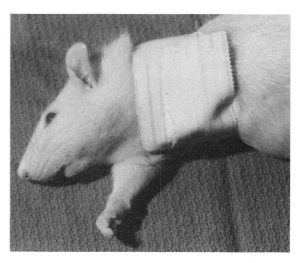

FIG. 8.15 After completion of the sling, the tape may be hardened with glue or have noxious substances applied to it.

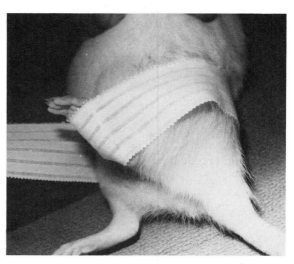

FIG. 8.16 A modified Ehmer sling is being applied to the left rear leg of a rat.

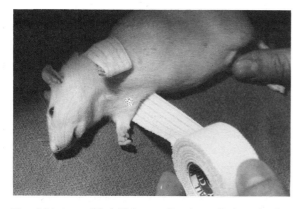

FIG. 8.14 A modified Velpeau sling is applied to the left foreleg of a rat.

animals such as rabbits may be treated with the same devices that are applicable to cats, including the use of bone plates.

Hindlimb paralysis in rabbits secondary to inappropriate handling and resultant spinal trauma deserves special mention. A careful neurological and radiological examination should be performed to determine the feasibility of

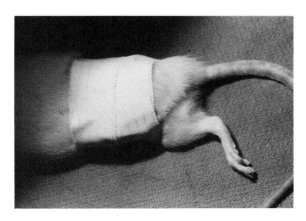

FIG. 8.17 Upon completion of the sling, precautions can be taken to discourage chewing.

restoring function. Laminectomy, vertebral body fracture repair, or modified spinal instrumentation can be attempted. In many cases, the spinal cord has either been severed or functionally transected resulting in neurotmesis (permanent paralysis). From clinical experience, dorsal laminectomies can be successful if spinal cord trauma is minor, but fractures or luxations, along with signs of severe neurotrauma, will probably require euthanasia. The syndrome is discussed in *Chapter 6*.

Amputations are required in some cases of trauma. Simple cases include tail amputation in gerbils subsequent to inappropriate handling. More complex cases would involve the amputation of limbs in the larger animals. In general, small mammals readily adapt to the loss of a limb. However, rabbits are unlikely to recover from the loss of a major portion of the rear leg. The decision to amputate should be carefully discussed with the owner and the particular species behaviour and ambulatory characteristics should be carefully considered.

When amputations are performed, the same principles that apply to dogs and cats are appropriate. Amputations are performed by incising muscles at the tendons of origin and insertion if possible. Closure should be planned so as to cushion the stump with muscle. Haemostasis and gentle tissue handling are imperative.

Successful treatment of internal trauma depends upon the appropriate diagnosis and rapid treatment. Because of diagnostic difficulties in small mammals, many cases of significant internal trauma will probably be fatal. Radiographic and sonographic examinations, in conjunction with techniques such as abdominocentesis, and thoracocentesis, should be performed, if indicated, at the earliest opportunity. Surgical procedures such as splenectomy, hepatic lobectomy or hollow organ repair can be performed as in dogs and cats.

Trauma surgery in small mammals can be a challenge. It is possible to be successful if aggressive medical and surgical management is instituted promptly.

Harderian Gland Removal

The Harderian gland is present in the orbit of most small mammals. Glandular secretions of lipids and protoporphyrins are normally spread over the pelage during grooming. Secretions may be increased in association with stress or other environmental factors. Excessive secretion has been implicated as one of the causative factors in facial dermatitis, a syndrome commonly referred to as 'sore nose' in gerbils (Thiessen and Pendergrass, 1982). Removal of the gland may be performed as part of the medical management of this syndrome (Kittrell and Thiessen, 1981).

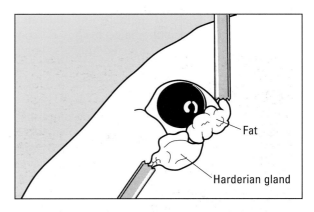

FIG. 8.18 The incision has been made in the conjunctiva of the eye and blunt dissection has been initiated. Note the associated fat pad at the lateral canthus which is preserved. The Harderian gland is being removed by blunt dissection after grasping with forceps. Note the size of the gland.

Technique

The gland is located in the ventral portion of the orbit near the lateral canthus, extending caudally towards the optic nerve.

To remove the gland, the conjunctiva is grasped with forceps and incised with either scissors or a scalpel blade. The reddish-brown gland is grasped with forceps, rolled out dorsally and bluntly dissected free of the surrounding tissues. Haemorrhage should be minimal and can be stopped with digital pressure using a moistened cotton applicator. Small incisions should not require sutures. However, conjunctival incisions enlarged during the dissection may require a few 5/0 absorbable sutures buried in the conjunctiva. The eye is treated prior to surgery with an ophthalmic ointment containing antibiotics and then every 8–12 h for 3–5 days post-surgically.

Dental Extractions

Overgrowth of the incisors and molars occurs in many small mammals, most notably the rabbit. Teeth in these species grow continuously throughout life and are continually eroded during mastication. Dental malocclusion is most often caused by congenital prognathism but may also be associated with trauma or infection. Anorexia is the most common clinical presentation but oral bleeding, especially if the molars are involved, may also be seen. Failure to treat dental disease leads to malnutrition and often death. Because dental malocclusion is considered highly heritable, affected animals should not be bred.

Technique

Extraction of incisors is readily accomplished using standard dental techniques (Brown, 1991) (Figs 8.19–8.22). Incisors are loosened with either a small root elevator or an 18 gauge hypodermic needle. Careful dissection and elevation of the tooth is continued to its root prior to extraction with dental forceps. With correct root elevation, the tooth should be loose enough for removal with minimal traction. The tooth root is bluntly rounded with a hollow tip. If the entire tooth has not been removed it will regrow

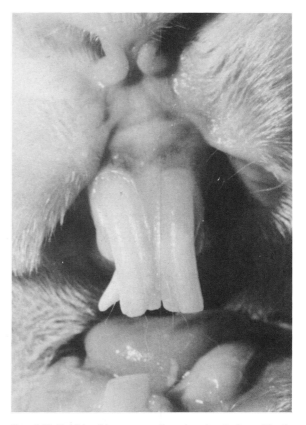

FIG. 8.19 Rabbit with overgrowth and malocclusion of both the upper incisors and peg teeth.

within 2 months. In the rabbit there is also a pair of peg teeth behind the upper incisors which must be removed in the same manner.

Haemorrhage is minimal with these techniques and can be controlled with digital pressure and gauze sponges. The cavity may be packed with haemostatic cellulose if necessary. Systemic antibiotics should be administered if infection is present.

If owners elect for palliative treatment, trimming or floating the teeth with sharp nail clippers, Rongeurs forceps, dental burrs or Dremmel drills can be performed. Complications associated with these techniques include fracture of the tooth, overheating of pulp tissues with the drill or burr and possible secondary trauma to the operator if pieces of the teeth become airborne. These techniques must be continued

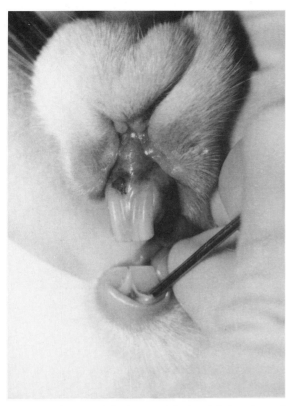

FIG. 8.20 The root of the lower left incisor is being elevated with an 18 gauge needle.

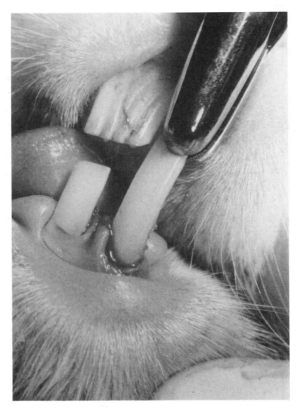

FIG. 8.21 Following elevation of the dental root, the tooth is gently extracted with dental forceps.

throughout life at approximately 6–8 week intervals.

Malocclusion of the molars is more difficult to diagnose and treat. Because of the small size of the oral cavity in many of these mammals, instrument manipulation and usage is difficult. Molars can be trimmed with Rongeurs or small files in the larger animals. With tooth extraction in rabbits, guinea-pigs and chinchillas, the opposing tooth must also be extracted because of continuous growth throughout life and the lack of apposing occlusal wear. It is theoretically possible to extract these teeth using an open surgical technique, however, the technique is not described and in cases of congenital malocclusion, removal of all molars may be necessary. This would require lifetime dietary modification. Care must be taken to avoid trauma to the tongue, soft palate and larynx during these procedures. The prognosis for treatment of maloccluded molars is more guarded than for the incisors and is frequently unrewarding.

Animals adapt well to the loss of incisors by using their lips to procure food. The absence of molars requires soft foods because of the loss of masticatory ability.

Bulla Osteotomy (Middle Ear Drainage)

Pasteurellosis in rabbits, mycoplasmosis in rats and streptococcal disease in guinea pigs can lead to otitis media. Middle ear disease is associated with a head tilt to the affected side and may lead to signs of inner ear involvement (rolling, anorexia) and death. Treatment with antibiotics is frequently unrewarding but anecdotal reports associate cures with their long-term administration. In chronic cases, bulla osteotomy and drainage of the tympanic bulla may be indicated.

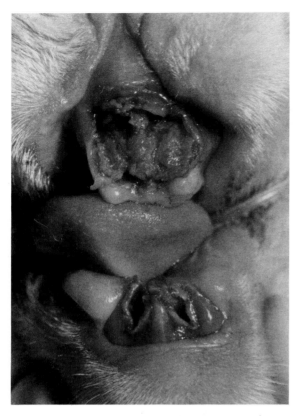

FIG. 8.22 Following extraction of the four incisors and two peg teeth, the cavities may be packed with haemostatic cellulose to control haemorrhage.

Technique

Bulla osteotomy is more commonly performed in rabbits because of a higher incidence of otitis media. Confirmation of tympanic bulla involvement should be obtained by otoscopic and radiographic examination prior to surgery. Although it is possible to approach the procedure through the oral cavity in some large animals, it is more practical to adopt a lateral approach.

The tympanic bulla can be palpated below the cartilaginous floor of the external ear canal. A vertical incision is made from the floor of the external ear to a point dorsal to the angular process of the mandible and the maxillary branch of the external jugular vein (Fig. 8.23). The parotid salivary gland must be atraumatically dissected cranially and ventrally to expose the

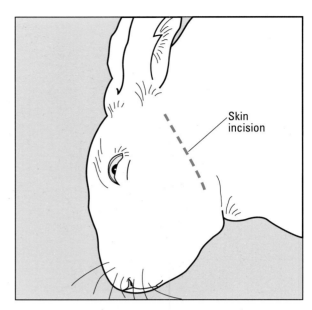

FIG. 8.23 The rabbit has been positioned in right lateral recumbency for a left bulla osteotomy.

bone of the elliptical tympanic bulla. Care should be taken to avoid trauma to the facial nerve (cranial nerve VII).

The ventral floor of the bulla is entered using a Steinmann pin or a burr, taking care not to penetrate too deeply (Fig. 8.24). In the rabbit, the auditory ossicles are dorsal and medial to the area of surgical invasion. Upon entering the cavity, purulent material may not be readily removed, because of the thickness of the exudate. The hole may be enlarged with Rongeurs forceps if necessary and the cavity should be flushed copiously with saline and antibiotics. The drainage site may be kept patent by implantation of a ventrally draining silicone tube drain until the character or quantity of drainage changes (3–5 days). Alternatively, some form of closed suction drainage using a butterfly catheter and red-topped vacuum blood collection tube may work after the bulla has been opened surgically. The tissues are closed routinely and the drain tube should be flushed daily if one is placed. It may be removed following cessation of the drainage. Small mammals will frequently scratch

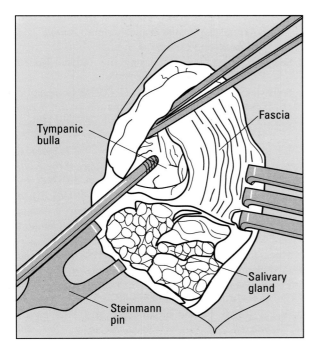

FIG. 8.24 Following dissection, the tympanic bulla is entered with an orthopaedic pin or burr.

out any type of drainage tube and the use of an Elizabethan collar should be considered. Systemic antibiotics must be administered during the entire course of treatment.

This procedure is associated with many postoperative complications including self-mutilation and cellulitis. Consequently, its use is best reserved for cases which do not respond to antibiotic therapy.

Summary

This chapter is not meant to be an exhaustive description of every possible surgical technique in rabbits and rodents. Many descriptions of surgical techniques and their development are found in research publications, rather than clinical journals. Consequently, the clinical outcomes of some surgeries have not been documented in controlled studies. In fact, much of the information available to veterinarians concerning rabbits and rodents is based upon anecdotal accounts from continuing education sources. This means that it may be incorrect or not universally applicable. It is vital for clinicians to use their diagnostic and surgical skills to make judgements as to the applicability of the surgical techniques described here. Before undertaking a surgical procedure, the veterinarian should be familiar with the general principles of surgery described here as well as the detailed descriptions of biology and diseases in the various species chapters.

References

Bojrab, M. J., Birchard, S. J. and Tomlinson, Jr, J. L. (eds.) (1990) *Current Techniques in Small Animal Surgery*, 3rd edn. Lea and Febiger, PA.

Brown, S. A. (1991) Surgical removal of incisors in the rabbit. *Journal of Small Exotic Animal Medicine* **1** 150–153.

Cunliffe-Beamer, T. L. (1993) Applying principles of aseptic surgery to rodents. *Animal Welfare Information Newsletter*, **4,** 3–6.

Flecknell, P. A. (1987) *Laboratory Animal Anaesthesia*. Academic Press, NY.

Fox, J. G., Cohen, B. J. and Loew, F. M. (eds.) (1994) *Laboratory Animal Medicine*. Academic Press, NY. pp. 207–240.

Fraser, C. M., Bergeron, J. A., Mays, A. and Aiello, S. E. (eds.) (1991) Management, husbandry and diseases of rabbits. In: *The Merck Veterinary Manual*, 7th edn, Merck and Co., Rahway, NJ. pp. 1057–1070.

Gentry, S. J. and French, E. D. (1994) The use of aseptic surgery on rodents used in research. *Contemporary Topics in Laboratory Animal Science* **33,** 61–63.

Gillett, N. A., Brooks, D. L. and Tillman, P. C. (1984) Medical and surgical management of gastric obstruction from a hairball in the rabbit. *Journal of American Veterinary Medical Association* **183,** 1176–1178.

Goring, R. L. (1994) Common orthopedic procedures of rabbits. *Proceedings of the North American Veterinary Conference*, 899.

Harkness, J. E. and Wagner, J. E. (1995) *The Biology and Medicine of Rabbits and Rodents*, 4th edn. Williams and Wilkin, Baltimore.

Harkness, J. E. (ed.) (1987) *Exotic Pet Medicine, Veterinary Clinics of North America, Small Animal Practice*, Vol. 17.

Holmes, D. D. (1984) *Clinical Laboratory Animal Medicine*, Iowa State University Press, Ames, IA.

Kittrell, E. M. W. and Thiessen, D. D. (1981) Does removal of the Harderian gland affect the physiology of the Mongolian gerbil (*Meriones unguiculatus*)? *Physiology and Psychology* **3**, 299–304.

Kraus, A. L., Weisbroth, S. H., Flatt, R. E. and Brewer, N. (1984) Biology and diseases of rabbits. In, *Laboratory Animal Medicine*, Fox, J. G., Cohen, B. J. and Loew, F. M. (eds) Academic Press, NY. pp. 207–240.

Leary, S. L., Manning, P. J. and Anderson, L. C. (1984) Experimental and naturally-occurring gastric foreign bodies in laboratory rabbits. *Laboratory Animal Science* **34**, 58–61.

Orosz, S. E. (1994) Anaesthesia and basic surgical principles. *Proceedings of the North American Veterinary Conference*, 802–803.

Quesenberry, K. E. and Hillyer, E. V. (eds.) (1993) *Exotic Pet Medicine I, Veterinary Clinics of North America, Small Animal Practice,* Vol. 23.

Quesenberry, K. E. and Hillyer, E. V. (eds.) (1994) *Exotic Pet Medicine II, Veterinary Clinics of North America, Small Animal Practice*, Vol. 24.

Romanovsky, A. A. (1993) Surgery in rodents: Risk of potential hypo- and hyperthermia. *Animal Welfare Institute Newsletter* **4,** 7.

Sedgwick, C. J. (1982) Spaying the rabbit. *Modern Veterinary Practice* **63**, 401–403.

Sedgwick, C. J. and Martin, J. C. (1994) Concepts of veterinary practice in wild mammals. In: *Exotic Pet Medicine II*, Quesenberry, K. E. and Hillyer, E. V. (eds.).

Swindle, M. M. (1993) Introduction to surgery of rabbits and rodents. In: *Proceedings of the North American Veterinary Conference*, pp. 803–804.

Swindle, M. M. and Adams, R. J. (eds.) (1988) *Experimental Surgery and Physiology: Induced Animal Models of Human Disease*. Williams and Wilkins, Baltimore.

Thiessen, D. D. and Pendergrass, M. (1982) Harderian gland involvement in facial lesions in the Mongolian gerbil. *Journal of American Veterinary Medical Association*, **181**, 1375–1377.

Waynforth, B. H. and Flecknell, P. A. (1992) *Experimental and Surgical Technique in the Rat*, 2nd edn. Academic Press, London.

Appendix I

Drug Dosages for Rodents and Rabbits

Please note that many of the dosages cited in this table are empirical as results of drug specific pharmacokinetic studies are not accessible or have not been conducted in these species. Allometric scaling, a technique which utilizes the animal's estimated metabolic rate versus body size to determine drug doses, may result in better efficacy. Part II of this table gives some examples of calculated drug doses and frequencies using this technique. An average animal weight for each species was used to calculate the specific minimum energy cost (SMEC) using the following formula: K [weight (kg)$^{0.25}$] where K is equal to 70. The SMEC multiplied by a dimensionless number specific to each antibiotic results in the dose and the frequency of administration. Note that the frequencies of administration are much higher than the conventional ones cited in Part I of the table. It may not always be possible or practical to administer therapeutic agents at such frequencies, therefore professional judgement should be used as to which dosage is appropriate for the situation.

LEGEND: c - chinchilla; g - gerbil; gp - guinea pig; h - hamster; m - mouse; r - rat; rab - rabbit

	PART I		
Drug	Species	Dose/Route/Frequency	Comments
Antibiotics/Antifungal			
Amikacin	c	2 mg/kg IV IM SC TID	
Amoxicillin	r	150 mg/kg IM SID	
Amphotericin B	h	1 mg/animal SC SID	5 days per week for 3 weeks
Ampicillin	g	2–10 mg/100 g SC TID	Not recommended in hamsters
	r	150 mg/kg SC BID	Nor guinea pigs Possible adverse effects
Cefaxolin	gp r	15 mg IM BID 60 mg/kg PO BID	Not recommended in hamsters

Appendix (Part I) continued →

PART I

Drug	Species	Dose/Route/Frequency	Comments
Cephaloridine	g,m,r	30 mg/kg IM BID	
	gp	25 mg/kg IM	
	h	10 mg/kg IM BID	
	rab	15 mg/kg IM SID	
Cephalexin	gp	15 mg/kg IM BID	
	r	60 mg/kg PO SID	
		15 mg/kg SC SID	
Chloramphenicol palmitate	c,h	30–50 mg/kg PO BID	For hamsters tx 5–7 days
	g,gp,m,r	50 mg/kg PO BID	
	rab	50 mg/kg PO SID or split BID	
Chloramphenicol succinate	c,g,h	30–50 mg/kg IM BID	
	gp	50 mg/kg IM BID	
	r	6.6 mg/kg IM BID	
	rab	30 mg/kg IM SID or divided BID	
Ciprofloxacin	gp	25 mg/kg PO IM SC BID	
	h	10 mg/kg PO BID	
	m,r	10 mg/kg PO BID	
	rab	10–20 mg/kg PO BID	
Dimetronidazole	g	0.25–1.0% in water	tx 5–7 days
	gp	20 mg/kg PO SC SID	tx 5 days
	h	7.5 mg/hamster PO TID	tx 14 days
		2 mg/ml in water	
	r	1 mg/ml in water	
Enrofloxacin	c,g,h	10 mg/kg IM SC PO BID	
	gp	10 mg/kg IM SID	
	m,r	10 mg/kg PO IM BID	May be painful as IM injection
	rab	10 mg/kg IM SC SID	

Appendix (Part 1) continued →

	PART I		
Drug	Species	Dose/Route/Frequency	Comments
Gentamicin	c	2 mg/kg IV IM SC TID	
	g,h,m,r	5 mg/kg IM SID (BID m,r)	
	gp	5–8 mg/kg SCSID	
	h	2–4 mg/kg IM SC TID	
	rab	2.5 mg/kg IM SC IV BID	
Griseofulvin	c,g,gp,rab,r	all 25–30 mg/kg PO SID	Prolonged treatment may be necessary
	h	20 mg/kg	
Metronidazole	h	7.5 mg/hamster PO	tx 5 day
Neomycin	g	100 mg/kg PO SID	tx 7 day
	gp	10 mg/kg PO BID	
	h,m	2 mg/ml water	tx 14 day
	rab	200–800 mg/l water	
Procaine Penicillin	r,m	40,000 IU/kg IM, SC	Not recommended in hamsters or guinea pigs
	rab	40,000 IU/kg SC, IM SID	Has been associated with fatal alteration of gut flora
Streptomycin	rab	50–100 mg/kg IM	Higher doses in rabbit may be toxic Not recommended in hamster or gerbil
Tetracyline/oxytetracycline	c	10 mg/ounce water	
	g	50 mg/kg PO BID	
		800 mg/l water	
	gp	50 mg/kg QID	
		5 mg/kg PO BID	
	h,m	400 mg/l water	Sweeten with 5% sucrose to ensure intake tx for 10 days
	r	10 mg/kg IM BID	
		1 mg/ml water bottle	
	rab	250–1000 mg/l water	> 250 mg/l may result in decreased water consumption
Tolramycin	gp	30 mg/kg SC BID	
Trimethoprim sulfadiazine	c,m,r	30–50 mg/kg IM SC PO BID	Route of administration depends on formulation used
	g,gp	30 mg/kg SC SID	
	h,rab	30 mg/kg PO SC IM BID	

Appendix (Part I) continued →

	PART I			
Drug	Species	Dose/Route/Frequency	Comments	
Tylosin	g	10 mg/kg IM SC	tx 5–7 days	
	h	20–80 mg/kg IM SID/BID	tx 21 days	
	h,m,r	66 mg/l water		
	r	10 mg/kg SC IM SID		
Antiparasitic Drugs				
Amitraz	g,h	3–6 topical treatments 14 days apart	0.66 ml to 1 pint water	
Amprolium	rab	0.5 ml of 9.6% soln/500 ml water	tx 10 days	
Carbaryl powder	h	5% dust or diluted 1:1 with talc	Do not use in young hamster	
Dichlorvos	h	resin strip	Leave above cage but beyond access for 3 days, remove for 3 days, then repeat	
Fenbendazole	gp	20 mg/kg SID PO	Effective against *Syphacia muris*, feed weeks 1 and 3 repeat in 2 weeks	
	r	150 mg/kg feed		
	rab	1 ml of 2.5% soln/5 kg PO		
Ivermectin	c,g,h,m,r	200–400 µg/kg SC	Topical administration for all rodents:	
	m,r	Drop behind ear for 2 txs. 1 drop Ivermectin diluted 1:100 in 1:1 propylene glycol/water		
	gp	500 µg/kg SC, PO	1:10 in water misted over cage 1 per week for 3 weeks	
	m,r	2–3 mg/kg PO		
	rab	400 µg/kg PO SC	Repeat 2 week intervals for 3 treatments	
Lasalocid	rab	120 ppm	Added to feed	
Lindane	gp	1% solution	Weekly	
	h	0.1% solution	One time treatment	
Niclosamide	g,h,m,r	100 mg/kg PO	Administer once, repeat in 7 days	

Appendix (Part 1) continued →

		PART I		
Drug	Species	Dose/Route/Frequency		Comments
Piperazine	g,r	2 mg/ml water		All rodents
	gp	100 mg/kg PO SID		tx for 7, off 5, tx for 7 days
	gp	4–7 mg/ml water		
	h	10 mg/ml water		
	rab	500 mg/kg PO adults		Repeat in 10 days
		750 mg/kg PO young		
Praziquantel	m,r	25–50 mg/kg		2 doses 7 days apart
	gp	10 mg/kg		once
	rab	5–10 mg/kg SC		
Robenidine	rab	66 ppm		Added to feed; will not eliminate hepatic coccidiosis
Ronnel	h	45 ml of 33.5% suspension in 250 ml propylene glycol		
Sulfadimethoxine	c	12.5 mg/kg PO BID		
		12.5% in drinking water for 5–7 days		1 ml of 5% suspension in 3 ml water
	h,r	20–50 mg/kg PO SID or in water		give for 7 days
	rab	20–50 mg/kg PO SID		
Sulfamethazine	gp,h	1 g/l water		tx 5 days
Sulfaquinoxalone	gp,h	1 g/l water		tx 14–21 days,
	rab	0.1% in drinking water		stop for 10 days, then repeat
	h	0.5 ml of 20% stock soln in 1 l water		
Thiabendazole	gp	100 mg/kg PO SID		tx 7–14 days
	h	0.1–0.3% in diet		tx 5 days
	m,r	200 mg/kg PO		Single tx
	rab	100–200 mg/kg PO		
Tolnaftate	gp	1% BID topical		
Miscellaneous Drugs				
Atropine	c	0.02–0.04 mg/kg SC		
	h	0.004–0.01 mg/100 g SC, IM		

Appendix (Part I) continued   →

	PART I		
Drug	Species	Dose/Route/Frequency	Comments
Bretylium tosylate	gp	20 mg/kg SC PRN	
Cholestyramine	gp	100 mg/ml in water	
	rab	2 g/day in 20 ml water	
Cyclophosphamide	gp	300 mg/kg IP SID	
Dexamethasone	gp	0.4 mg/kg SC SID	
	h	0.6 mg/kg SC IM IP	
	rab	0.5–2 mg/kg IV IM IP SC	
Diphenylhydantoin	g,gp	25–50 mg/kg BID PO	
Diphenylhydramine	gp	5 mg/kg SC PRN	
Dopamine	gp	0.08 mg/kg IV PRN	
Ephedrine	gp	1 mg/kg IV PRN	
Epinephrine	gp	0.003 mg/kg IV PRN	
Heparin	gp	5 mg/kg IV PRN	
Human chorionic gonadotropin	gp	1000 units IM PRN	
Hydralazine	gp	1 mg/kg IV PRN	
Insulin	h	2 units SC	Used in glucose tolerance study
Isoproferemol	gp	0.06 mg/kg IM PRN	
Metaclopromide	rab	0.2–1 mg/kg PO SC IV IM BID	
Oxytocin	g,h	0.2–3 units/kg SC IM	
	gp	1–3 IU/kg IM PRN	
Phenobarbital	g	10–20 mg/kg	To control seizures

Appendix (Part I) continued →

PART I			
Drug	Species	Dose/Route/Frequency	Comments
Prednisone	gp rab	2 mg/kg IM SID 2 mg/kg IM SC SID	
Primidone	gp	25 mg/kg PO BID	
Vitamin and Nutritional Supplements			
Calcium gluconate	gp	1 mg/kg PRN	
Calcium carbonate	gp	4 mg/kg PO SID	
Magnesium hydroxide	gp	4 mg/kg PO SID	
Potassium chloride	gp	0.5–1.0 mg/kg PO IM SID	
Vitamin A	gp,h	50–500 IU/100 g IM	
Vitamin B complex	h rab	0.002–0.02 ml/100 g IM 0.02–0.4 ml/kg IM SID	
Vitamin C	gp h	50–100 mg/kg IM PO SID 2–20 mg/100 g IM SID	
Vitamin D	h	20–40 IU/100 g IM	
Vitamin E	gp	5–10 mg/kg SID IM	
Vitamin K	gp h	3 mg/kg SC SID 1–10 mg/kg IM	

Appendix (Part I)

PART II

	*SMEC	Ampicillin		Cephalexin		Enrofloxacin		Ivermectin
		mg/kg	Frequency per day	mg/kg	Frequency per day	mg/kg	Frequency per day	mg/kg
Rabbit 4 kg	49	123	4×	12	4×	6	2×	0.49
Guinea pig 650 g	78	195	6×	20	6×	9	4×	0.78
Hamster 100 g	124					15	6×	1.24
Gerbil 80 g	132	330	10×	34	10×	16	7×	1.32
Mice 35 g	162	405	12×	41	12×	19	8×	1.62
Rat 350 g	91	227	7×	23	7×	11	5×	0.91
Chinchilla 500 g	83	207	6×	21	6×	10	4×	0.83

*SMEC=Specific Minimum Energy Cost.

References for Introduction

Hainsworth, F. R. (1981) *Animal Physiology Adaptations in Function.* Reading, Addison-Wesley, pp. 160–163.

Schmidt-Nielsen, K. (1984) *Scaling—Why is Animal Size so Important?* Cambridge: Cambridge University Press, pp. 90–98.

Sedgwick, C. M. (1994) Concepts of veterinary practice in wild mammals in exotic pet medicine II. Veterinary Clinics of North America: Small Animal Practice. K. E. Quesenberry and E. V. Hillyer (eds.)

Morris, T. H. (1995) Antibiotic therapeutics in laboratory animals. *Laboratory Animals* (in press).

Chinchilla References

Hagen, K. W. and Gorham, J. R. (????) Dermatomycoses in fur animals: Chinchilla, ferret, mink and rabbit. *Veterinary Medicine, Small Animal Clinician* **67**(**1**): 43–48.

Hoefer, H. L. (1994) Chinchillas. *Veterinary Clinics of North America*: *Small Animal Practice* **24**(**1**): 103–111.

Jenkins, J. R. (1992) Husbandary and common diseases of the chincillas (*Chinchilla laniger*). *Journal of Small Animal Exotic Medicine* **2**: 15–17.

Kennedy, A. H. (1970) *Chinchilla Diseases and Ailments.* Clay Publishing Company. Bewdley, Ontario, Canada.

Webb, R. A. (1991) In: *Manual of Exotic Pets* Benyon, P. H. and Copper J. E. (eds.) pp. 15–22. British Small Animal Veterinary Association.

Gerbil References

Harkness, J. (1994) Small rodents. *Veterinary Clinics of North America*: *Small Animal Practice*, **24**: 89–120.

Holmes, D. (1984) *Clinical Laboratory Medicine,* Iowa State University Press, Ames, Iowa.

Jacobson, E. K., Kollias, G. V. and Peters, L. J. (1983) Dosages for antibiotics and parasiticides used in exotic animals. *Compendium or Continuing Education in Practice Veterinary* **5**: 315.

Russell, R. J., Johnson, D. K. and Stunkard, J. A. (1981) *A Guide to Diagnosis, Treatment and Husbandry of Pet Rabbits and Rodents.* Veterinary Medicine Publishing, Lenexa, Kansas.

West, C. (1991) Gerbils. In: *Manual of Exotic Pets*, Beynon PH, Cooper JE eds. pp. 31–38, Gloucestershire, UK.

Guinea Pig References

Anderson, L. C. (1987) Guinea pigs husbandary and medicine. *Veterinary Clinics of North America*: *Small Animal Practice* **17**: 1045–1060.

Borchard, R. E., Barnes, C. D. and Etheridge, L. G. (1991) *Drug Dosage in Laboratory Animals*: *A Handbook*, 3rd edn, Teleford Press, Inc., Caldwell, N.J.

Collins, B. R. (1994) Common diseases and medical management of rodents and lagomorphs. *Veterinary Clinics of North America*: *Small Animal Practice* **24**: 261–316.

Flecknell, P. A. (1991) Guinea pigs. In: *Manual of Exotic Pets* (Beynon, P. H. and Cooper, J. E., eds), British Small Animal Veterinary Association, Gloucestershire, UK, pp. 51–62.

Gordin, F. M. *et al.* (1985) Activities of perfloxacin and ciprofloxacin in experimentally induced Pseudomonas pneumonia in neutropenic guinea pigs. *Antimicrobial Agents Chemotherapy*, **27**: 452–4.

Harkness, J. E. and Wagner, J. E. (1989) *The Biology and Medicine of Rabbits and Rodents*, 3rd edn, Lea & Febiger, Philadelphia, PA.

Hawk, C. T. and Leary, S. L. (1994) *Drug Information and Formulary for Laboratory Animals.* In press.

McKellar, Q. A. (1989) Drug dosages for small mammals. *In Practice* **1989**: 57–61.

McKellar, Q. A., Midgley, D. M., Galbraith, E. A., Scott, E. W. and Bradley, A. (1992) Clinical and pharmacological properties of ivermectin in rabbits and guinea pigs. *Veterinary Record* **130**: 71–73.

Murphy, S. G., LoBuglio, A. F. (1977) L2C leukemia: a model of human acute leukemia. *Ped Prod.* **36**: 2281–2285.

Schiff, J. B. *et al.* (1984) Comparative activities of cirofloxacin ticarcillin and tobramycin against experimental *Pseudomonas aeruginosa* penumonia. *Antimicrobal Agents Chemotherapy* **26**: 1–4.

Schumann, S. M. (1989) Individual care and treatment of rabbits, mice, rats, guinea pigs, hamsters and gerbils. In: *Current Veterinary Therapy X*: *Small Animal Practice* (Kirk, R. W., ed) WB Saunders Co., Philadelphia. PA. pp. 738–765.

Richardson, V. O. G. (1992) *Diseases of Domestic Guinea Pigs*, Blackwell Scientific Publications, Oxford, UK.

Hamster Antibiotic References

Flynn, B. M., Brown, P. A., Eckstein, J. M. *et al.* (1989) Treatment of *Syphacia obvelata* in mice using ivermectin. *Lab. Anim. Sci.* **39**: 461–463.

Harkness, J. E. (1994) Small rodents. *Veterinary Clinics of North America*: *Small Animal Practice* **24**: 89–102.

Harkness, J. E. and Wagner, J. E. (1983) *The Biology and Medicine of Rabbits and Rodents*. 2nd edn. Lea & Febiger, Philadelphia.

Holmes, D. D. (1984) *Clinical Laboratory Animal Medicine*. Iowa State University Press, Ames IA.

Schuchman S. M. (1989) Individual care and treatment of rabbits, mice, rats, guinea pigs, hamsters, and gerbils In: *Current Veterinary Therapy* Kirk R. W. (ed) Vol. X, pp. 738–765. WB Saunders Co., Philadelphia, PA.

Small, J. E. (1987) Drugs used in hamsters with a review of antibiotic-associated colitis. In: *Laboratory Hamsters* Van Hoosier G. L. Jr, McPherson C. W. (eds). Vol. pp. 179–199. Academic Press Inc, Orlando FL.

Wagner, J. E., Earrar P. L. (1987) Husbandry and medicine of small rodents. *Veterinary Clinics of North America*: *Small Animal Practice*. **17**: 1061–1087.

Rabbit References

Brown, S. (1993) Rabbit drug dosages. *Rabbit Health News* **10**: 6–7.

Hillyer, E. V. (1994) Pet rabbits. *Veterinary Clinics of North America*: *Small Animal Practice* **24(1)**: 25–65.

Okerman, L. (1988) *Diseases of Domestic Rabbits* Blackwell Scientific Publications, Oxford, England.

Okerman, L. (1994) *Diseases of Domestic Rabbits*, Second Edition. Blackwell Scientific Publications, Oxford, England.

Walden, N. B. (1990) *Rabbits. A Compendium* (The T G Hungerford VADE MECUM series for Domestic Animals: Series C.13) Post Graduate Foundation in Veterinary Science, University of Sydney, Sydney South NSW, pp. 37, 38, 40, 67.

Rat and Mouse References

Baker, H. L., Lindsey, J. R., Weisbroth, S. H. (1980) *The Laboratory Rat, Vol. II*: *Researach Applications*. Academic Press.

Coghan, L. G., Lee, D. R., Psencik, B. and Weiss, D. (1993) Practical and effective eradication of pinworms (*Syphacia muris*) in rats by use of fenbendazole. *Laboratory Animal Science* **43**: 481–487.

Diggs, H. E., Feller, D. J., Crabbe, J. C., Merrill, C. Farrell, E. (1992) Effect of chronic ivermectin against *Trichosomoides crassicauda* in naturally infected laboratory rats. *Laboratory Animal Science* **42**: 620–622.

Flynn, B. M., Brown, P. A., Eckstein, J. M. and Strong, D. (1989) Treatment of *Syphacia obvelate* in mice using ivermectin. *Laboratory Animal Science* **39**: 461–463.

Fox, J. G., Cohen, B. J. and Loew F. M. (1984) *Laboratory Animal Medicine*, Academic Press.

Huerkamp, M. J., (1993) Eradication of pinworms from rats being kept in ventilated cages. *Laboratory Animal Science* **43**: 86–90.

National Researach Council (1992) *Recognition and Alleviation of Pain and Distress in Laboratory Animals*. National Academy Press, Washington DC.

Wayneforth, H. B. and Flecknell, P. A. eds. (1992) *Experimental and Surgical Technique in the Rat*, 2nd edn, Academic Press.

Appendix II

List of Abbreviations

ACC	antibiotic-associated colitis
BID	twice daily
CPE	cytopathic effect
DIC	disseminated intravascular coagulation
g.b.w.	grams body weight
Hap V	hamster papovavirus
HCG	human chorionic gonadotropin
ICLO	intracellular campylobacter-like organisms
IM	intramuscular
IO	intraosseous
IP	intraperitoneal
IV	intravenous

LCM	lymphocytic choriomeningitis
LCMV	lymphocytic choriomeningitis virus
MECA	metastabilised chlorous acid/chlorine dioxide
NSAIDs	non-steroidal anti-inflammatory drugs
PI	proliferative ileitis
PO	per os
PVM	pneumonia virus of mice
SC	subcutaneous
SID	once daily
SV5	Simian Virus 5
TID	every 8 hours
tx	as required

Index